Demographic Transition in China

Studies on
Contemporary China

Art and Ideology in Revolutionary China *David Holm*

Studies on Contemporary China
The Contemporary China Institute, based at the School of Oriental and African Studies (University of London), was established in 1968. Throughout its existence, it has been a national focus for research and publications on 20th-century China. This new series, which is edited at the Institute, seeks to maintain and extend that tradition by making available the best work of scholars throughout the world. Future volumes will embrace a wide variety of subjects, including China's social, political and economic change, intellectual and cultural developments, and foreign relations.

Volumes in the Series
Art and Ideology in Revolutionary China *David Holm*

Demographic Transition in China

Fertility Trends since the 1950s

PENG XIZHE

CLARENDON PRESS · OXFORD
1991

Oxford University Press, Walton Street, Oxford OX2 6DP
Oxford New York Toronto
Delhi Bombay Calcutta Madras Karachi
Petaling Jaya Singapore Hong Kong Tokyo
Nairobi Dar es Salaam Cape Town
Melbourne Auckland
and associated companies in
Berlin Ibadan

Oxford is a trade mark of Oxford University Press

Published in the United States
by Oxford University Press, New York

British Library Cataloguing in Publication Data
Peng, Xizhe
Demographic transition in China: fertility trends since the 1950s
1954.—(Studies in contemporary China)
1. China. Population
I. Title II. Series
304.60951
ISBN 0–19–828715–1

Library of Congress Cataloging in Publication Data
Peng, Xizhe.
Demographic transition in China: fertility trends since the 1950s/
Peng Xizhe.
(Studies on contemporary China)
Includes bibliographical references (p.) and index.
1. Fertility, Human—China. 2. Demographic transition—China.
3. Marriage—China. 4. Birth control—China. 5. China—Population policy. 6. China—Population. I. Title. II. Series: Studies on contemporary China (Oxford, England).
HB1064.A3P46 1991 304.6'32'095109045—dc20 90–14220
ISBN 0–19–828715–1

Typeset by Cambrian Typesetters, Frimley, Surrey
Printed in Great Britain by
Biddles Ltd
Guildford & King's Lynn

Acknowledgements

THE research on which this book is based was conducted by the author for a Ph.D. degree in Demography at the Department of Population Studies in the London School of Economics and Political Science. This work was supported by fellowships awarded by the United Nations Fund for Population Activities (1983–6) and the Population Council in the United States (1986–7). The Population Investigation Committee provided a grant for data processing.

It is impossible to thank properly all those people who have helped me in the preparation and completion of my work. I feel deeply indebted to Professor John Hobcraft for his encouragement and supervision. This research would never have have been completed without his academic and personal support. Particular thanks are due to C. Langford for his generosity and help throughout various stages of this work. I benefited greatly from Dr C. Wilson. His valuable comments and editorial help are greatly appreciated. Substantial help was received from other staff of the department. Computing advice was obtained from the staff of the Computer Service of the London School of Economics. I should like to thank all of them most sincerely.

In the final preparation and revision of this book, the Contemporary China Institute (CCI) of the London School of Oriental and African Studies has been very supportive. Financial help from the Institute is acknowledged. I owe special thanks to Dr R. F. Ash and the late Professor K. R. Walker for their valuable comments and help in getting this book published. While this manuscript was being prepared for the Press, news came of the tragic death of Professor Kenneth Walker. That this book should have found its way to publication owes much to the encouragement and advice which I received from Professor Walker. I should like to put on record here the very special debt which I owe him, personally as well as professionally. Thanks are also due to many friends for their help in improving my proficiency in English and editorial assistance. Any remaining errors are my own responsibility.

I would also like to express my warm appreciation to the Institute of Population Research at Fudan University in the People's Republic of China, and many Chinese colleagues for their material and personal support.

Both my family and my wife's family have encouraged me to take the time to complete this book. To them I owe more thanks than can plainly be expressed. It is to my wife Lu Bo who shared the stresses and strains related to writing this book with great understanding and tolerance, that I dedicate this book with gratitude and affection.

Contents

List of Figures

List of Tables

Abbreviations

ASFMR	Age-Specific First-Marriage Rate
ASFR	Age-Specific Fertility Rate
CBR	Crude Birth-Rate
CCCP	Central Committee of the Communist Party
CDR	Crude Death-Rate
GPVIA	Gross Product Value of Industry and Agriculture
MAFM	Mean Age at First Marriage
NIR	Natural Increase Rate
PCEBC	Per Capita Expenditures for Birth Control
PTFR	Partial Total Fertility Rate
TFR	Total Fertility Rate
TMR	Total First-Marriage Rate
WFS	World Fertility Survey

1

Introduction

In the middle of 1987, the global population reached its five-billion mark. This statistic highlights the urgency of population control throughout the world. Rapid and accelerating population growth is indeed one of the most salient features of the contemporary world. Not until 1850 did the world's population reach one billion. Thereafter it took little more than 75 years to add the second billion and a further 35 years for the third billion. After reaching the three-billion mark in 1960 and four billion in 1974, it took only 13 years to increase another billion to the world's total. Despite the recent decline in the global growth rate, especially in less-developed countries (due almost entirely to a fall in China's birth rate),[1] the annual increment to the world's total population continues to increase. More than 90 per cent of this increase occurs in the Third World.[2]

Although there are differences of opinion amongst scholars, it is widely believed that rapid population growth has an adverse effect on socio-economic development in today's less-developed countries. There is an increasing awareness that excessive population growth is a major obstacle to improvements in living standards, social welfare, education, etc. The more interested we are in planning for the future and in improving human life on earth, the more concerned we should be with population issues.[3]

I. A Brief History of China's Population Growth

China's population issue has attracted great attention, not only because of its immense size, which now amounts to more than one billion, but also because of its rapid change since the founding of the People's Republic in October 1949.

Although China was one of the first countries in the world to calculate its population, there were very few historical statistics available. Moreover, the territories of the various dynasties differed and the objects of the population accounts varied (e.g. some counted in terms of households and some in terms of able-bodied men).[4]

Nevertheless, we do know that China's population grew very slowly and almost no consistent trend can be traced until the eighteenth century. In the year AD 2, the population counted by the Han Dynasty was about 60 million. For the next sixteen centuries, the population fluctuated drastically, but demonstrated virtually no growth.[5] The period 1749–1851 witnessed a rapid population growth under the early Qing rulers, when stable political and favourable economic conditions generally prevailed.[6] China's population doubled in a century and an average annual growth rate of 0.9 per cent was estimated.

The population growth during the next century slowed down mainly due to societal unrest. During the last several decades of the Qing Dynasty, a series of rebellions coupled with natural disasters resulted in millions of deaths. Before 1949 China's population growth was characterized by a high birth-rate, a high mortality rate, and a low natural increase rate. The estimated crude birth-rate for China's rural population in 1929–31 was about 41 per thousand, which was balanced by a similar crude death-rate.[7] This situation led to an approximately zero population growth. Over the period 1840–1949, China's population rose from 412 million to 542 million, an average annual growth rate of 0.25 per cent.[8]

Since 1949 mortality conditions have substantially improved. A sharp mortality decline took place during the 1950s. By 1957 China's crude death-rate had already been halved from pre-1949 levels. In 1970 China reported its national crude death-rate as 7.6 per thousand population. This was without doubt a significant achievement.

The birth-rate, however, did not decline simultaneously. As late as the early 1970s China's birth-rate remained at the pre-1949 level. Consequently, the first 20 years of the People's Republic witnessed a rapid population growth. Increasing from 541 million in 1949, China's total population reached 830 million in 1970, an annual growth rate of 2.16 per cent.

The rate of population growth fell off gradually from the early 1970s, owing to marked fertility decline. The downward trend of the crude death-rate continued over the 1970s, although the change was modest. By the early 1980s the national figure of natural increase rate had dropped to around 12 per thousand. In a short period of three decades, China had experienced a rapid demographic transition.

However, this rapid demographic change did not occur homogeneously across the country. There are marked regional differentials in mortality and fertility. Table 1.1 presents the birth-, death-, and natural

TABLE 1.1. *Reported crude birth-, death-, and natural increase rates for China by province*

Province	1954			1981		
	CBR	CDR	NIR	CBR	CDR	NIR
Beijing	40.09	8.24	31.85	17.55	5.78	11.77
Tianjin	44.35	7.82	36.53	18.60	6.10	12.50
Hebei	34.89	10.19	24.70	23.99	6.05	17.94
Shanxi	36.55	14.60	21.95	20.31	5.64	14.67
Nei Monggol	40.87	11.15	29.72	23.11	5.77	17.34
Liaoning	43.76	8.00	35.76	18.53	5.32	13.21
Jilin	48.14	10.38	37.76	17.67	5.32	12.35
Heilongjiang	42.51	10.54	31.97	19.79	4.95	14.84
Shanghai	52.74	7.12	45.62	16.14	6.44	9.70
Jiangsu	36.72	12.06	24.66	18.47	6.10	12.37
Zhejiang	35.01	11.47	23.54	17.93	6.27	11.66
Anhui	42.55	16.44	26.11	18.73	5.20	13.53
Fujian	35.18	10.72	24.46	22.07	5.87	16.20
Jiangxi	32.66	14.22	18.44	20.42	6.54	13.88
Shandong	37.65	11.70	25.95	18.84	6.26	12.58
Henan	41.10	13.19	27.91	20.64	6.01	14.63
Hubei	31.86	15.95	15.91	20.17	7.33	12.84
Hunan	39.61	17.52	22.09	21.11	7.03	14.08
Guangdong	35.09	12.72	22.37	24.99	5.54	19.45
Guangxi	36.39	15.20	21.19	27.25	5.61	21.64
Sichuan	39.86	15.43	24.43	17.96	7.02	10.94
Guizhou	33.69	12.10	21.59	27.89	8.48	19.41
Yunnan	37.38	16.48	20.90	25.36	8.60	16.76
Xizhang	—	—	—	31.05	9.92	21.13
Shaanxi	34.95	11.05	23.90	20.35	7.10	13.25
Gansu	32.55	11.10	21.45	20.12	5.72	14.40
Qinghai	37.93	11.43	26.50	26.65	7.48	19.17
Ningxia	—	—	—	29.65	6.08	23.57
Xinjiang	29.78	16.06	13.72	29.08	8.41	20.67
CHINA	37.97	13.18	24.79	20.91	6.36	14.55

Note: — data not available.

Source: Hu and Li 1986.

growth rate for every province in the mainland of China for the selected years.

In the early 1950s the table shows that the natural increase rate varied greatly between provinces: from the highest of 45.62 per thousand in Shanghai to the lowest of 13.72 per thousand in Xinjiang. There were ten provinces where the natural increase rate exceeded 26 per thousand, almost all of them located in the northern part of China. Such a rapid natural growth in the northern provinces and great cities, if correct, was the result of high fertility combined with lower mortality, which may reflect the effects of different processes of urbanization and industrialization at that time.

Three decades later, while most provinces experienced decline in natural population growth, there was little change in the natural increase rate in some southern and northwestern provinces. Shanghai's natural increase rate was below 10 per thousand in 1981, but the rate in Ningxia remained as high as 24 per thousand.

In a broad sense, China follows the classical model of demographic transition. However, this uneven progress of the transition in China's provinces deserves more research. In this book, the focus is on one of the major components of demographic changes: fertility transition.

II. Selected Theories of Fertility Transition

Population growth is a combined product of three demographic variables: fertility, mortality, and migration. Among them, fertility, in most instances, is the prime determinant of population growth and composition. Therefore, to understand fertility is to understand not only a major portion of all demographic behaviour, but a fundamental element in social structure and the human condition.[9] For this reason, human fertility has been the primary focus of population studies since Malthus.[10] With the world-wide decline in levels of mortality, the analysis of childbearing and family formation has become more dominant in population studies than ever before.

A large number of theories are available on this subject, and they developed in different directions or orientations. However, it cannot be said that much progress has been made with respect to understanding the mechanism of fertility decline, despite decades of intensive research.[11] Here is not the right place for an academic debate, but a brief survey of major relevant theories may help us to understand the issue better.

Demographic transition is the most important theoretical idea in social demography.[12] Basically, the classical theory states that both the mortality and fertility of a population will decline from high to low levels as a result of socio-economic development.[13] The transition process passes a series of stages from an initial stage of high fertility and mortality, and very slow population growth, to an end state of near zero rate of natural increase and stable population, as a result of very low fertility and mortality rates. In between, there are intermediate stages characterized by rapid population growth, or population explosion, essentially because the great improvement in mortality occurs first, while the decline in fertility lags behind. Since the proposition of the demographic-transition theory, great efforts have been made to challenge or re-examine this classical formulation.

Caldwell believes that the demographic-transition theory is faulty and has proposed his 'wealth-flow' theory.[14] He argues that industrialization is not a necessary condition for fertility decline. Instead the nucleation of families, which is mainly motivated by westernization, is regarded as a major pre-condition. He points out that the underlying determinant of fertility decline is the changing direction of intergenerational wealth flow. In all traditional societies, he claims, high fertility is accompanied by a wealth flow from the younger to the older generation. Once the direction of the wealth flow has reversed, fertility will start to decline. Mass education is viewed by him as one of the fundamental forces in the course of fertility transition.

Several other approaches have been employed in studying fertility transition. Based on the institutional context of reproduction, McNicoll argues that a significant shift in the institutional setting and cultural environment in which fertility decisions are made is a sufficient condition for changes in fertility behaviour.[15] In other words, an individual's reproductive behaviour is strongly influenced by the surrounding institutional arrangements, such as family type, the kin-system, community organization, and so on.

Some scholars use a rational decision-making model to analyse individuals' fertility behaviour in terms of costs and benefits of childbearing.[16] Others believe that population questions are all macro questions and should be studied at the societal level. Several theories stress influences working only through the demand for children.[17] In contrast, others focus on the supply side or stress the cost of fertility regulation. An attempt has also been made to combine demand, supply, and regulation cost. Changes associated with modernization would affect fertility decisions via their impact on one or more of these three variables.[18]

Some believe that by taking care of the people, the population will take care of itself.[19] They claim that the best contraceptive is development.[20] Others maintain that availability of family-planning services is the key to rapid fertility reduction in a developing country.[21] They hold that family-planning programmes have significant, independent effects over and above the effect of socio-economic effects on fertility transition.[22]

Beyond debates on these underlying causal factors of fertility change, there has been a continuing stream of research related to the proximate determinants of fertility. Here there is much common ground among demographers.[23] Changes in nuptiality, breastfeeding, contraceptive use, abortion, and other biological factors are directly associated with fertility levels and trends. However, the roles of these proximate variables in demographic transition vary greatly, in size and sometimes even in direction, between countries.[24]

Much empirical research has been carried out in the past two decades and has facilitated our understanding of the matter. The World Fertility Survey (WFS) demonstrates that fertility declines in the less developed countries have been largely the result of greatly increased fertility control through modern contraception, which is closely associated with the organized family-planning programme.[25] Although the classical demographic-transition theory is basically the summary of experiences of European countries, one of the consistent findings of the European Fertility Project is that non-socio-economic variables, such as religion, language, ethnicity, and region, explain much of the variability in marital fertility decline in Europe, even after conventional socio-economic variables have been taken into account.[26]

It seems that no single, fully articulated, reformulated theory is yet justified. Nevertheless, all previous research provides necessary building blocks for the creation of a general fertility theory. The Chinese experience will certainly contribute a lot to this process.

III. Objective and Organization of the Book

Fertility transition, as defined by Easterlin, is the combined process of fertility decline and the shift to deliberate fertility control.[27] Making use of recent information on China's population and socio-economic development, this book documents and analyses the fertility transition in China since 1949. Utilizing some of the current demographic techniques, it describes the fertility levels, trends, and differentials in terms of regional and rural–urban residence. Provincial patterns in the timing and pace of fertility transition are examined and an attempt has been made to trace possible explanations.

China is such a large country that there are considerable differentials among different provinces in their levels of development, local customs and cultural tradition, ethnic composition, etc. Equally important to this study is the recognition that although all provinces are under strong central guidance to operate population programmes, the local accomplishment of these policies and institutions created to reduce fertility vary enormously between regions. As we will see in the later chapters, success or failure of policy implementation is to a large extent determined at the local, especially provincial, level. Furthermore, reproductive behaviour varies substantially, not only between regions, but also in terms of acceptance of or resistance to change among women with different educational background, occupation, place of residence, etc. It is believed, therefore, that only after these fertility differentials have been reasonably ascertained, can one proceed to a full understanding of fertility transition in China. In short, one of the major objectives of this study is to analyse fertility differences, especially diversities between regions.

The introductory chapter reviews selected theoretical frameworks in studying fertility transition. The chapter also discusses the data sources and major fertility indices used for the analysis.

Since fertility decline in China is closely associated with and facilitated by well-organized programmes, a historical review of the evolution of China's family-planning programme and its local performance is logically an important part of the book. The population programme is studied within its political and social context. Because the provincial authority is the most important administrative unit that is encouraged to modify the central policies in order to adapt to the local situation, the success or failure of government policy on population control is assessed basically at the provincial level.

The importance of socio-economic conditions on fertility transition is analysed in Chapter 3. On the one hand, this search for explanations examines a number of provincial indicators of socio-economic development through different stages of the transition. In addition, the relationship between women's status and their fertility behaviour is tested. Beyond that, a qualitative study is made of the effects of the institutions on fertility differentials.

A major part of the book, Chapters 4–6, involves a thorough demographic analysis of fertility levels and trends for China as a whole and for each of its 28 provinces, separating the rural from the urban population. This is accompanied by a similar analysis of changes in nuptiality patterns. Xizhang and Taiwan are excluded from this study due to the nature of the data source.[28] While Chapter 4 reports the national trends in fertility and nuptiality, Chapters 5 and 6 present the results for the urban and rural population respectively. Chapter 6 also embraces the rural–urban comparison.

The concluding chapter sums up the major findings and policy implications of the study. It discusses the recent development of China's fertility transition in the context of China's current economic and political reform. The chapter also presents briefly the author's personal view of China's future population prospects.

In summary, this is an empirical work and does not assert the primacy of any single theoretical framework. As a matter of fact, theory by itself can only direct us to the right questions, it can not provide answers.[29] This study yields valuable insights into factors affecting the fertility transition within China and provides a basis for judging the relative merits of those different views about fertility transition.

IV. The Data

The major source of demographic data used in this study is China's 1982 Fertility Survey, which was officially named as China's National One-Per-Thousand-Population Fertility Sampling Survey. Conducted by the State Family Planning Commission, this retrospective survey provides invaluable information on China's fertility and nuptiality changes over the last several decades.

This survey was a stratified-cluster sampling survey. China's 1982 Census listing was used as the sample frame. The stratification of urban and rural population was settled by using the address code of the Census. Eight hundred and fifteen rural production brigades and urban resident committees were randomly selected as sample units with a total sample population of just over one million, or one per thousand of the national total population.[30]

Within the sample population, all women aged 15–67 were interviewed about their marital and fertility histories. Contraceptive practice and women's socio-economic backgrounds were also included in the survey questionnaire. Sampling and non-sampling errors were rigorously controlled throughout every stage of the survey.[31] Interviewers were well trained, and propaganda and mobilization of the masses were carried out extensively.

This survey was successfully undertaken with a relatively high accuracy. Although misreporting is inevitable, analyses suggest a very low level of error in data collection in the survey. After careful examinations of the consistency of the survey and census data. Coale claims that 'with some minor exceptions, then, the fertility and nuptiality information taken from the census and survey can be accepted as of high quality; as such, they provide the basis for a valid history of recent trends in China.'[32]

Unfortunately, only tabulated results of the survey are available to

TABLE 1.2. *Sample sizes and sample units of China's 1982 Fertility Survey by province*

Province	Sample size			Sample units
	Total	Urban	Rural	
Beijing	3103	1941	1162	7
Tianjin	3044	1719	1325	6
Hebei	17030	1575	15455	53
Shanxi	7681	955	6726	30
Nei Monggol	6257	1843	4414	16
Liaoning	12513	4836	7677	22
Jilin	6744	1892	4852	14
Heilongjiang	9599	3133	6466	23
Shanghai	4416	2888	1528	6
Jiangsu	21019	3447	17572	41
Zhejiang	11705	1440	10265	44
Anhui	14357	1662	12695	32
Fujian	7414	826	6588	17
Jiangxi	9509	1094	8415	24
Shandong	23409	1559	21850	88
Henan	21717	1992	19725	50
Hubei	15638	2419	13219	38
Hunan	16727	1939	14788	50
Guangdong	17692	3020	14672	32
Guangxi	10512	973	9539	17
Sichuan	30114	4385	25729	85
Guizhou	7841	1108	6733	27
Yunnan	10088	1254	8834	16
Shaanxi	8956	1545	7411	35
Gansu	5732	1057	4675	19
Qinghai	1489	283	1206	6
Ningxia	1290	387	903	4
Xinjiang	4418	1241	3177	13
NATIONAL TOTAL	310014	52413	257601	815

the author, which to some extent limits the choice of research methodologies and the scope of the analysis. Nevertheless, full utilization of this information enables us to document and analyse fertility transition in China and its provinces in great detail.

The total number of respondents in the survey is 310,014, which is quite exceptional compared with many other surveys such as the World Fertility Survey. This is no less true for most individual provinces. For example (see Table 1.2), in the survey more than 30,000 women were interviewed in Sichuan province alone. The sample size for each province, on average, is more than 10,000. But this is not the case for some small provinces due to the method of single-stage proportional sampling. This is especially true as the sample is further broken down into the rural and urban population. As a result, stochastic variations are much greater in the fertility and nuptiality measures calculated for individual provinces than for China as a whole, and vary between provinces. The effects of small sample size are more obvious for the urban populations. Moreover, because people who live in one place show a statistical tendency to resemble each other more than people who live far apart,[33] the implication of clustering on analysis should be borne in mind. Sampling error caused by the clustering seems to be larger in major municipalities and small provinces, due to the small number of sample units.

Moreover, the extent of reporting errors varies between provinces. It is believed that misreporting was more severe in some interior provinces due in part to low education level and local customs. Variability in annual rates, therefore, should be treated with caution. Nevertheless, the original data will be used with as little adjustment as possible in order to document the genuine fluctuations.

In addition to the data source discussed above, this study also makes use of data from China's 1953, 1964, and 1982 population censuses as well as a mass of government statistics. In the past several years, with the recovery of China's statistical system, statistical yearbooks and the like have been published for most provinces in China. Basic information on women's status, contraceptive use, and general socio-economic development in the region can therefore be obtained, although these data are often not systematic and not free from errors. Since the early 1980s the Chinese Population Information Centre has begun to publish its annual handbook on Chinese population issues, which contains very detailed and valuable information on China's population policy, family-planning regulations, and local achievements, etc. This is one of the major sources for the present study, especially for the discussion of recent development of the family-planning programme. These statistics, in many instances, can be used for internal research only and are not available to foreign researchers. Beyond these, this study investigates various relevant literature written in Chinese language, and fragmentary information is gathered as the analysis progresses.

V. Major Demographic Indices

In demographic terms, fertility relates to the number of live births a woman has actually had. There are many measures of fertility, and perhaps the simplest and most frequently used one is the crude birth-rate. The crude birth-rate is the ratio of the number of live births during a given year to the mean population of that year. This rate is very easy to calculate and understand, and very useful in estimating the growth rate for a population. However, like many other crude rates in demography, the analytical utility of the crude birth-rate is limited, which is mainly because of the effect of the specific composition of a population. The size of the birth-rate will depend on the relative size of these groups at fertile ages. This shortcoming becomes crucial in comparative fertility analysis.

Considering the features of the major data source of the study, a set of interrelated demographic indices is used in this work to describe and compare the trends in fertility and nuptiality over time. These indices are basically the conventional measures and little indirect or modelling technique is employed.

The basic index of fertility is the Age-Specific Fertility Rate (ASFR), which is calculated by relating the number of live births occurring to women of a given age to the total number of women of that age. A set of these rates serves as a basis for detailed comparisons which are not affected by differences between the populations for age–sex composition. China's 1982 Fertility Survey provides us with the necessary information to calculate these age-specific rates for each of the twenty-eight provinces under study, separating the rural from the urban population for the time period from the 1940s to the early 1980s with some truncation in the earlier years. While comparison of these sets of age-specific rates for a given population between different time points can tell us the age pattern of fertility changes, comparisons between different population groups, usually between provinces, demonstrates the spatial patterns of such changes.

On this basis, total fertility rate (TFR) can be calculated very simply by summing up the ASFRs for a given period. Total fertility rate is the measure of fertility that is probably most widely used by demographers because it is a single-figure measure and independent of age structure. The TFR can be viewed as the number of children a woman would have if she survived to age 50 and experienced exactly the ASFRs for the year in question throughout her reproductive life.[34] For most purposes of this study, the TFR is treated as the prime indicator of fertility.

The upper-age limit of the 1982 Fertility Survey in China was set at 67 years old. This means that it is possible to calculate complete sets of age-specific fertility rate only from 1964 onward based on the information collected in the survey. Before that date, only truncated fertility rates for younger ages are available. In order to take advantage of the measure TFR, partial total fertility rate (PTFR) is employed in this study for the analysis prior to 1964. The PTFR is a similar measure to the TFR. The difference is that the former sums up age-specific fertility up to and including age 39, the latter up to age 50.

Broadly speaking, the study of fertility can be conducted through period or cohort measures. As the period analysis studies events occurring during a particular period of time, the cohort study considers the experience of one group of women over time. This means that the period fertility analysis describes the experience of a synthetic cohort, while the cohort analysis summarizes the actual experience of a real cohort. The computing procedure for cohort fertility rate is basically the same as for calculating period fertility rate. The cohort total fertility rate, or the complete family size, can be interpreted as the average number of children a woman in the particular cohort (e.g. birth or marriage cohort) has borne by age 50. Similar to that, the index of average number of children born to women at certain ages, which can be obtained directly from the Fertility Survey or by cumulating the ASFRs for the successive ages belonging to the same cohort, show us the fertility progress of a cohort through the childbearing ages. As the major concern of this research is to analyse fertility trends in given population groups by their yearly performance, and because of the data requirement of a fairly long, consistent time series in cohort analysis, period measures are most frequently used in the work.

Fertility rate may be further refined by restricting the base population to married or ever married women. Then a set of marital fertility rates can be estimated using the same procedures as those described above. Analysis based on these marital fertility rates eliminates the influence of variations or changes in nuptiality patterns, and separates the effect of marriage from the effect of changes in the level of fertility within marriage upon overall fertility.

There are good reasons for studying nuptiality itself. However, since the major interest of this study is fertility transition, marriage is merely studied in terms of its relationship to childbearing. In a country like China, first marriage marks the time point when a woman first becomes exposed to the risk of childbearing. Therefore, the mean age at first marriage (MAFM) is the major indicator we use in analysing changes in nuptiality patterns. From our major data base, information on the number of marriages, broken down by age and year, are available. Then the calculation of the MAFM is straightforward as a weighted average of the ages at first marriage, where the weights are numbers of marriage incident. An overwhelming majority of Chinese women get married before reaching their early 30s. For the sake of simplicity, our calculation for the MAFM only includes women up to age 32. The exclusion of women who get married at age 33 and over seems to reduce the MAFM slightly, but will not distort the general picture at all.

In addition to the MAFM, age-specific first-marriage rates (ASFMR) are calculated in an analogous way to the Age-Specific Fertility Rate. Since the first marriage is a non-repeatable event, the cumulated ASFMR up to certain ages for given cohorts is regarded approximately as the proportion of women ever married at those ages in the corresponding period, and used to estimate the age-specific period marital fertility rate. On the other hand, the total first marriage rate (TMR) is estimated simply by summing up the ASFMRs for the given time period as we did in calculating the total fertility rate. It equals the proportion that would ever marry in a hypothetical cohort subject to the marriage rates of the year in question.[35] The trend of TMR indicates changes in marriage occurrences over time. As in calculating the MAFM, women who get married after 32 years old are left out in computing the ASFMR and the cumulated ASFMR and the TMR as well.

In the ensuing chapters, fertility and nuptiality will be described primarily in terms of these demographic indices just mentioned. By and large, conventional statistical and demographic methods are employed in the following chapters. In cases where some new concept, index, and analytical method are involved, their definitions and usage will be shown in the relevant places.

NOTES

1. World Bank, *World Development Report* (Oxford: Oxford University Press, 1984).
2. United Nations, *World Population Prospects: Estimates and Projections as Assessed in 1984*, as *Population Studies*, No. 98 (1986).
3. S. F. Hartley, *Population: Quantity vs. Quality* (Englewood Cliffs, NJ: Prentice-Hall, 1972), 2.
4. Editorial Committee of China Handbook, *Life and Lifestyle* (Beijing: China Handbook Series, Foreign Languages Press, 1985).
5. Shou Jinghua, 'Interview with a Specialist on Population', *Beijing Review*, 22 (46), 16 Nov. 1979.
6. Ho Ping-ti, *Studies on the Population of China, 1368–1953* (Cambridge, Mass.: Harvard University Press, 1959).
7. G. Barclay, A. Coale, *et al.*, 'A Reassessment of the Demography of Traditional Rural China', *Population Index*, 42 (4), 606–35 (1976).
8. Liu Zheng, 'Population Planning and Demographic Theory', in Liu Zheng, Song Jian, and others, *China's Population: Problems & Prospects* (Beijing: New World Press, 1981), 3.

9. L. H. Day, *Analysing Population Trends: Differential Fertility in a Pluralistic Society* (New York: St. Martin's Press, 1983), 2.
10. J. Matras, *Population and Societies* (Englewood Cliffs, NJ: Prentice-Hall, 1973), 292.
11. R. Freedman, 'Theories of Fertility Decline', in K. Mahadevan, P. J. Reddy, and D. A. Naidu (eds.), *Fertility and Mortality: Theory, Methodology and Empirical Issues* (New Delhi: Sage Publications, 1986), 30–6.
12. S. E. Beaver, *Demographic Transition Theory Reinterpreted* (Lexington, Mass.: D. C. Heath and Company, 1975).
13. See e.g. W. S. Thompson, 'Plenty of People', *American Journal of Sociology*, 34 (1929), 959–75; F. W. Notestein, 'The Economics of Population and Food Supplies', *Proceedings of the Eighth International Conference of Agricultural Economists* (London, 1953); A. J. Coale and E. M. Hoover, *Population Growth and Economic Development in Low-Income Countries: A Case Study of India's Prospect* (Princeton, NJ: Princeton University Press, 1958), 12–13.
14. J. C. Caldwell, 'Toward a Restatement of Demographic Transition Theory', *Population and Development Review*, 2 (2), 231–66 (1976); also id., *Theory of Fertility Decline* (London: Academic Press, 1982).
15. G. McNicoll, 'Institutional Determinants of Fertility Change', in C. Hohn, and R. Mackensen (eds.), *Determinants of Fertility Trends: Theories Re-examined* (Liege: Ordina Editions, 1982), 147–68.
16. See e.g. P. E. Hollerbach, 'Fertility Decision-making Process: A Critical Essay', in R. A. Bulatao, and R. D. Lee (eds.), *Determinants of Fertility in Developing Countries* (New York: Academic Press, 1983), ii. 340–80.
17. See e.g. P. H. Lindert, 'Child Costs and Economic Development', in R. A. Easterlin (ed.), *Population and Economic Change in Developing Countries* (Chicago: The University of Chicago Press, 1980), 5–69.
18. R. A. Easterlin, and E. M. Crimmins, *The Fertility Revolution: A Supply–Demand Analysis* (Chicago: The University of Chicago Press, 1985).
19. Action Pack, Distributed by the World Population Year Secretariat of the United Nations Fund for Population Activities, 1974.
20. K. Singh, 'Statement Made at the World Population Conference', Bucharest (Aug. 1974), Mimeo.
21. R. T. Ravenholt, and John Chao, 'Availability of Family Planning Services—The Key to Rapid Fertility Reduction', *Family Planning Perspectives*, 6 (4), 217–23 (1974).
22. B. Berelson, W. P. Mauldin, and Z. Sykes, 'Conditions of Fertility Decline in Developing Countries 1965–1975', *Studies in Family Planning*, 9 (5), 89–147 (1978).
23. J. Hobcraft, 'The Proximate Determinants of Fertility', in J. Cleland, and C. Scott (eds.), *The World Fertility Survey: An Assessment* (London: Oxford University Press, 1987), 796–837.
24. R. Freedman, 'Fertility Determinant', in Cleland and Scott (eds.), *World Fertility Survey*, pp. 773–95.
25. Freedman, 'Theories of Fertility Decline', cited in n. 11, above.
26. A. J. Coale, and S. C. Watkins (eds.), *The Decline of Fertility in Europe* (Princeton, NJ: Princeton University Press, 1986).
27. R. A. Easterlin, 'Modernization and Fertility', in Bulatao and Lee (eds.), *Determinants of Fertility in Developing Countries*, ii. 565.
28. A discussion on Tibet population can be found in Wang Ke *et al.*, 'Demographic

Transition and Current Population Situation of Chinese Tibetan', *Population Research* (English edition), 2 (3), July 1985.
29. A. Mason *et al.*, 'Population Growth and Economic Development: Lessons from Selected Asian Countries', *Policy Development Studies*, No. 10 (1986), UNFPA.
30. Xiao Zhenyu, 'The Design of 1982's Fertility Sampling Survey in China', in China Population Information Centre, *Analysis on China's National One-Per-Thousand-Population Fertility Sampling Survey* (Beijing, 1984), 11–23.
31. Li Bohua, 'Assessment of the Accuracy of a Sampling Survey', in China Population Information Centre, *Analysis on China's National One-Per-Thousand-Population Fertility Sampling Survey* (Beijing, 1984), 24–31.
32. A. J. Coale, *Rapid Population Change in China 1952–1982* (Washington, DC: National Academy Press, 1984), 38.
33. C. Scott, and T. Harpham, 'Sample Design', in Cleland and Scott (eds.), *World Fertility Survey*, pp. 309–46.
34. C. Newell, *Methods and Models in Demography* (London: Belhaven Press, 1988).
35. Coale, *Rapid Population Change in China 1952–1982*, cited in n. 32, above.

2

The Development of Provincial Family-Planning Programmes

It is widely accepted that China's rapid fertility decline is largely due to its very successful family-planning programme. The evolution of the programme can be traced back to the mid-1950s and has been marked by fluctuation, mainly caused by political upheavals. In addition, the implementation of these programmes was not easy. Tremendous difficulties and problems were encountered, especially at local levels. As a result, its outcome varied widely according to time and location.

One of the prominent features of China's family-planning programme is its decentralized policy implementation. Although the policy initiative began with the central government, its implementation relies to a large extent on local authorities. Special regulations regarding family planning have been issued by provincial authorities. Therefore, throughout the last several decades the provincial patterns of China's fertility transition have been closely connected with the development of provincial family-planning programmes.

In this chapter, the experiences of family-planning programmes at the provincial level are reviewed and their impacts on fertility transition are assessed. The evolution of birth control in China has a very long history. This study, however, is confined to the period starting in 1949, which is believed to be most relevant to the fertility transition at provincial levels.

I. Review of China's Population Policy

China's population policy has embraced two major strands. On the one hand, great efforts have been made to reduce mortality rates through developing health services and improving living standards. China has succeeded in achieving this development goal. On the other hand are attempts at the control of the population growth. This study will be concerned with the latter.

Mao Zedong's Views of Birth Control

In a country like China, the opinions and attitudes of the top leaders have a strong influence on national policy-making processes. Mao Zedong, the late chairman, played an extremely important role as an ideologist, a balancer, and an innovator until his death in 1976.[1] As with other issues, Mao's view of birth control changed over the years, greatly affecting the development of national and provincial family-planning programmes. This chapter, therefore, begins with a brief review of Mao Zedong's attitudes towards birth control and family planning.

Mao Zedong was first known to have expressed his ideas on population in 1949, when the Communist Party took over the national power. In September 1949, in reply to the white paper on the United States relations with China given by the US government, Mao repudiated Acheson's demographic interpretation of the origin of the Chinese revolution and revealed his own assessment of China's population affairs. He declared that to have a large population 'is a good thing' for China, and 'even if China's population multiplies many times, she is fully capable of finding a solution, the solution is production.'[2] In this declaration, Mao Zedong also proposed the famous thesis that people are the most precious of all things in the world. These views dominated China's population issues until 1952, and their influence was still very strong several decades later.

After the 1953 census, Mao's opinions gradually began to change, probably under the influence of both increasing pressure from growing population and an open debate that was held on the issue at that time. In a government draft directive called 'National Programme on Agricultural Development' which was released in 1956 and reportedly formulated and drafted under his direct personal guidance, birth control for the first time appeared in an official government document: 'It is necessary to publicize and promote birth control and planned parenthood in all densely populated areas.'[3]

One year later, Mao Zedong again showed his concern over population problems. In his famous speech to the Supreme State Conference 'On the Correct Handling of Contradictions among the People', Mao pointed out that 'we have this large population, it is a good thing, but of course it also has its difficulties.' Meanwhile, he criticized other people who went around 'grumbling that there are too many people'.[4] Several months later, Mao once again endorsed birth control in his October speech to the enlarged Third Plenary Session of the Eighth Central Committee of the Chinese Communist Party. He directed that family planning should be promoted particularly in densely populated regions. He said that 'as far as procreation is concerned, the human race has been in a state of total anarchy and has failed to exercise control.' In addition, he proposed 'there should also be a ten-year programme for family planning' and 'complete realization of family planning in the future'.[5] There can be no doubt that such a public endorsement of birth control by Chairman Mao facilitated the formulation and implementation of the family-planning programme.

However, Mao's view on birth control remained inconsistent over the next few years, especially in 1958 when he launched the Great Leap Forward. In an article written for the party journal *Red Flag*, Mao referred to the large population as 'the decisive factor' in the Leap.[6] He was critical, in a meeting held in Chengdu, of propaganda about over-population, since it could create a pessimistic atmosphere. He stressed that a large population was a good thing and that China could control its population growth when the total population reached around seven- or eight-hundred million.[7]

After the massive demographic crisis in 1958–62, an unprecedented birth boom occurred. The population pressure was increasingly perceived by the government. In a talk with Edgar Snow in January 1965, Mao once again agreed with birth control and asked Chinese scientists to invent a simple oral pill for contraception.[8]

Thereafter, Mao gradually realized the urgency of the need to promote family planning. In 1971 the State Council issued a directive which stated among other things that 'birth control is an important matter that Chairman Mao has advocated for many years.' Mao's quote, 'to allow anarchy in human reproduction is not to be tolerated. It is necessary to practise family planning', was cited as the guideline of the campaign. It is also said that in 1973 Mao suggested the establishment of the State Council Family Planning Office. Furthermore, considering the strong influence of feudal ideology over birth control, Mao indicated that simply making the contraceptives available free of charge was not enough. He asked family-planning personnel to deliver birth-control services to people's homes.[9] At the end of 1974 Mao Zedong gave the instruction (maybe the last on birth control before his death) to promote the national economy and slow down population growth. 'Population growth must be controlled.'[10]

From this brief review, we can see that in the early years, Mao's views of the population issue were very optimistic and mainly ideological. Later, taking a more realistic view, his opinion gradually inclined towards the advocacy of birth control. In spite of Mao's attitudes, in general his views endorsed birth control and had a positive effect on the promotion of China's family-planning programme.

The Evolution of China's Population Policy

Immediately after the founding of the People's Republic, the government paid great attention to restoring the national economy and restructuring the social order. The government was fully occupied in reconstruction and was too busy to promulgate or even consider a clear-cut population policy.[11] The new marriage law was passed and enforced in 1950. However the main aim of the campaign for implementation of the new law was to reform the traditional marriage system and the prevailing unequal status of women in society rather than population planning.[12]

The Soviet Union's thought and policies concerning population were accepted by the Chinese government and masses as the orthodox socialist ones. 'Mother heroine' was widely propagated through the media, and awards and financial assistance were offered to families which had multiple births.[13] Moreover, the pronatalist tendency pursued by the State was evident in other social and economic policies. For example, according to 'The Regulation of Labour Insurance' passed by the State Council in 1951, female workers or male worker's wives could receive a birth subsidy from their employers. Free medical care for expectant mothers and for mothers and their infant children was provided.[14] More importantly, sterilization and induced abortion were rigorously restricted by the government. In short, the population policy, if one did exist, was pronatalist in that period.

The period of the First Five-Year Plan, 1953–7, witnessed a great increase of concern about population growth. There were open debates on this issue, especially among relevant scholars and officials.[15] The government Administration Council, predecessor of the State Council, directed the health department to help the public with contraception as early as 1953. Meanwhile the relevant regulation about abortion was under revision.[16]

In 1954 the vice-chairman Liu Shaoqi, then second only to Mao, declared in a forum on birth control that birth control should be promoted and not opposed. In reply to a letter written by the Ministry of Health, the Centre for the first time issued a directive on birth control in March 1955.[17] Proper control over childbearing was advocated. It was reported that China started to manufacture contraceptives in 1955.

Nineteen fifty-six was the year when the first family-planning programme started. On August 6, the Ministry of Health issued a 'Regulation on Contraception', which was accompanied by an extensive campaign to provide general information on birth control. In September the same year, Premier Zhou Enlai in his 'Report on the Proposals for the Second Five-Year Plan for the Development of the National Economy', given at the Eighth National Congress of the Chinese Communist Party, pointed out that 'a due measure of birth control is desirable'. Giving birth in a planned way was confirmed as a part of the Party's Eighth Congress's line.[18] This could be viewed as an official endorsement of birth control.

Many measures were also taken to facilitate birth control after that. Late marriage was widely publicized as a means of reducing population growth, although the rationale centred on the mother's health and changing the traditional family institution. A joint directive was issued by the ministries of Health and Commerce to expand the supplies of contraceptives and reduce the sale price. Restrictions on induced abortion and sterilization were relaxed. Despite strong opposition, clinical abortion was allowed to be carried out up to the tenth week of pregnancy, independent of the age of the pregnant women or the number of her children. The Chinese Medical Association set up a Birth Control Technical Guidance Committee to co-ordinate research on contraception and to provide technical guidance.[19]

During this campaign, birth control depended largely on public health organizations and personnel. Although it was reported that a government office was established to take charge of the matter, there was no evidence available on its operation.[20] The Ministry of Health was fully responsible for this issue. Newspapers and periodicals were utilized to disseminate the birth-control knowledge. The *People's Daily* published its first editorial article on birth control in March of 1957.[21] Major mass organizations, such as China's Women's Federation and the All China Federation of Trade Unions, were all involved in the campaign.

However, the population debate of 1957, which was closely tied to the short-lived Hundred Flowers Campaign initiated in 1956, was soon silenced. As early as summer 1957, during the Anti-rightist campaign, all propositions concerning birth control were identified with 'Malthusianism'. People supporting birth control were criticized, the most notable being Ma Yinchu, the author of 'New Population Theory'.[22] Although official support for birth control was never withdrawn, the climate of opinion once again turned steadily against the campaign.[23]

With the launching of the Great Leap Forward and Communization movements in 1958, the first birth-control campaign was nipped in the bud, although no change in population policy was officially announced. Even so, it paved the way for the later programmes. For instance, restrictions on contraceptive use were lifted, and abortion and sterilization were legalized in 1957. Research into birth-control methods was encouraged. The introduction of the vacuum aspiration abortion method, which made abortion safer, was one good example.

Between 1958 and 1961, China was preoccupied first by the Leap and then by overcoming the economic crisis. Birth control was virtually abandoned. 'The more people, the more views and suggestions, the more intense the fervour, and the greater the energy' was one of the slogans of the Leap. Thus the question was not whether China was over-populated but rather whether China had enough manpower to meet the needs of its socialist construction. In this period, birth-control guidance committees and contraceptive factories all ceased to function. Although contraception guidance was still available from doctors, it was dependent solely on the patient's medical need and health conditions. Enormous increases in mortality and declines in fertility were the demographic consequences of the Great Leap Forward and the nation-wide natural calamities.[24]

Nevertheless, the Great Leap and Communization did create better social conditions for the enforcement of birth control than the old system. The new structure of the rural communes in particular de-emphasized family and kinship authority over the individual, which allowed the implementation of family-planning measures without any great sensation in later years.

In 1962, with the nation recovering from the chaos of the Great Leap, sharp fertility compensation emerged. Alarmed by this, and aware of the bitter lesson that the relationship between population and food supply was not as optimistic as previously thought, people began turning their attention to the subject of birth control again. The second birth-control campaign started officially with the issuing of the directive on promoting family planning by the Central Committee of the Communist Party (CCCP) and the State Council in December 1962. In that directive, the State Council called on the various localities to promote birth-control measures earnestly and to bring childbearing into the orbit of state planning. The State Council set up a special agency, the Family Planning Staff Office,[25] to take charge of birth control. Soon, corresponding agencies were established at the local levels.

A population target had still not been set. However, slogans such as 'two children are just right, three are too many, and four is an error' indicated the government's desire to limit the family size. For the first time, supplies of contraceptives were distributed free of charge in some areas and under certain circumstances. Restrictions on induced abortion were further relaxed. Birth-control supplies could be imported duty-free.[26] Meanwhile, some other relevant social welfare policies were also revised to be in favour of birth control. In many provinces, for instance, birth subsidies were only provided to mothers who were bearing a first or second child; higher order births were no longer eligible for such benefits. Nevertheless, many policies continued to hinder the implementation of family planning. Food grain, private plots, and housing land, for example, were all allocated on a per capita basis in the rural areas. In the cities, living subsidies for low wage-earners with large families were another factor which retarded birth control.

In the 1950s China perceived birth control mainly in terms of maternal and infant welfare. The main aims of birth control were to protect women and children and to bring up and educate the younger generation in an appropriate way. In the second family-planning campaign, although these rationales remained, consideration was also given to the interests of the masses and the nation. Marriage and birth were no longer purely personal affairs, since government and society had to provide maintenance, education, and employment. Therefore, family planning was regarded as serving the health and welfare of the entire people and socialist construction. This campaign focused on the urban population.

Just as the second birth-control campaign was about to bring down population growth, the start of the 'Cultural Revolution' in the summer of 1966 disrupted the programme.

The major targets of the Cultural Revolution were 'Capitalist-roaders', 'Bourgeois academicians', and those who held bourgeois ideology.[27] At first, the movement was dominated by Red Guard activities; but soon everyone was mobilized to take part in the movement. Debate and fighting between those 'revolutionary rebels' who took over the power from the government and Party bureaucrats and their opponents increased and led to widespread violence and social disturbance. As with other government organs, the work of family-planning agencies came to a standstill and their personnel were dismissed. Advocates of birth control became associated with the 'Capitalist-roaders'. The networks for manufacturing and distributing contraceptives were disrupted, so that supplies of contraceptives were cut off. Control over the age at marriage broke down, and the practice of early marriage became widespread throughout the country. This can be seen from the falls of the mean age at first marriage. Virtually no family-planning programme existed during this period.

After 1969 confusion gradually gave way to order. Reorganization and restructuring of the Party and the administrative bureaucracy got under way. The government was alarmed by the soaring growth in population, and reactivated the family-planning campaign.

Family planning finally began to be promoted in earnest in 1971 with the issue in July of the State Council Directive (Number 51, 1971)—the personal initiative of Premier Zhou Enlai. Unlike previous campaigns, the goal of the third campaign was very clear. The specific requirements for the campaign were summed up later as three norms, 'Wan, Xi, and Shao', which means later marriage and childbearing, longer birth interval, and fewer children.

The standard age for late marriage was set at the provincial level rather than by the central government. Therefore, it varied from one region to another. Generally speaking, the recommended marriage age in urban areas was 27 for men and 25 for women, and 25 for men and 23 for women in the rural areas. The legal minimum marriage age remained 18 for women, as it had been set by China's 1950 marriage law. One of the major measures used to promote late marriage was control over marriage registration. This worked very well, in part thanks to the organization of Chinese society and the influence of Chinese traditions.

The policy required a four-year interval between first and second births. In practice, a longer interval was encouraged. The emphasis of the campaign was on 'fewer births'. The real definition of 'fewer' had in the mean time undergone a downward movement. In general, the ideal number of children was considered to be two.

In 1973 the State Council set up a leading group for family planning. Local family-planning activities revived with the direct participation and supervision of Party leaders. Population targets were for the first time formally included in national economic planning. Contraceptives were supplied free of charge nation-wide in 1974 after a circular issued by the State Council's Family Planning Leading Group and other departments.

At first, measures aimed at achieving the target of 'two children per family' were limited almost exclusively to ideological education and persuasion as in the previous campagins. During this period, the realization of population targets depended almost entirely on government propaganda and the people's voluntary co-operation. Later, measures and regulations that could be enforced efficiently were formulated, mainly at the local level. Material incentives and sanctions were also imposed.

Chinese delegations began to appear at international population forums.[28] At home, more than five national conferences on family planning were held by the State Council between 1972 and 1978. Population research was also revived after 20 years silence.[29]

After the death of Mao Zedong and the fall of the 'Gang of Four' in 1976, China's politics entered a new stage. The attention of the government and the Party shifted to economic development. The 'Four Modernizations', of industry, agriculture, scientific research, and defence, were announced as the highest priority task instead of political struggles. The effects of population growth on the overall development were more seriously realized by the government, and more attempts were made to promote the family-planning programme. In 1978 family planning was for the first time confirmed in legal form and became an article of the new Chinese Constitution.[30] The State Council Family Planning Leading Group was reorganized and given more authority.

By the end of 1978 China's birth control seemed to have been very successful in slowing population growth. The natural increase rate had decreased from 23.4 per thousand in 1971 to 12 per thousand in 1978. However, it was clear that when the large cohorts borne in the 1950s and 1960s gradually reached the age of marriage and childbearing, the population growth would inevitably soar, even if all those newly married couples were to give birth only to two children. In order to speed up the process of modernization, 'one child per family', a new family-planning policy far more ambitious than any previous ones, was announced by the government.

The major motivation behind the policy was economic considerations. According to the government's long-term plan, the per capita GNP should be increased from about 250 US dollars[31] in 1979 to 800–1,000 dollars by the end of this century. To achieve this goal, the population target by the year 2000 was set at 1.2 billion. In August 1978 vice-premier Chen Muhua, then the head of the State Family Planning Commission, provided the statistical rationale for the new campaign. She concluded that even if every couple only had two children the population target could still not be attained. Hence, some couples would have to have only one child.[32] Earlier, the national goal had been that 80 per cent of all couples in cities, and 50 per cent in the rural areas, should have only one child. Later, the target of the single-child family shifted to 95 per cent in the cities and 90 per cent in the countryside.[33]

This time, the government's intervention was much stronger than ever before. The Central Committee of the Communist Party issued an open letter in September 1980 to all members of the Party and the Communist Youth League asking them to take the lead in responding to the new policy and set a good example to the rest of the population.[34] Besides the family-planning personnel, leaders at all levels were urged to take charge of the issue. Intensive mass education and propaganda campaigns were conducted. The media were fully mobilized to take part in the campaign.

However, resistance to the policy was strong, especially in rural areas. Political and social pressures were employed and an elaborate set of incentive and disincentive measures had to be developed. Although persuasion and education are the main official methods of birth control, coercive measures were reportedly used at local levels when simple persuasion did not work.

According to China's 1982 Census, 77.6 per cent of urban women pledged to have only one child and were accordingly issued with the single-child certificate. The figure for the rural areas was only 31.3 per cent. For the country as a whole, it was reported that by 1982, 19.5 million, about 67 per cent of all eligible couples, had pledged to have only one child.

More recently, the rigorous policy has been modified and implemented along more pragmatic lines to make it easier to carry out the programme. On 13 April 1984 a Central Document (No. 7) was issued. The critical importance of family planning was reaffirmed, but local family-planning offices were given more autonomy in devising regulations and setting targets in accordance with local conditions. The basic principles of the policy, as stated by Wang Wei the head of the State Family Planning Commission at that time, were that family planning should serve the overall development plan, birth-control regulations should be enforced in accordance with the local conditions, and the programme should be implemented upon the public co-operation or mass line.[35] Such a modification is known by Chinese as 'blocking up the big breach, meanwhile opening a small hole'.[36] Bearing a second child is, in fact, permitted for a large proportion of rural couples, though the policy of one couple, one child is still strongly recommended by the government. Since then, there has been no major change in government's policy towards population control.

In May 1986 the Party Central Committee issued its Document No. 13, calling on local governments to learn from past experience, overcome mistakes and perfect population policy.[37] Following the appointment of Peng Peiyun as minister of the State Family-Planning Commission in January 1988, several important meetings were held by the Politburo of the CCP in order to re-examine China's population policy. China's low level of economic development and the importance of the family unit in socio-economic activities were among the factors which were taken into account. China's international image was a further major consideration. The outcome of these meetings was to introduce greater flexibility into population policy. The modified measures emphasize the promotion of later marriage and late child-bearing in order to generate fewer but healthier births. In cities and those areas considered economically and culturally well developed, the policy of one child per couple was to be maintained and consolidated. Meanwhile, the policy of allowing the 'only girl household' to produce a second child after an interval of several years was to be put into effect in most rural areas.[38] This approach was regarded not only as an effective means of controlling population growth, but also one that was more palatable to the public.

There have been regional variations in the formulation and implementation of the population programme. In general, birth-control regulations for urban residents have been more or less stable during the 1980s. With few exceptions and subject to prior approval, each family living in China's urban areas was permitted to have only one child. Changes or modifications mostly affected the countryside. By the end of 1988, in eighteen provinces peasant families with just one daughter were permitted—after an interval—to have a second child. In a further six provinces or autonomous regions, every peasant family was to be allowed to have two children, regardless of the sex of the first child. However, in provinces such as Jiangsu and Sichuan, such concessions were introduced only within limited geographical areas. Furthermore, the regulation of one child per couple for the majority of peasant families in the suburbs of the three major municipalities remained intact. By contrast, couples within minority nationalities have generally been allowed to have two or more children.

II. The Development of Provincial Family-Planning Programmes

The Chinese political system is highly centralized. Nevertheless, decentralization has gradually emerged since the late 1950s as one of its primary administrative characteristics.[39] Policy-makers at the national level, in fact, expect the regional administrators to adapt national policies to local conditions. This is also the case where family planning is concerned. One of the advantages of this pattern is that it allows local government a voice in the implementation of the birth-planning policy. On the other hand, wide local variations in the degree of compliance with national policy result.[40]

Birth Control in the 1950s

In the 1950s most of the work relevant to birth control was conducted by local health authorities and personnel. However, Birth Control Guidance Committees, sometimes called Birth Control Committees, were set up in many provinces, such as Hunan and Tianjin. These committees usually consisted of the heads of various government departments and mass organizations. The heads of the provincial health department, in some cases even the provincial Party secretary, chaired the committee, depending on the importance attached to birth control by local leaders. The task of these committees was to co-ordinate and regularize the various activities associated with the promotion of birth control.[41] They were, therefore, not given authority to take full responsibility for the work. At lower levels, birth control was more prominent in urban than rural areas. Birth Control Guidance Committees were reportedly set up in most urban areas. By contrast, such guidance committees only existed in city suburbs and densely populated rural areas.

Hunan was publicized widely at that time as a model province for birth-control efforts. It was said that except for the minority and mountainous areas, all cities and counties in the province had set up organizations to deal with birth-control propaganda and guidance.[42]

In some provinces, directives or official instructions were issued. For example, Hunan province issued a joint directive from the Women's Federation, Trade Union, Education, and Health Departments to call on publicizing contraceptive knowledge and help women to control and overcome the difficulties brought about by large families.

No general numerical target for population growth was established since birth control at that time was orientated towards health concerns. However, in the case of Shanghai this was only partly true. Birth control attracted great attention during the third session of the Second Municipal Congress in 1957. Protecting the city from over-population was given equal importance with women and children's health care. An annual birth-rate lower than 20 per thousand was also suggested as the target of the city's population growth for the Second Five-Year Plan period (1958–62).

Following directives issued by the central government, birth control was widely propagated, especially in the cities. Exhibitions, one of the most important means of birth-control propaganda at that time, were held in many large cities. These exhibitions were reported to be very successful in attracting large numbers of viewers. This was possibly the first time that the public could openly learn about contraception. These exhibitions did receive some criticism for showing very detailed animated diagrams,[43] probably due to the traditional Chinese reluctance to discuss sexual matters in public.

Beijing organized a ten-month exhibition between 1956 and 1957, and reportedly more than 0.83 million people visited it, about 40 per cent of its total population at that time.[44] In Jilin, a city in Jilin province with a population of around half a million in the mid-50s, a three-month exhibition on birth control attracted about 16.6 per cent of its population. In Guangzhou, the capital of Guangdong province, 0.4 million people visited an exhibition.

Besides exhibitions, various other methods of propaganda were employed. In addition to newspapers and periodicals, many pamphlets on birth control were published and distributed in order to disseminate contraceptive knowledge. Propaganda meetings were convened. It was recorded that the number of people involved in those various kinds of birth-control propaganda amounted to 8 and 8.6 million in Guangdong and Hunan provinces respectively.

Training of birth-control personnel, including propagandist and medical staff, formed another important aspect of the first birth-control campaign. In Hunan province about 59,000 people were trained to be propagandists for birth control in 1957 alone. In Guangdong province the figure was more than 30,000. Medical staff were also trained to perform birth-control operations, such as sterilization and abortion. According to partial statistics, 422 doctors in Hunan province took part in such training in 1957 alone.

No systematic data are available on provincial differentials in the birth-control campaign and the prevalence of contraception in the 1950s. Nevertheless, we do know that in some provinces, such as Guizhou, there was no large-scale propaganda for birth control, and the Birth Control Technical Guidance Committee did not exist until 1963. Another example is Gansu province. In a speech given at the Chengdu Conference in 1958, Mao Zedong singled out Gansu and some other sparsely populated provinces as examples of areas where birth control was not necessary. This speech to a large extent hindered the progress of the family-planning campaign in the province.

Moreover, the first birth-control campaign was characterized by more talk than real action. The network for contraceptive services had not yet been built up. During the 1950s the only available modern birth-control methods were those for external-use, including sterilization, abortion, condoms, diaphragms, and contraceptive jellies and foams. Even in provinces where extensive propaganda was carried out, birth-control operations performed there were very insignificant. For instance, in 1958, only 6,000 people accepted male or female sterilization and induced abortion in Guangdong province, less than 1.8 operations in every 10,000 population.[45] The number of those operations performed in Hunan province in 1957 was a little higher at 8,000, about 2.4 per 10,000 of the province's total population. Tianjin seems to have taken a more efficient action: the annual average of these three birth-control operations between 1956 and 1962 amounted to 4,000, or a proportion of 12 per 10,000 population. IUD insertion in the 1950s was much less popular than the three operations mentioned above. The effective oral contraceptive was reported to have developed in 1957, but there was no widespread use of any oral contraceptive until late 1969.[46]

In conclusion, the first birth-control campaign was more prominent at the national than at the provincial level, and it involved more propaganda than real action. Because the significance of birth control was on maternal and child health and women's liberation, the impact of the campaign on limiting population growth was almost invisible. As it was the first serious attempt to alter values that had been central to Chinese culture for millennia, difficulties were unavoidable.[47]

Furthermore, the supplies of contraceptive facilities were very limited. As stated by Coale, one of the main pre-conditions of marital fertility decline is that effective techniques of fertility reduction must be known and available.[48] This was certainly not the case in China in the 1950s. Not all couples, even in the big cities, had access to modern contraceptive services. It was reported that the total supply of contraceptives at that time was sufficient to meet the needs of only 2.2 per cent of all couples of reproductive age.[49] Moreover, the western-trained doctors who could perform birth-control operations, which were then still a complicated procedure, were in extreme shortage. As a result, fertility levels in almost all provinces remained unchanged in both rural and urban areas. Shanghai may be the exception where the initial fertility decline began in the late 1950s. Modern urban life-style and easy access to contraceptives may have been be largely responsible for this early transition.

Despite that, the campaign in the 1950s did disseminate the knowledge of birth control and those trained birth-control personnel became the backbone of the later campaigns.

Birth Control in the 1960s

The second birth-control campaign started in late 1962. Government played a more important role in this campaign than ever before. The State Council set up its family-planning leading group in 1963. Shortly after that, provincial committees were reorganized or set up (see Table 2.1). At first, names of those committees varied between provinces. Late in 1964 they were unified as Family Planning Committees—an indication that birth control was now to be implemented in a planned way.

The composition of the committees testified to the importance attached to them. In the 1950s the responsibility for birth-control affairs, such as education and propaganda, rested entirely in the hands of public-health personnel. Now the political cadres were required to share this responsibility and the Party was put in charge of its implementation.[50] The committee for Shanghai was made up of officials from the municipal Party committee, the municipal council, other local government agencies and mass organizations, together with some medical experts. In Guangdong province the leader of the provincial Communist Party chaired the committee. By contrast, the committee in Gansu was under the supervision of its provincial Cultural and Educational Office.

Under the provincial Family Planning Committee, there was the provincial Family Planning Staff Office, responsible for day to day administration. In the 1960s such staff offices were usually branches of the Department of Health. Birth-control officials were specialized. The Family Planning Committees were also commonly set up at municipal and county level. The regional differentials in administrative network for birth control, however, were considerable at the grass-roots level, especially in rural areas. It was reported that 40 per cent of communes and 20 per cent of all brigades set up family-planning leading groups in Shanxi province. The situation in Hunan province was reportedly better. Almost every commune and brigade had set up a family-planning office by the mid-1960s, or at least had someone special in charge of these affairs. Such a pattern extended down to the production team, China's basic socio-economic unit in rural areas at this time.

There was no general requirement for the campaign. However, 'two is best, three is too many' was the slogan proposed in Hunan, Guangdong, and Hebei provinces.[51] In Beijing the slogan was simply 'too many children is not desirable'. Although the national and societal interests were introduced, the main significance of birth control was still seen in terms of benefits to individuals.

Later marriage was regarded as one of the main measures of the planned-birth campaign. The government did not set a national standard for later marriage. However, the recommended marriage ages for men and women, at least in Guangdong and Hunan, were 28 and 25 respectively in urban areas, and two or three years lower for rural youngsters. The requirement for a longer birth interval, which was commonly set at four years, was also proposed in many provinces. Later marriage and delayed childbearing were put into practice more efficiently in urban areas, where the government control and socialization processes were more effective.

In addition, many other social policies were revised nation-wide to facilitate the campaign. For example, birth subsidies for births of higher parity were abolished, married youths were given very restricted opportunities to enter universities for higher education, etc. Therefore, the second birth-control campaign witnessed, in embryonic form, reproductive norms which came to prevail in the 1970s.

During the early stages of the second campaign, the focus was still on the urban population. Intellectuals and cadres were the main targets of the campaign. According to the instruction given by Hunan provincial government, the work of planned birth should have followed the sequence of 'party member first, non-member later, cadres first, masses later, city first, village later, and pilot area first, other places later'. This strategy was adopted in many other provinces as well. As a result, the campaign had very little effect on the rural population. It is reported that only 20 per cent of the counties in Guangdong carried out the programme at that time.

Medical care for the rural population improved greatly, but was still poor. Whereas in 1957 there were 0.59 doctors (including both Western-trained and Chinese traditional medicine) for every 1,000 population living in rural areas, by 1964 the figure had increased to 0.82.[52] Travelling birth-control medical teams, mostly from large cities, were sent to rural areas to promote birth control. It was reported that five birth-control medical teams with 600 personnel from Shanghai worked in its outskirts between 1963 and 1965, and 70,000 birth-control operations were performed by them. Such experiences were paralleled in many other provinces. However, services provided by these mobile teams could not meet the needs of the large rural population, especially those living in the remote areas. In fact, only after the establishment of the rural health-care network several years later, did means of birth control really reach the hands of the rural population.

The means of propaganda employed in the first campaign were also used in the 1960s but on a larger scale. Trained propagandists in

Shanghai amounted to one-quarter of a million, which means that there was approximately one propagandist among every 8.5 women of childbearing age. About 1.2 per cent of the total population of Guangdong province (i.e. half a million people) were trained there as propagandists. There were less than 2 propagandists out of every 1,000 population in Shanxi province,[53] compared with 22 in Shangai.

In the 1950s the cost of contraceptives, as well as birth-control operations, was paid by the individual. Tianjin was the first place to provide free contraceptives in July 1963. Following that, Shanghai, Guangdong, and Qinghai, together with some other provinces, announced that birth-control facilities were going to be available free of charge. In many other provinces, such as Gansu, the prices of contraceptives and operations were reduced. It was not until the early 1970s that the cost of birth control was totally subsidized by the State.

Data on government spending on birth control in 1965 are available although the real coverage of the budget is not very clear. Nevertheless, per capita expenditure on birth control has been estimated for each province and can be viewed as another indicator of the local commitment to birth control. Because details of the population's sex and age composition in 1965 are not currently available for each province, the provincial total population has to be used as the denominator for calculation. Results are shown in Table 2.1.

It can be seen that the birth-control expenditure varied considerably between provinces, ranging from 12 cents per person in Shanghai down to 1 cent per person in Guizhou province.[54] The national average at that time was 4.1 cents per person. A geographical pattern also emerged from the comparison: all fourteen provinces with above the national average expenditure, except Shaanxi and Nei Monggol, are situated along China's eastern border. Per capita expenditure was highest in the three large municipalities. On the other hand, the financial support from local governments for family planning was far smaller for those living in the vast central and western parts of China. In any case, these figures were provincial averages. It is certain that most of this money was spent in urban areas. The rural population benefited far less than their urban counterparts from the government expenditure.

The relationship between population density and per capita expenditure is not explicit, though the eastern provinces are generally densely populated. The population density in many central provinces, such as Henan, was much higher than the national average. But birth-control spending there was far below the national average. In contrast, although provinces such as Jilin were sparsely populated, they spent

TABLE 2.1. *Indicators of birth control in the 1960s by province*

Province	Total population (1)[a]	Population density (2)[b]	Set up office (3)[c]	Per capita expenditure (4)[d]	Ratio of: Operations (5)[e]	Ratio of: Propagandist (6)[f]
Shanghai	1094	1745	1963.5	12.0*	16.43	22.85
Beijing	776	452	1963 s	9.5*	17.84	
Tianjin	336	553	1963.1	8.1*	20.70	
Heilongjiang	2134	43		7.8*		
Jilin	1639	84	1963.5	6.3*	4.13	
Shandong	5711	363		5.9*		
Hebei	4724	210	1963.4	5.8*	5.70	7.41
Fujian	1760	138	1964 f	5.2*		11.36
Liaoning	2808	185		5.1*		
Nei Monggol	1296	10		5.0*		
Shaanxi	2144	101		4.9*		
Jiangsu	4624	434	1964 f	4.5*	12.50	
Zhejiang	2957	278		4.2*		
Guangdong	4231	191	1963.10	4.1*	6.00	11.82
Shanxi	1872	116		3.5		1.67
Hubei	3505	180		2.6		
Hunan	3901	177	1962.10	2.4	2.75	
Guangxi	2445	101		2.4		
Ningxia	227	32		2.2		
Sichuan	7137	120		2.1		
Anhui	3286	224		1.8		
Yunnan	2161	52		1.8	0.52	
Qinghai	230	3	1963 s	1.7		
Henan	5240	301		1.6		
Gansu	1346	28	1963 s	1.6		
Jiangxi	2209	126		1.4		
Xinjiang	789	5		1.1		
Guizhou	1821	97	1963 s	1.0	1.31	

[a] Year-end population in 1965, in 10,000s.
[b] Population density refers to 1964, person/km^2.
[c] Refers to the time when the family planning committee was set up. f (s) indicates the first (second) half of the year.
[d] Per capita expenditure on birth control in 1965, in cents (Renmin Bi)
= total family planning budget/total population
* indicates the figure is above the national average
[e] The number of operations per 1,000 population. Operations include tubectomy, vasectomy, insertion of IUD, and induced abortion. The average number of operations between 1962–5 is used as the numerator, except Yunnan where the figure refers to 1963 alone. The denominator is the total population in 1965.
[f] Refers to propagandists per 1,000 population.

Sources: Cited in n. 38; and also State Family Planning Commission of PRC, *Quanguo jihuashengyu ziliao huibian (Collection of Family Planning Statistics), 1983.*

relatively large amounts on birth control. The eastern provinces were and still are the most prosperous regions in China. This seems to suggest that expenditure on birth control in the mid-1960s was closely linked to the development level of provincial economy. It is also likely that the relatively better infrastructure of communications in the eastern region allowed the government policy to be carried out more effectively.

During the 1960s the four birth-control operations—tubectomy, vasectomy, insertion of IUD, and induced abortion—were the most commonly used birth-control methods. Oral contraceptive pills were still at the experimental stage. No data are available on provincial birth-control prevalence in the 1960s. However, the number of those four operations per thousand of the population has been estimated for several provinces and is included in Table 2.1.

These operations seem to have been far more popular in the three major municipalities than any other provinces. In the southwestern provinces, Yunnan and Guizhou, the figures were very small.

This finding is not surprising as the second campaign was in general based in urban areas, and the suburbs of these big cities were served efficiently by mobile medical teams. These estimates are provincial averages. Separation of the rural from the urban population is only possible in a few provinces. Hence, the real achievements in provinces with a dominant rural population are to some extent concealed.

Hunan's case can be taken as an example. In 1965 the four operations performed in cities accounted for 47 per cent of the province's total operations, although the urban population only accounted for 10.4 per cent of the total population of the province. This means that there were 21.7 operations in every one thousand of Hunan's urban residents, a similar ratio to that in the three large municipalities.

The rural–urban differential in Hebei province was less extreme, operations amongst the 9 per cent of the population living in urban areas accounting for 38.6 per cent of the province's total birth-control operations in 1966. Compared to other provinces, the ratio of the four operations in Jiangsu, where 85 per cent of the population were rural residents, was much higher and only just behind the three big cities. This comparison suggests the diffusion of family-planning programmes to the vast rural areas occurred earlier in Jiangsu than in many other provinces.

The results of birth-control efforts in the urban areas were very impressive. As we will show in the later chapters a sustained decline in urban fertility began in virtually every province around the mid-1960s.

There is a very close relationship between birth-control expenditure and provincial fertility level in the 1960s. The correlation coefficient between the total fertility rate in the late 1960s and the government expenditure on birth control is as high as 0.85. This is a clear indicator of the important role played by the government in bringing down the population growth. It may also reflect the importance of birth control diffusion during the early stage of the fertility transition.

The family-planning programme virtually came to a halt during the chaotic period of the Cultural Revolution. The marriage boom, combined with the absence of publicity and supply of contraceptives, contributed to a high birth-rate, especially in 1968 and 1970. The general trend towards low fertility was maintained in urban areas, but the effects of birth control were insignificant in the rural areas, although an initial decline in rural fertility can be found in the rural districts of major municipalities and some eastern provinces.

It is interesting to note, however, that the idea of birth control persisted, despite the attack of 'revisionist' and 'capitalist' socio-economic policies. As soon as the confusion began to diminish, family planning once again received attention. For instance, as early as January 1968, the Shanghai Municipal Revolutionary Committee, the apparatus of political and administrative authority during the Cultural Revolution, issued a notice on strengthening birth control and advocating later marriage. A similar notice was also reportedly issued in Tianjin, where the Family Planning Committee even resumed work for a short while. In Hunan a provincial conference of family-planning work was said to have been convened in April 1969. In spite of these activities, the family-planning programme remained largely dormant and was not reactivated until the early 1970s.

Another very important event during the Cultural Revolution was the establishment of the rural-health network. In as early as 1965, Mao Zedong criticized the Ministry of Health as an urban overlord, and insisted that medical and health work should put the focus on the rural areas.[55] Following Mao's proclamation, especially during the Cultural Revolution, China's health network underwent a massive reorganization. The 'barefoot doctor' is a Chinese innovation. Although barefoot doctors only received several months of primary medical training, they did provide basic health care to peasants when they returned to their villages. The introduction of barefoot doctors into the family-planning campaign in the early 1970s became one of the key factors responsible for the success of the campaign at that time.

The 'Wan, Xi, Shao' Campaign

The third nation-wide birth-control campaign was launched after the restoration of order in the early 1970s. Premier Zhou Enlai personally initiated the programme. A State Council Directive (Number 51) issued in July 1971 formally marked the beginning of the campaign. In that Directive, the leading cadres at various levels were called on to strengthen leadership, and to conduct penetrating propaganda and education on birth control.

Organization

With the restoration of state apparatus, the State Council Family Planning Leading Group was set up in 1973 with Hua Guofeng as its head, and the offices at provincial level were correspondingly re-organized. Shortly afterwards, Offices of Family Planning were established at all lower administrative levels, from municipal to commune revolutionary committee. Family Planning Small Groups were also set up at grass-roots levels, such as the resident neighbouring committee in urban areas and the production team in rural areas. A nation-wide family-planning network was under construction. In some provinces, the resumption of the family-planning programme started even earlier. Guangdong, and reportedly, Hunan and Jiangsu re-organized their programme networks in 1970. With the simplification of bureaucratic organizations, birth-control staff were usually attached to offices under the health department and held a relatively lower position in the bureaucratic hierarchy. For example, family-planning personnel in Jiangsu at first belonged to the Staff Office for Prevention of Snail Fever.

However, nation-wide implementation of the policy did not come until at least a few years later, since political struggle and rebuilding the Party and government system were given priority. In many provinces the early 1970s was a period of recovery for family planning. In fact, mainly due to the aftermath of the shattering events of the Cultural Revolution in some provinces, much more time was spent in restoring government functions. It was reported that the administrative function in Guizhou province was hardly realized until 1974, which impeded the implementation of the family-planning campaign. Until 1975 virtually no work was conducted in forty (about half) of the province's counties.

One of the features of family planning in the first half of the 1970s was its close linkage to the on-going political movements, such as criticizing Lin Biao (the former vice-chairman of the CCP) and Confucius, the movement to criticize the so-called right deviationist wind to reverse correct verdicts, etc. Family planning was treated as a political task. The uneven progress amongst provinces and regions was often attributed to the strength of the local Party leadership, and is believed to be connected with the degree of provincial political stability and the authority of local leadership.

Three reproductive norms, known as 'later, longer, and fewer', were summed up in 1973 at the First National Report-back Meeting on Family Planning Work and guided the new campaign thereafter. Some provinces were always slightly late to follow the national trend. Jiangsu and Hebei formally proposed 'later, longer, and fewer' in 1973, Jilin did so in 1974, and Guizhou province as late as 1978. The power to set these norms was in the hands of the provincial authorities. For instance, in the early 1970s the age of later marriage was set at 25 for women in urban areas and 23 in rural areas in Beijing, Hunan, Jilin, and some other provinces, but 23 for urban women in Jiangsu and Hebei provinces. An interval of 3 to 5 years between births was commonly regarded to be ideal. Two children per couple was widely accepted to be the target for the small family.

Since the mid-1970s, the leadership for family planning has been strengthened. The State Council Family Planning Committee was reorganized again in 1978. It was then headed by vice-premier Chen Mu-hua. More personnel were recruited or transferred, which made it possible for there to be at least one full-time staff member in every rural commune's Family Planning Committee. Guangdong was one of the leading provinces: more than 3,000 part-time staff were transferred to be full-time cadres for family planning at grass-roots levels in 1978. This was regarded as a national model.

Annual targets of the natural increase rate in the various provinces have been set by the State Council Family Planning Staff Office since the mid-1970s. Each province upon receiving its target, allocated birth quotas for the lower administrative units under its direct jurisdiction. This procedure was repeated down the line to the basic family-planning units.

Accompanying this process was the tactic of group birth control, which was characterized by 'self-proposal and group evaluation'.[56] A prominent feature of the Chinese family-planning programme is its community basis, not only in providing services, but also in setting population growth targets. The strategy used for the programme was still the mass line, or as Wolf has it, the government and the community pitted against the individual.[57] Although the final decision on birth control had to be made by couples themselves, social pressure was obviously an important factor.

In a country like China where the majority of population live in rural areas and a large proportion of the rural population is illiterate,[58] these small group study meetings served as a very important means to disseminate birth-control knowledge, and as noted by Salaff,[59] to establish psychological and social support for members to practise family limitation. Hence, the success of the programme relied to a large extent on the persuasion and other activities of the grass-roots-level community leaders. Birth quotas were allocated to the eligible couples, and this was viewed as a guarantee for fulfilling the target set by the higher level. Non-complying individuals were under great pressure from the group to use contraceptives or to postpone marriage. The programme administrators and workers were also under great pressure to show significant success or continued progress in their work, since their career advancement largely depended on it.

Though the central government has repeatedly stressed the importance of persuasion, local cadres have often resorted to coercive measures in order to meet numerical targets. The extent of coercion seems to be closely linked with the prevailing political atmosphere and general level of education. Despite that, the success of the family-planning programme in China is still decisively dependent on the voluntary co-operation of the populace rather than on coercion.

Birth-Control Expenditure

In addition to Tianjin and Shanghai, many more provinces began to provide contraceptives free of charge in the early 1970s. Hebei province took the step in December 1972, and Henan in 1974. Contraceptives were first supplied freely throughout the country in 1974 after the issue of a Directive by the State Council. Since then, expenditure on procurement of contraceptive supplies and on reimbursement for the four birth-control operations made up a large part of the provincial annual budget for family planning, the other parts covering the propaganda and educational activities, manpower training, and research.[60] During the 1970s, as the campaign progressed, the annual expenditure on family planning gradually increased, providing financial support for the programme. Considerable provincial diversities have always existed. The estimated per capita expenditures for birth control (PCEBC) for each province throughout the 1970s are presented in Table 2.2.

On one hand, these figures can be viewed as the financial input of the provincial programme. On the other hand, they can be treated as

TABLE 2.2. *Per capita expenditure on birth control (PCEBC) in the 1970s*[a]

Province	1971–3	1974–6		1977–9		1971–9
	PCEBC	PCEBC	Rise (%)	PCEBC	Rise (%)	Total PCEBC
CHINA	27.9	43.8	57	57.5	31	129.2
Beijing	36.6*	46.5*	27	24.0	–48	107.1
Tianjin	20.1	33.6	67	51.9	54	105.6
Hebei	54.3*	53.7*	–1	65.7*	22	173.7*
Shanxi	37.2*	51.3*	38	57.1	11	145.6*
Nei Monggol	34.5*	45.6*	32	51.5	13	131.6*
Liaoning	35.6*	45.1*	27	62.2*	38	142.9*
Jilin	33.7*	53.7*	59	62.2*	16	149.6*
Heilongjiang	31.2*	59.5*	91	58.4*	–2	149.1*
Shanghai	21.6	18.3	–15	25.3	38	65.2
Jiangsu	28.5*	36.9	29	48.1	30	113.5
Zhejiang	33.9*	35.7	5	54.6	53	124.2
Anhui	21.0	36.6	74	51.2	40	108.8
Fujian	28.2*	40.0	42	72.3*	81	140.5*
Jiangxi	13.0	40.4	211	67.2*	66	120.6
Shandong	33.9*	57.2*	69	71.3*	25	162.4*
Henan	24.5	45.0*	84	62.7*	39	132.2*
Hubei	33.0*	39.6	20	53.1	34	125.7
Hunan	27.8	44.2*	59	57.0	29	129.0
Guangdong	28.1*	46.7*	66	56.6	21	131.4*
Guangxi	16.1	20.3	26	33.2	64	69.6
Sichuan	22.3	48.8*	119	63.7*	31	134.8*
Guizhou	10.5	33.3	217	56.5	70	100.3
Yunnan	10.9	30.4	179	43.6	43	84.9
Shaanxi	27.8	49.5*	78	67.4*	36	144.7*
Gansu	32.5*	60.7*	87	74.7*	23	167.9*
Qinghai	21.8	35.7	64	40.2	13	97.7
Ningxia	38.3*	32.0	–16	33.4	4	103.7
Xinjiang	5.4	11.5	113	21.0	83	39.7
MEAN	27.23	41.14		53.08		121.50
ST.D.	10.38	12.02		14.79		31.34

[a] Measured in cents (Renmin Bi). The exchange rate between Renmin Bi and US dollar was around 1.97:1 in 1975. The average of the province's total population in the corresponding period is used as the denominator.

* indicates the figure is higher than the national average.

Source: Estimated from data in *Collection of Family Planning Statistics, 1983*, compiled and published by State Family Planning Commission (Beijing, June 1983).

partial indicators of the programme's achievements, since *ceteris paribus* greater success might be expected to have led to the provision of more birth control services and the expenditure of more money.

Several interesting features can be seen from Table 2.2. In general, the expenditure per head increased year by year and across the country. However, the speed and the timing of such increases varied greatly from province to province. In the early 1970s the regional pattern of expenditure in 1965, which was discussed in the earlier section, remained valid. Provinces along the eastern border, with the exceptions of Shanghai and Tianjin, spent much more on family planning. This seems to suggest that the birth-control policy was implemented earlier in the eastern regions. The PCEBCs for China's two key municipalities, Shanghai and Tianjin, were not as much above the national average as was to have been expected because of the success of their family-planning campaigns.

This phenomenon deserves attention and some possible explanations have been investigated. Shanghai and Tianjin took the lead in birth control in the first two campaigns. By the 1970s birth control had become so well understood by the public that it was no longer necessary to conduct large-scale propaganda and training, and the budget could be concentrated on the birth-control services. In addition, since the social infrastructure was far superior in those two cities, their budgets may well have been used more efficiently than in many other provinces. Furthermore, since the early 1970s, China's birth-control services in the vast rural areas have been closely connected with the rural co-operative medical network. Barefoot doctors and rural medical clinics were the backbone of the birth-control campaign.[61] The rural-health service was basically maintained by local communities, and depended largely on the local economic situation. Therefore, the effectiveness of the programme in more affluent areas was also attributable largely to the existence of well-established rural-health networks. Actual per capita expenditures on birth control in those areas were accordingly much higher than the index PCEBC indicated.

The per capita expenditure on birth control increased in all but three provinces in the mid-1970s. Although the absolute values were still not so high as others, the increase of the PCEBC in 5 provinces, Guizhou, Sichuan, Yunnan, Jiangxi, and Xinjiang, was really impressive. Expenditure on birth control more than doubled in these provinces—no doubt the result of a late start and subsequent catching-up from a low PCEBC base in the early 1970s.

Birth-control spending continued to increase through the late 1970s, while the regional differentials diminished. In 1971–3 the highest provincial PCEBC was 10 times the level of the lowest one. The figure was down to 5 in the mid-1970s, and fell again to 3 in the late 1970s. This may have resulted from the unification of the campaign, but also perhaps reflected the diffusion of local experience and lessons.

In the 1970s provinces with large minority populations were consistently among those with low expenditure per head. This doubtless reflects the special status of minority nationalities *vis-à-vis* population policy. There are 8 out of 29 provinces in the mainland of China where the minority population exceeds 10 per cent of the province's total, including Xinjiang, Guangxi, Yunnan, Guizhou, Qinghai, Ningxia, Nei Monggol, and Xizhang. Measures for planned population growth were not demanded of these minorities, as in the case of the populous Hans. Indeed, the ultimate aim at that time was to promote the population growth for some of the less populous minority groups, and provide birth-control services only to those with minority status who requested it, while growth of the majority Han population was strictly controlled.[62] Xinjiang is an extreme case where the PCEBC was consistently the smallest in the country. For the whole of the 1970s the per capita expenditure on birth control for people living in Xinjiang only amounted to 40 cents, which was less than one-third of the national average of 130 cents.

On the other hand, the adjacent areas with three northeast provinces plus Hebei and Shandong were constantly among the national highest quarter. In these areas, family planning seems to have been carried out earlier and consistently more efficiently.

Achievements

Shanghai still took the national lead in birth control in the 1970s. It was reported that as early as 1971, 72 per cent of all married couples at fertile ages were already using contraceptives. The prevalence rate rose to 83 per cent in 1973, 86 per cent in 1975, and 97 per cent in 1979. The use of IUD insertion and the oral pill increased sharply. In 1971 only 13.5 per cent of couples who were using contraceptives reported that they took pills, and 7.15 per cent used an IUD. By 1975 pill-takers and IUD-users accounted for 21 per cent and 13.7 per cent of all contraceptive-users respectively.[63]

The regional differentials in birth control were great, even among large cities. Available data show that in 1973, the contraceptive-prevalence rate was 83 per cent for Shanghai as a whole, while the same rate for Beijing was 70 per cent for the urban population, and 60 per cent in its rural districts. Prospects in remote provinces and rural areas seem to have been far less bright. The contraceptive-prevalence rate in

Shanxi was 49.6 per cent in 1972. Further inland, it was reported that as late as 1975, only one-third of women exposed to the risk of pregnancy were protected by some kind of contraceptive in Guizhou province.

The four birth-control operations still accounted for a large proportion (more than 40 per cent) of all birth-control methods, though the oral pill was rapidly gaining in popularity. In 1972 the percentage of the four birth-control operations to the total population, was 21.58, 17.85, and 8.87 in Shandong, Shanxi, and Yunnan provinces respectively.

All these figures suggest that the differentials in the progress of the family planning were considerable in the early 1970s. These differentials were due in part to lack of qualified family-planning personnel. In Guizhou province in the early 1970s there were only 49 full-time staff in charge of the province's family-planning programme. Out of the 570 hospitals in this province, only 153 were capable of conducting birth-control operations.

In the late 1970s a system of measures for evaluating the performance of the programme was diffused to all provinces. The system was designed to measure the extent to which eligible couples in a given unit complied with the requirements of the family-planning programme. The main indices are the Late Marriage Rate, the Birth Limitation (equivalent to contraceptive prevalence) Rate, and Planned Birth-Rate. The Planned Birth-Rate is a Chinese innovation, which is defined as percentage of births with birth quotas to all births. The programme's statistics are not free from error. The main problem is over-reporting, which is mainly caused by the demand on field workers to achieve specific targets. In spite of that, those statistics do provide systematic data for an examination of provincial differentials in family planning. In Table 2.3, these three indices are presented for all provinces in 1979. A distinction is further made between urban and rural population.

It should be pointed out that these indices, especially the planned birth-rate and the later marriage rate, are not always good measures for direct comparison of regional differences, because of local variations in these norms. For instance, urban women in Hebei, Jiangsu, Jilin, and Liaoning who married at age 24 were classified as late marriage, whereas, the norm in Shanghai and Beijing was 25. In addition, these norms have been revised from time to time. Therefore, these measures should be used with caution in analysing regional diversity.

From Table 2.3 one can see that the achievements of the programme were outstanding. The contraceptive prevalence rate in China is far higher than in many other developing countries and approaches the level of developed countries.[64] There is considerable regional variability in contraceptive practice. Roughly speaking, the family-planning

TABLE 2.3. *Indices of birth-control achievement, China 1979* (in %)

Province	Late marriage			Contraceptive use			Planned births		
	Total (1)	Urban (2)	Rural (3)	Total (4)	Urban (5)	Rural (6)	Total (7)	Urban (8)	Rural (9)
CHINA	86.0	93.7	82.7	79.8	87.2	78.7	65.1	79.6	63.7
Beijing	97.9	96.5	83.4	86.6	89.5	83.3	84.0	90.1	79.3
Tianjin	97.9	98.2	97.5	85.7	89.2	82.8	71.1	92.4	61.8
Hebei	96.0	98.2	95.5	84.4	85.9	84.3	77.8	78.7	77.7
Shanxi	83.0	90.0	82.0	80.0	88.0	78.0	65.6	72.1	64.6
Nei Monggol	73.7	94.5	70.0	73.0	84.4	70.5	51.4	76.5	48.6
Liaoning	90.6	97.6	86.2	86.4	89.5	84.9	74.4	85.6	70.5
Jilin	80.6	90.5	76.8	80.7	85.7	79.3	67.0	84.3	62.9
Heilongjiang	79.7	89.6	75.9	84.3	87.9	83.1	73.5	84.4	70.6
Shanghai	94.0	83.9	96.5	97.3	99.9	95.0	87.6	97.0	82.7
Jiangsu	92.5	97.2	91.5	87.7	86.2	88.0	73.4	79.9	72.8
Zhejiang	77.6	88.4	76.7	78.9	80.2	78.8	59.7	66.0	59.3
Anhui	88.1	94.9	86.9	76.9	81.5	76.4	62.0	81.0	61.0
Fujian	67.7	89.3	63.5	82.4	88.2	81.1	46.5	61.4	45.2
Jiangxi	71.9	91.5	62.5	77.4	88.5	76.4	53.3	74.9	52.1
Shandong	95.1	98.9	94.6	85.4	88.8	85.1	80.3	89.9	79.5
Henan	95.7	96.4	95.0	75.7	85.9	74.9	62.6	78.0	61.8
Hunan	84.1	90.2	83.1	78.6	90.2	77.5	72.0	65.3	72.6
Hubei	85.5	97.5	84.2	82.1	88.3	81.6	63.2	78.4	62.3
Guangdong	81.5	94.7	67.0	73.4	84.1	71.9	62.7	75.8	61.4
Guangxi	—	—	—	58.9	80.0	57.8	52.3	65.9	51.9
Sichuan	94.7	96.2	94.4	88.5	88.8	88.4	75.1	81.0	74.2
Guizhou	71.5	91.0	69.1	67.2	81.0	66.2	48.9	71.7	48.0
Yunnan	77.2	89.6	75.4	55.8	75.8	54.6	55.3	64.2	54.9
Shaanxi	83.1	94.1	81.9	84.7	88.4	84.1	61.8	75.7	60.5
Gansu	89.0	96.0	87.0	82.0	86.0	81.0	62.0	73.0	60.4
Qinghai	45.0	82.5	11.0	45.2	81.9	38.5	27.2	66.9	23.0
Ningxia	72.1	82.5	56.4	60.4	71.6	56.0	39.7	66.4	30.1
Xinjiang	89.1	94.7	86.3	80.3	89.5	76.0	70.5	88.3	66.7

Note: — means data are not available.

Source: State Family Planning Commission, *Collection of Family Planning Statistics, 1983*.

campaign has been implemented much better in cities and towns than in the countryside, better in the eastern than in the western provinces, better in the northern than in the southern regions, with central China lying in between. The three major municipalities were still well ahead of other provinces. Among provinces, Hebei, Shandong, Jiangsu, Liaoning, and Sichuan formed the top quarter by all three measures. More than 84 per cent of all fertile women in these provinces were practising birth control in 1979. In contrast, provinces in the western, except Sichuan, and southern parts of China made up the lowest third.

Contraceptives were used moderately in provinces with high proportions of national minorities, such as Qinghai, Ningxia, Guangxi, Guizhou, and Yunnan. As was mentioned earlier, this was due in part to the fact that family-planning programmes had been enforced much less strongly among national minorities. Guangdong and Hunan did quite well in the first two birth-control campaigns, at least in terms of propaganda. However, their leading positions were surpassed in the 1970s, and Guangdong was persistently among the worst.

In the 1970s intra-uterine devices (IUD) were the most popular contraceptive methods used by Chinese women, and accounted for about one-half of all contraceptive methods. Female and male sterilizations were the second most popular. However, the pill and condom were more common in urbanized areas, and the greater the degree of urbanization the less the IUD was used. Such an association is attributed to the fact that urban areas have more efficient contraceptive distribution systems.[65]

The distribution of 'later marriage' follows a similar pattern. As we will show in forthcoming chapters, resistance to later marriage was stronger in places where early marriage prevailed in the past. In rural areas of Qinghai province, only 11 per cent of marriages satisfied the norm of later marriage, and 56 per cent in Ningxia autonomous region. The later marriage rates were very low in Fujian and Jiangxi where local marriage customs remained very strong. It is interesting to note that the later marriage rate in Shanghai's urban districts (0.84) was lower than that in its rural area (0.96). This may be caused by the very high age criterion for later marriage for Shanghai's urban population.

As far as the planned birth-rate is concerned, it can be seen that about one-third of total births in 1979 were outside birth quotas. Regional variations were very marked and the situation was worse in rural areas. Shanghai held the best record nation-wide: 83 per cent of all rural births took place within the quotas. Despite the fact that birth control in minority areas was carried out very moderately, a large proportion of births occurred outside the birth plan there. Among the lowest quarter, where the planned birth-rate in the rural areas was below 55 per cent, were Qinghai, Ningxia, Fujian, Guizhou, Nei Monggol, Guangxi, Jiangxi, and Yunnan.

These varying performances of the 'Wan, Xi, Shao', campaign resulted in considerable regional variations in fertility transition throughout the 1970s. The geographical distribution of contraceptive prevalence, later marriage, and planned births, and that of the fertility

TABLE 2.4. *Correlation coefficients between birth-control expenditure, family-planning measures, and the TFR*

	1	2	3	4	5	6
1. Expenditure 1965	—	0.090	0.417	0.585	0.600	−0.731
2. Expenditure 1970s		—	0.245	0.328	0.155	−0.316
3. Late marriage rate 1979			—	0.780	0.860	−0.733
4. Contraceptive prevalence 1979				—	0.836	−0.856
5. Planned birth rate 1979					—	−0.794
6. Total fertility rate 1979						—

rate, corresponded closely: the correlation coefficients between these three measures and the Total Fertility Rate in 1979 were −0.856, −0.733, and −0.794 respectively (see Table 2.4). This close relationship between contraceptive prevalence and total fertility remained in the early 1980s ($r = -0.859$ in 1981).[66] All these figures confirm the importance of the family-planning programme on fertility transition.

The One-Child Campaign

By the end of the 1970s the fertility transition in urban areas was virtually complete in almost every province. Sharp fertility declines had been recorded in the rural areas of the eastern provinces, whereas fertility levels remained very high in most of the interior provinces.

The rather ambitious one-child policy was first put forward in the second half of 1978. Following the issue of the open letter from the Communist Central Committee in September 1980, the campaign was carried out vigorously. There was no national standard or legislation, although some attempts had been made in this direction.[67] Instead, the implementation of the compaign was largely reliant on local commitment.

The entire country was mobilized to carry out the campaign. Birth-control activity was regarded as one of the main tasks of all branches of the Communist Party at all levels. The organization of the family-planning programme was extended and strengthened. Every possible means of propaganda was utilized.

In accordance with the instruction of the central government, provincial stipulations were published. Basic principles of provincial regulations were the same, but the concrete requirements and incentive packages varied to match local economic and social conditions. Economic incentives for family planning had been used in previous programmes. In the one-child campaign, a more complicated package of the incentive and disincentive was introduced. This may be viewed as an attempt by the government to balance the economic costs and benefits of raising children.[68]

Eligible couples were required to apply for the one-child certificate if they pledged to have no more children. Upon obtaining the certificate, the couples and their child were offered benefits specified by local regulations. In contrast, couples who continued to bear two or more children without early approval were exposed to heavy penalties.

The package of benefits and penalties varied from province to province, and differed between rural and urban areas, as well as between counties and communes within the province. In addition, these regulations were modified over a period of time. It is impossible to document the varying stipulations in detail. Nevertheless, a rough generalization can be made as follows:

Benefits:

A monthly nutrition or welfare allowance in cash or in workpoints from the time of birth of the child or the time when the parent obtained the one-child certificate until the child reached certain age (usually 14). 5 *Yuan* per month was a fairly common figure.

Preferential treatment was given to single-child families in the allocation of public/state-owned housing in urban areas. In rural areas, the single child was counted as 1.5–2 persons in the allocation of the private plot and housing land. In rural communes the single child was also entitled to an adult grain ration.

Paid or extra paid maternal leave.

Priority access to free medical, educational, and kindergarten facilities. Highest priority in job assignment when child grows up.

Penalties:

Deduction of a fixed percentage of salary (usually about 10 per cent for an unapproved second child, and more for any child born afterwards), or deduction of workpoints, for a certain period (commonly 7–14 years).

No paid maternal leave for third or higher parity births.

Children born outside the plan were not covered by state or collective health schemes. Per capita allowances for grain, private plot, and housing land would be withdrawn in rural areas.

Single fines for extra births.

Regulations concerning economic sanctions varied widely. For instance, one of the punishments for a second unapproved child was a 5 per cent monthly deduction from parents' wages in Zhejiang and Fujian provinces, but a 10 per cent deduction in Beijing, Hebei, Liaoning, Jiangsu, Gansu, and Qinghai, and 20 per cent in Henan province. Furthermore, the period of the deduction ranged from 3 years in Shanghai to 14 years in Hebei, Henan, Liaoning, Gansu, and Ningxia. In Heilongjiang province, the economic sanction was simply a single payment (the minimum fine was 1,200 *Yuan*).

The implementation of these economic incentives and disincentives was very flexible, especially in the vast rural areas. Since many peasants live at a marginal subsistence level, heavy penalties or rewards were thought unnecessary or unenforceable. Furthermore, the allocation of economic benefits placed a heavy burden on the units which were responsible for it, especially in the poor rural communes.[69]

Perhaps more important are the exceptional conditions under which a couple could have a second child. These exceptions were more or less standard within a province, but varied between provinces. In some special circumstances, couples in both cities or countryside areas were entitled to bear their second child upon approval. These special circumstances have been in general common to all provinces.

In Table 2.5, the special conditions under which, as of 1984, a second child was allowed are presented for the majority of China's provinces. Some of these conditions are very subtle in conception and can be interpreted differently. To clarify the study, they are grouped according to basic principles.

In general, only the first few categories are valid for the urban population and they are basically the same across the country. The others are only applied to the rural population. In other words, the single-child policy has been carried out very strictly in urban areas, but less so in rural areas.

Regulations in some provinces were more detailed than in others. Attention should be paid to the category of 'real difficulties' which permitted rural couples to have a second child. This was the most flexible factor in the single-child policy and varied significantly between provinces. In Guangdong province, for instance, rural couples with a single female child were allowed to give birth to another child, if they encountered 'real difficulties'. This is clearly associated with strong son preference in that region. Moreover, the definitions of these articles were vague enough to give local cadres considerable flexibility in their interpretation. They were given the authority to approve second births. These regulations were used as the guidelines for the campaign. The

TABLE 2.5. *Provincial regulations on second child by 1984*

Province	Reasons for allowing a second child														
	1	2	3	4	5	6	7	8	9	10	11	12	13	14	15
Gansu	+	+	+	*	+		*			*		*	*	*	+
Guizhou	+	+	+		+	*				*		*	*	*	+
Sichuan	+	+	+	+		*	*			*		*	*	*	+
Guangdong	+	*	+				+	+	+				*		+
Hubei	*	*	*	*		*	*			*	*	*	*		
Anhui	+	+	+	*	+	*	*			*		*	*		
Jilin	*	*	*	*						*		*	*	*	
Hunan			+	+	+										+
Jiangxi	+	+	+		+	+	+			+			+	+	
Fujian	+	+	+	*		+	*	*	*		*	*			+
Shanghai	+	+	+			*				*		*	*	*	
Qinghai	+	+	+												
Shanxi	+	+	+	+	+	+	+			+	+	+	+	+	
Nei Monggol	+	+	+		+										
Henan	+	+	+	*		*	+			+	*	*	*		
Liaoning	+		+	*	+	*		*		*		*	*		
Jiangsu	+	+	+	*		*				+	*	*		+	
Shandong	+	+	+	*	*	+	*	*		+	+	*	+	*	
Ningxia	+	+	+												
Tianjin	+	+	+	*		*		*		+		+	+	*	
Guangxi	+	+	+	*	+	*	*	*	*	*		+	*		+
Beijing	+	+	+	+	+	+	+			+		*	+		
Heilongjiang	+	+	+	*	+	+				+		*	+		*
Zhejiang	+	+	+	*	+	*	*	*	*	*	*			+	
Hebei	+	+	+	*	+	+	+	+		+		+	*	*	

Note: 1. A couple's first child suffers from a non-hereditary disease or disablement and is unable to become an able-bodied labourer.
2. Pregnancy occurs after a couple who have remained childless for many years adopted a child.
3. One spouse in a second marriage has never had children and the other has one child from a previous marriage.
4. One or both spouses are returned overseas Chinese.
5. Both spouses are minority nationalities.
6. One spouse is handicapped to a specified degree.
7. A peasant couple lives in a mountainous area where population is sparse.
8. One spouse is a fisherman or fisherwoman.
9. One spouse has been working in mining continuously for over 5 years.
10. One or both spouse is an only child.
11. Only one son has been born to a family for at least two consecutive generations.
12. Only one of the male children in a family is able to reproduce.
13. In a rural family with no sons, one of the daughters marries uxorilocally.
14. One of the spouses is the offspring of a martyr.
15. Rural couples with real difficulties.

\+ indicates that the conditions were introduced before May 1983.
* indicates that the conditions were introduced in 1984–5.

Sources: Handbook of Chinese Population Information, 1983 and 1985; *Chinese Population Monographs* for relevant provinces; *Economic Yearbook of Anhui Province, 1984.*

provincial success of the campaign largely depended on the interpretation and implementation of the stipulations.

The Chinese authorities claimed that the policy was implemented flexibily.[70] On the one hand, through these special conditions, the policy adapted to the strong Chinese traditions concerning family lineage. On the other hand, special privileges were given to minority groups, returned overseas Chinese, etc. consistent with government policy towards these groups. Furthermore, disadvantaged groups, such as those living in poor and remote areas, were given a chance to improve their situation by having an extra child. On the whole, as noted by Greenhalgh,[71] the principal considerations of those regulations were to preserve the patrilineal family and reduce gross inequalities.

The single-child policy was not in general implemented in minority areas. The above regulations only applied to the majority Han population. The policy towards ethnic minorities was aimed at voluntary rather than compulsory compliance for the majority Han population. However, the government gradually came to the view that family-planning programmes should also be carried out in those minority nationalities with more than 10 million population in total. For couples who belonged to those minorities with a smaller total population, the new policy was that two children per family was the norm, and some could have three; but that four should be avoided.[72] In Xinjiang some couples with minority status were allowed to have four children, depending on their individual circumstances. Minority nationalities in some parts of Ningxia and Sichuan were allowed to have a third child. Restrictions on the Han population in minority regions were also relaxed. In Ningxia rural couples of Han nationality were merely encouraged to have one child, but in reality a two-children rule applied.

Despite the government's continual reiteration that the policy must be applied on a voluntary basis, occurrences of local coercion were widely reported. This was due in part to heavy pressure from higher levels on the local grass-roots family-planning workers. As the campaign progressed, the economic incentives in a unit were linked to the fulfilment of the birth-control targets. This meant that the welfare of the entire unit would be affected by couples who ignored the birth quota. Some local authorities resorted to forced abortion and sterilization to keep births within the quota set down by higher authorities. In addition, some over-zealous cadres were eager to show their achievements, which might improve their promotion prospects.

These harsh events are of course unpleasant, and the government frequently condemned such work methods. However, if social and political pressure are in some cases necessary to prevent birth-rates from 'soaring' in certain over-populated districts and provinces, so are the remedies.[73] No systematic information is available on this matter.

Partly as a result of these provincial diversities in policy formulation, but also because of regional differences in the acceptance of and resistance to the policy, the results of the single-child campaign varied considerably between provinces. Table 2.6 presents the percentage of couples holding one-child certificates according to province, in selected years. It should be noted that the definition of ratios in 1979 is the same as in 1980, but differs from that of 1984 (see notes to the table).[74] These figures can not be directly compared.

Table 2.6 demonstrates the regional and rural–urban differentials very clearly. Nineteen seventy-nine was the first year of the single-child campaign. However, in one-third of provinces more than 70 per cent of couples with one child in the urban areas pledged to have no more, and held single-child certificates. Except for Sichuan and Hunan these provinces were mostly situated along the eastern coast. By contrast, the percentages in provinces situated in the south coast and western part of China were generally lower. Guangdong was one of the earliest provinces to proclaim a one-child policy with a programme of incentives and disincentives in 1979.[75] Nevertheless, its record was among the poorest in the country. Only 11 per cent of eligible couples in Guangdong's urban areas were issued the certificates.

The differences amongst the rural population were more remarkable. In 1979 whilst 78 per cent of eligible couples in Sichuan province accepted the one-child certificates, fewer than 3 per cent of couples in Guangxi, Guangdong, Henan, Guizhou, and Fujian provinces did so.

There were great rural–urban differences. Even in Tianjin, the third largest municipality in China, only 24 per cent of rural couples obtained the certificates in 1979, compared to 86 per cent amongst the urban population. However, in Sichuan province which had one of the highest acceptance rates for a single child, there was little difference between the rural and the urban population. These regional and rural–urban differences may reflect not only timing factors, but also difficulties, in the implementation of the policy.

One year later, in 1980, 57 per cent of all eligible couples in China were presented with one-child certificates, 51 per cent of the rural and 83 per cent of the urban population. Regional differentials were reduced, but still existed on a large scale. Apart from provinces with a large proportion of ethnic minorities, acceptance of the one-child certificates in Fujian, Jiangxi, Anhui, and Guangdong was very low. In these four provinces, couples holding the one-child certificates

TABLE 2.6. *Percentage of couples holding one-child certificates*[a]

Province	1979			1980			1984		
	Total	Rural	Urban	Total	Rural	Urban	Total	Rural	Urban
CHINA	3.97(5.20)	34.6	64.0	57.1	51.0	82.9	18.25	12.87	30.93
Beijing	52.8(10.41)	22.4	69.9	83.5	65.0	92.7	43.26	31.41	52.09
Tianjin	56.4(11.01)	23.7	85.7	83.3	66.8	96.4	41.66	23.39	59.37
Hebei	72.8(11.73)	71.5	80.7	78.7	75.9	93.1	18.93	14.17	29.77
Shanxi	7.3(0.93)	5.5	15.7	76.8	78.0	69.0	12.51	8.07	20.78
Nei Monggol	11.0(1.09)	7.7	24.1	35.1	31.1	50.8	12.95	7.33	21.01
Liaoning	68.2(12.11)	54.0	91.8	91.8	87.9	97.6	35.83	26.46	47.22
Jilin	15.3(2.04)	5.4	45.0	50.6	34.9	84.1	27.25	20.40	35.86
Heilongjiang	54.3(7.41)	51.9	58.2	82.4	76.9	94.1	24.37	15.61	32.78
Shanghai	87.2(8.43)	71.5	93.6	74.8	61.6	85.1	53.32	44.90	60.16
Jiangsu	65.3(12.18)	62.0	86.6	76.1	73.5	90.6	30.41	26.55	43.39
Zhejiang	18.5(2.59)	15.1	53.7	39.0	35.4	75.4	18.70	14.29	33.02
Anhui	8.2(0.91)	6.7	21.3	17.1	12.0	47.4	9.22	4.74	27.57
Fujian	5.5(0.75)	2.3	27.7	15.5	8.6	60.1	7.34	2.39	16.47
Jiangxi	(0.49)			21.3	16.7	44.1	4.56	1.35	15.38
Shandong	58.9(9.98)	56.5	80.0	88.3	87.2	96.5	27.99	23.40	33.55
Henan	2.8(0.40)	1.6	16.3	25.8	18.8	75.4	18.42	15.76	33.33
Hubei	14.2(2.00)	8.7	56.1	42.6	33.5	85.9	14.41	8.11	23.95
Hunan	34.8(4.31)	28.8	81.5	40.2	33.4	84.1	8.25	4.20	23.59
Guangdong	3.2(0.40)	1.9	11.0	21.9	14.0	61.7	7.47	1.27	20.83
Guangxi	1.9(0.16)	0.7	12.6	6.5	2.8	43.2	4.48	1.01	14.51
Sichuan	79.5(11.92)	78.4	84.1	81.1	79.6	91.1	25.34	22.08	39.80
Guizhou	3.5(0.26)	1.7	19.3	10.5	6.5	28.8	4.24	1.33	14.88
Yunnan	14.0(0.81)	5.4	68.8	16.7	9.7	64.7	5.07	1.51	17.44
Shaanxi	12.9(1.56)	6.4	43.6	79.7	76.2	95.0	14.59	10.01	24.88
Gansu	22.3(2.15)	18.9	38.6	25.0	17.3	81.8	8.63	4.32	26.07
Qinghai				13.3		39.2	5.68	1.99	17.81
Ningxia				6.9	3.0	18.7	4.45	0.38	13.96
Xinjiang	29.2(0.03)	15.0	29.8	39.1	26.9	57.1	6.96	4.00	12.88

[a] Figures for 1979 and 1980 refer to couples holding one-child certificates as percentage of all couples with one child; figures for 1984 refer to ever married women obtaining one-child certificates as percentage of all ever women at reproductive ages; the definition of figures in brackets for 1979 is the same as for 1984.

Source: Data for 1979 and 1980: *Collection of Family Planning Statistics, 1983*. Data for 1984 from *Handbook of Chinese Population Information, 1985*. Both were compiled and published by China's Population Information Centre, Beijing.

accounted for about 20 per cent of all eligible couples, whereas in Beijing, Tianjin, Liaoning, Heilongjiang, Shandong, and Sichuan provinces more than 80 per cent of such couples were issued with the certificates. On the whole, the single-child programme was carried out more efficiently along the east coast and in the north of China, but the achievements on the south coast and west provinces were poor.

The regional pattern persisted in 1984, although the index was different. More than half of all the married women of reproductive age accepted one-child certificates in Shanghai, and more than 40 per cent in the two other major cities, Beijing and Tianjin, more than a quarter in Liaoning, Jiangsu, Shandong, Jilin, and Sichuan. There were nine provinces, including Jiangxi, Guangxi, Guizhou, Yunnan, Qinghai, Ningxia, Xinjiang, Guangdong, and Hunan, in which less than 10 per cent of all couples at fertile ages held the certificates. Since the denominator of the calculation is all ever married women aged 15–49, the index not only indicates the success of the single-child campaign, but also reflects the achievement in the previous programmes. Furthermore, the single-child policy underwent a nation-wide modification after the issue of the government Document No. 7 in the Spring 1984, so that figures in 1984 may be also affected by this policy relaxation.

It is reported that by May 1986, there were 32 million only-children younger than 13 years old in China, accounting for 3 per cent of the national total.[76] Potential achievement in the birth-control programme remains very marked in provinces in the western and southern parts of China. On the other hand, further sharp advance in the three major municipalities and eastern provinces seems to be unlikely.

III. Future Prospects for China's Family-Planning Programme

In the foregoing sections, we have documented the broad features of the Chinese family-planning programme and its achievements at both the national and the provincial levels. We have not, however, examined the operational details of the programme, since much has been written on this subject.

The necessity of the one-child policy may be open to discussion. Attention has been paid to the social consequences of the policy. There are alternatives.[77] The long-term future of the Chinese family-planning programme seems bright, but there are still tremendous difficulties in the short term.

The Chinese government is strongly committed to family planning. Population control is regarded as a basic national policy and viewed as one of the crucial elements which will determine the fate of the four modernizations.[78] The network of contraceptive services has been established and has worked effectively. Research on contraceptive methods is well sponsored. Knowledge of birth control has been widely understood, and the importance of population control for national development, as well as for individual well-being, has been accepted by the populace. As the process of the modernization continues, the resistance to birth control and the small family will, one hopes, disappear.

However, this is not to say that the future programme can be implemented easily. As a side-effect of the political and economic reforms of the past few years, the early advantage of combining the family-planning programme with administrative authority is disappearing, especially at the grass-root level. The commune system has been abolished or reorganized. Individual households have become the basic economic unit once again. Reform in urban areas is also under way. The administrative function of the Party apparatus is diminishing. In the course of this dramatic institutional change, a certain number of local officials have taken a wait-and-see attitude.[79] Such organizational changes, combined with differing interpretations of the Government's 1984 No. 7 document, have been accompanied by a retreat in the one-child programme. In Table 2.7 information on provincial performance of the family-planning programme in the most recent years is presented in terms of late-marriage rate, contraceptive-prevalence rate, and one-child certificate holder rate.

Since the implementation of the new marriage law in 1981, women who get married at an age three or more years older than the legal age for female marriage, which is set at 20, are classified as late marriage. This is a criterion much lower than that commonly enforced in the later 1970s. Even so, it can be seen that almost all of the provinces have experienced a downward trend with respect to the late-marriage rate. In 1986 about 54.12 per cent of first-time brides were aged 23 or over for China as a whole, compared with more than 86 per cent in 1979 and 65 per cent in 1983.[80] It is estimated that in 1986 the number of marriages which took place before the bride reached the legal marriage age accounted for about 15 per cent of all first marriages in China's countryside.[81] The estimated mean age at first marriage in 1986 is 22.54 years compared to 23.12 in 1979. It is plausible to say that the momentum of getting married earlier continued throughout the first half of the 1980s. Among the top quarter of provinces where the rate

TABLE 2.7. *Provincial performance of family-planning programmes, 1984–1986*

Province	Late-marriage rate (%)				Contraceptive prevalance (%)				One-child certificate rate (%)[a]			
	1984	1985	1986	Change[b]	1984	1985	1986	Change[b]	1984	1985	1986	Change[b]
CHINA	58.86	55.20	54.12	–4.74	85.82	85.80	85.61	–0.21	18.25	18.14	17.90	–0.35
Beijing	77.29	71.93	71.38	–5.91	81.92	85.25	87.07	5.15	43.26	47.23	49.16	5.90
Tianjin	68.50	63.25	65.75	–2.75	87.07	87.45	88.60	1.53	41.66	45.31	45.96	4.30
Hebei	58.24	52.84	51.46	–6.78	85.53	86.60	87.08	1.55	18.93	18.23	17.46	–1.47
Shanxi	59.20	59.30	60.11	0.91	87.78	87.75	88.73	0.95	12.51	11.17	11.66	–0.85
Nei Monggol	61.80	64.06	65.18	3.38	85.77	87.03	87.82	2.05	12.95	12.43	12.26	–0.69
Liaoning	51.22	48.35	55.17	3.95	88.51	87.34	85.66	–2.85	35.83	36.25	33.34	–2.49
Jilin	65.57	60.92	58.02	–7.55	88.74	87.73	88.51	–0.23	27.25	27.73	27.63	0.38
Heilongjiang	71.21	67.48	59.92	–11.29	91.63	91.52	89.32	–2.31	24.37	25.13	24.34	–0.03
Shanghai	81.16	76.77	74.50	–6.66	88.53	86.30	86.48	–2.05	53.32	53.98	56.25	2.93
Jiangsu	76.06	67.92	64.12	–11.94	90.55	90.68	89.51	–1.04	30.41	31.38	31.91	1.50
Zhejiang	56.93	54.92	55.70	–1.23	89.64	90.25	89.58	–0.06	18.70	18.81	18.44	–0.26
Anhui	67.24	66.93	66.70	–0.54	88.70	89.46	87.19	–1.51	9.22	9.39	9.14	–0.08
Fujian	44.21	42.15	39.98	–4.23	87.02	85.93	86.87	–0.15	7.34	7.65	8.06	0.72
Jiangxi	38.80	37.83	38.09	–0.71	79.78	79.24	80.35	0.57	4.56	4.66	4.92	0.36
Shandong	70.59	68.12	64.64	–5.95	91.51	91.24	89.30	–2.21	27.99	26.61	24.83	–3.16
Henan	83.22	80.38	75.03	–8.19	90.78	89.77	87.91	–2.87	18.42	17.64	15.58	–2.84
Hubei	64.12	59.71	59.88	–4.24	87.07	86.75	86.15	–0.92	14.41	13.59	14.05	–0.36
Hunan	47.39	46.07	44.08	–3.31	87.91	88.33	87.61	–0.30	8.25	8.25	9.82	1.57
Guangdong	69.21	67.90	68.27	–0.94	89.21	85.58	85.46	–3.75	7.47	7.58	7.84	0.37
Guangxi	40.77	41.91	43.26	2.49	69.83	72.88	75.65	5.82	4.48	4.55	4.78	0.30
Sichuan	41.44	29.42	28.78	–12.66	88.03	87.41	87.40	–0.63	25.34	24.73	24.07	–1.27
Guizhou	48.86	48.70	47.66	–1.20	75.33	75.74	76.96	1.63	4.24	4.56	4.74	0.50
Yunnan	34.57	33.36	33.28	–1.29	67.40	68.74	70.01	2.61	5.07	5.36	5.69	0.62
Shaanxi	60.80	56.45	54.72	–6.08	84.63	82.29	84.47	–0.16	14.59	13.52	13.05	–1.54
Gansu	24.41	24.69	29.18	4.77	81.84	82.30	84.92	3.08	8.63	8.21	10.59	1.96
Qinghai	37.57	31.66	31.34	–6.23	73.75	68.76	70.69	–3.06	5.68	5.83	5.95	0.27
Ningxia	25.88	31.26	30.33	4.45	75.73	78.08	79.14	3.41	4.45	5.44	5.99	1.54
Xinjiang	46.13	42.53	45.10	–1.03	41.50	50.58	52.94	11.44	6.96	7.51	7.34	0.38
MEAN	58.72	55.68	55.43	–3.030	87.07	86.68	86.97	–0.155	13.68	12.98	12.66	0.330
ST.D.	16.32	15.49	14.46	4.850	10.47	9.02	8.12	3.233	13.52	14.12	14.22	1.961

[a] $\text{One child certificate rate} = \dfrac{\text{No. of couples holding one-child certificate}}{\text{Total No. of ever married women at reproductive ages}}$

[b] $\text{Change} = \text{Rate}_{1986} - \text{Rate}_{1984}$

Source: Chinese Population Information Centre, *Handbook of Chinese Population Information*, 1985, 1986, and 1987.

dropped by more than 6.5 percentage points are Sichuan, Jiangsu, Heilongjiang, Henan, Jilin, Hebei, and Shanghai. In Sichuan and Jiangsu, the two model provinces in terms of family-planning work, the late-marriage rate declined by 12.66 and 11.94 points respectively during 1984–6.

The table also indicates that the regional differences in late-marriage rate have remained more or less constant over time. The highest rate of late marriage can still be found in the three big municipalities, in Shandong, Jiangsu, Anhui, Guangdong, and Henan provinces. This suggests the persistence of local marriage traditions. We will return to this point in later chapters.

Changes in contraceptive practice seem to have been more moderate. The absolute number of people practising birth control increased over time. In 1986 there were 145.89 million Chinese using contraceptives, a figure 6.65 million more than in 1985. Nevertheless, the contraceptive-prevalence rate declined very slightly from 85.82 to 85.61 for China as a whole during this three-year period. This may be partly caused by changes in age composition of ever married women at reproductive ages, since the contraceptive-prevalence rate is a measure of weighted average similar to other crude rates in demography. With the decline in late-marriage rate and a large cohort reaching marriageable ages, the proportion of young women who are newly married but have not had their first child to total ever married women at fertile ages increases. It was reported that the yearly increment in the total number of first marriages was 0.8 million in 1985, 0.56 million in 1986, and 0.08 million in 1987.[82] Birth control is much less practised among those young and newly married women, in contrast to those in their late 30s who have experienced childbearing.[83] Thus, changes in age composition of women exposed to the risk of childbearing would affect the comparison of our contraceptive-prevalence rate over time.

In spite of some recent fluctuations, the prevalence rate in an overwhelmingly majority of provinces, however, increased during the period 1979–86. This may be attributed to wide publicity of birth-control knowledge and easy access to contraceptive services. Recent modification of the management of the contraceptive supply system seems to have had no major impact on the outcome of the programme. The regional diversities in contraceptive practice are relatively small compared to the two other measures. The lowest contraceptive-prevalence rate can once again be found in those provinces with a large proportion of minority populations.

So far as the one-child certificate rate is concerned, the picture is not always bright. Provinces can be grouped roughly in accordance with their proportions of ever married women who pledged to have only one child to total ever married women at childbearing ages in 1984. The first group consists of 9 provinces where the proportion of one-child certificate holders exceeds 0.24. The third group is composed of those where the proportion is less than 0.09. The second group is in between. It is interesting to note that during 1984–6, among the first group, the proportion continuously rose in Beijing, Tianjin, Shanghai, and Jiangsu provinces, but dropped or fluctuated in the rest. The rate declined slightly in all of the 8 provinces belonging to the second group, where the percentage of one-child certificate holders was between 9 and 24 in 1984. By contrast, all of the 11 provinces in which less than 9 per cent of ever married women were issued one-child certificates in 1984 improved their record in 1986, although some of the changes were very modest. These findings suggest that while the most advanced provinces continued to strive towards the one-child-per-family norm and the backward regions slightly improved their achievements, the performance of the one-child programme measured by the rate in a large number of provinces deteriorated over time. Setbacks in rural areas are largely responsible for such a trend. It is reported that there were some 30.51 million couples holding one-child certificates in 1986. This is a figure 1.06 million higher than that in 1985. In the cities and towns, the figure increased by 1.17 and 0.53 million respectively, while the absolute number of couples with one-child certificates dropped by 0.64 million in rural areas. This is partly due to the relaxation of birth-control effort and also owing to the recent adjustments of local regulations on the one-child programme: the policy was strengthened in some provinces but eased in others. Except for conditions mentioned in Table 2.5, more couples in China's countryside have been allowed to have their second births. By the end of 1985 it was reported that rural couples in the entire area of Guangdong and Guangxi, southern Zhejiang, and a large part of Shandong could have a second child if the first one was a girl. A second child has been permitted, no matter what the sex of the first child, throughout Ningxia, and, after a four-year interval, in parts of Shanxi, Guangxi, and Guangdong. Couples who are living in the remote areas have been given permission to give birth to a second child in Gansu, Sichuan, Shaanxi, and some other provinces.[84] By contrast, the birth of a second child is more strictly controlled in Shanghai and Jiangsu provinces.

On the whole, the future programme will be reliant more on people's voluntary acceptance and less on strong social pressure. However, for the great majority of Chinese couples, family size preference has not been reduced below two children[83] and the future implementation of the one-child campaign will therefore remain difficult.

The economic reform, especially the implementation of the rural responsibility system, has been very successful in terms of economic growth and improvement of peasants' living standards. But it has also greatly reduced the importance of the economic incentive and disincentive in planning births.[86] Under current economic conditions, the labour force is still the decisive factor for family welfare, and this stimulates more births. It is difficult at the present time to surmise the long-term demographic implications of the Chinese rural reforms.

One of the main shortcomings of previous programmes is that they concentrated on educational persuasion and improvement of contraceptive services, but did little to remove the fundamental obstacles of birth control, such as old-age security and traditional family norms. Of course, societal changes cannot be effected within a very short period, and the direct role played by family planning is limited. Nevertheless, the future success of population control in China will largely depend on these changes.

The difficulties in population control have been evident in the past few years. The birth-rate has increased and age at marriage declined, and these changes have attracted the government's attention. Several pilot experiments have been undertaken, such as the Contracted Responsibility System, which was initiated in Bose city of Guangxi Autonomous Region; the life-insurance policies for only children; and the establishment of some specialized organizations.[87] While much attention has been paid to improving the working style or methods and to reducing the coercive incidents in the last several years, no effective measures for population control have been taken yet. The future family-planning programme should be modified to adapt to the changing situation, especially changes in institutional settings. The crucial problem is to maintain, and if possible improve, the present standard of services in advanced areas, while greater efforts should be made to promote birth control in remote areas, including minority areas. Further, the family-planning programme should be more closely linked to fundamental social changes.

Confronted with its immense population and large child-bearing capacity, China cannot follow the slow pattern of European fertility transition. It must use every reasonable means to curb population growth. The success of the Chinese family-planning programme will not only benefit more than one billion Chinese, but will also be important in reducing the population pressure of the whole world.

NOTES

1. P. H. Chang, *Power and Policy in China* (University Park: Pennsylvania State University Press, 1975).
2. Mao Zedong, *Selected Works of Mao Tse-tung* (Beijing: Foreign Languages Press, 1975–7), iv. 452.
3. *Hong Qi (Red Flag)*, No. 6 (3 June 1978).
4. Mao Zedong, 'On the Correct Handling of Contradictions among the People', in *Selected Works of Mao Tse-tung*, v. 384–421.
5. Mao Zedong, 'Be Activists in Promoting the Revolution', in *Selected Works of Mao Tse-tung*, v. 486–8.
6. See *Hong Qi (Red Flag)*, No. 9 (1958), 1–3.
7. Si Chengli, 'Mao Zedong tongzhi dui jihuashengyu de gongxian (Comrade Mao Zedong's Contribution to Birth Control)', *Xibei Renkou (Northwest Population)* No. 3 (1984).
8. Ibid.
9. Zhang Chunyuan, 'Mao Zedong de renkou sixiang (Mao Zedong's Population Thought)', *Jingji Kexue (Economic Sciences)*, No. 6 (1986).
10. Wu Cangpin, 'Zhongguo shengyulu xunsu xiajiang de lilun jieshi (Theoretical Explanation of the Rapid Fertility Decline in China)', *Renkou Yanjiu (Population Research)*, No. 1 (1986), 11–16.
11. Hou Wenruo, 'Population Policy', in Liu Zheng *et al.*, *China's Population: Problems & Prospects* (Beijing: New World Press, 1981), 55–76.
12. E. Croll, *The Politics of Marriage in Contemporary China* (Cambridge: Cambridge University Press, 1981).
13. See e.g. Zhang Naigong and Zhou Ning 'Wosheng sanshinianlai renkou fazhan de huigu he jingyan jiaoxun (Review and Lessons of Population Growth in the Past 30 Years in our Province)', *Zhejiang renkou tongxun (Newsletter of Zhejiang Population)*, Feb. 1980.
14. Zhang Xinxia, 'Jianguo yilai woguo shengyu zhengce de yanbian (The Evolution of our Country's Population Policy since the Founding of the People's Republic)', *Shangdong Renkou (Shandong Population)*, No. 3 (1984).
15. Details of these debates can be seen in H. Yuan Tien, *China's Population Struggle: Demographic Decisions of the People's Republic 1949–1969* (Columbus: Ohio State University Press, 1973).
16. Hou Wenruo, 'Population Policy', cited in n. 11, above.
17. Editorial Committee, *Wenxian yu yanjiu (Document and Research)* (Beijing: People's Publish House, 1983), 152.
18. Zou Ping, 'The Review and Discussion of Changes in China's Population Policy during the Early Years of the People's Republic', *Population Research (English edition)*, 4 (4), 1–8 (1987).
19. Chen Pi-Chao, 'The Politics of Population in Communist China: A Case Study', Ph.D. diss. (Princeton University, 1966).
20. L. L. Chu, *Planned Birth Campaign in China 1949–1976* (Honolulu: East–West Centre, Case Study No. 5, 1977).
21. See 'Childbearing should be Properly Controlled', *Renmin Ribao (People's Daily)*, 5 Mar. 1957.
22. Ma Yinchu, former president of Beijing University, the author of 'New Population Theory' (in *People's Daily*, 5 July 1957). He was eventually denounced in 1960 as

neo-Malthusian and removed from his university post and positions in other socio-political institutes. He was rehabilitated in 1979. See *Beijing Review*, 22 (31), 3–4 (3 Aug. 1979).

23. Tien, *China's Population Struggle*, p. 231.
24. See Xizhe Peng, 'Demographic Consequences of the Great Leap Forward in China's Provinces', *Population and Development Review*, 13 (4), 639–70 (1987).
25. The actual meaning of 'family planning' in the Chinese language is to some extent different from its usage in the West. Therefore, some authors translated the name of the agency as Planned Birth Staff Office. See e.g. Chu (1977); Chen (1966). In this thesis the officially used term of Family Planning Office is used. But the difference should be borne in mind.
26. See *Ta Kung Pao*, 21 Jan. 1962.
27. See *Decision of the Central Committee of the Chinese Communist Party Concerning the Great Proletarian Cultural Revolution* (Beijing: Foreign Languages Press, 1966).
28. 'At the U.N. ECAFE: China Explains her Views on the Population Question', in *Beijing Review*, 16 (17), 16–17 (27 Apr. 1973).
29. Liu Zheng, 'Zhongguo renkoukexue de fazhan yu chengjiu (The Development and Achievements in China's Population Science)', *Renkou Yanjiu (Population Research)*, No. 1 (1985).
30. *Constitution of the People's Republic of China*, Art. 25. See *Renmin Ribao (People's Daily)*, 6 Dec. 1982.
31. China's per capita Net Material Product was estimated as 215 US dollars in 1979 and 246 dollars in 1980. See United Nations, *National Accounts Statistics: Analysis of Main Aggregates, 1982*, UN ST/ESA/STAT/SER.X/2, p. 9.
32. Chen Muhua, *People's Daily*, 11 Aug. 1978.
33. Ibid. 14 Feb. 1980.
34. See *People's Daily*, 26 Sept. 1980.
35. Wang Wei, 'Guanyu jihua shenyu gongzou wenti (On Family-Planning Work)', a speech given at the Party School of the CCCP on 15 Nov. 1985. See *Zhongguo renkou zi liao shouce (Handbook of Chinese Population Information), 1986*, 4–11.
36. Zhang Xinxia, op. cit., in n. 14 above.
37. Wang Wei, *Handbook of Chinese Population Information* (Beijing: China Population Information Centre, 1987), pp. 13–19.
38. Peng Peiyun, 'Grasp the work of family planning by unifying thinking and stabilising the policy', *China Population Newsletter*, vol. 65, No. 2 (1989), pp. 2–5.
39. J. R. Townsend, *Politics of China* (Boston: Little, Brown & Company, 1980).
40. Unless specified, main sources of provincial data used hereafter are as follows: Chapter 14 of the provincial volumes of *Zhongguo renkou chongshu (Chinese Population Monographs)* for Shanghai, Hebei, Jiangsu, Hunan, Gansu, Beijing, Tianjin, Jilin, Guizhou, and Shanxi; Li Hanbo, 'Guangdongsheng jihua shengyu gongzuo fazhan de jige jieduan (The Development Phases of the Family-Planning Programme in Guangdong Province)', *Guangdong Renkou (Guangdong Population)*, No. 2 (1984); Propaganda Dept. of the Party Committee of Qinghai, *Qinhai in the Past 35 Years, 1949–1984* (Xining: Qinghai People's Press, 1985); Editorial Committee, Economic Yearbook of Fujian Province, 1985, (Fuzhou: Fujian People's Press, 1985); *Renkou Kexue (Population Science)*, No. 1 (1981); Research Office of the Party Committee in Sichuan Province, Zhonggong SichuanshengWei yanjiuShi, *Sichuan Shengqing (A General Survey of Sichuan Province (Chengdu, 1984)*; Family Planning Commission of Shandong, *Shandongsheng renkou,*

jihuashengyu ji youguan jichu ziliao (Basic Information on Shandong's Population and Family Planning), 1985.

41. Chen Pi-Chao, 'Politics of Population in Communist China', p. 250.
42. *People's Daily*, 28 Dec. 1957.
43. L. Chu, *Planned Birth Campaign in China*, p. 59.
44. *People's Daily*, 21 Aug. 1957.
45. It is ideal to use the number of women, or all married couples, in reproductive age as the denominator. However, because the information is not adequate enough, we have to use the province's total population for the calculation.
46. L. Chu, *Planned Birth Campaign in China*, p. 89.
47. J. S. Aird, 'Population Policy and Demographic Prospects in the People's Republic of China', in *People's Republic of China: An Economic Assessment* (Washington, DC: Joint Economic Committee, US Congress, 1972), 220–331.
48. A. J. Coale, 'The Demographic Transition', in *Proceedings of the International Population Conference 1973* (Liege: IUSSP, 1973), 53–72.
49. 'Strengthen the Work of Supplying Contraceptives', *Ta Kung Pao*, 5 Feb. 1958.
50. J. Kaufman, *A Billion and Counting: Family Planning Campaigns and Policies in the People's Republic of China* (San Francisco: San Francisco Press, 1983), 23.
51. Ren Lizhong, 'Hebeisheng jihuashengyu gongzuo sanshinian de huigu (Review of Family-Planning Programmes in Hebei Province in the Past 30 Years)', *Hebei Renkou (Hebei Population)*, No. 4 (1984).
52. *Handbook of Chinese Population Information, 1985*, p. 307.
53. There were altogether 31,000 propagandists in Shanxi province at that time.
54. Measured in Chinese currency Renminbi, 100 cents = 1 *Yuan*.
55. *Beijing Review*, 21 Feb. 1975, p. 9.
56. Chen Pi-Chao, *Population and Health Policy in the People's Republic of China* (Washington DC: Interdisciplinary Communications Program, Occasional Monograph Series No. 9, 1976).
57. A. P. Wolf, 'The Preeminent Role of Government Intervention in China's Family Revolution', *Population and Development Review*, 12 (1), 101–16 (1986).
58. According to 1982 Population Census, in China's rural areas, 49% of all women (21% of men) aged 12 and over were illiterate or semi-illiterate. See *10 Percent Sampling Tabulation of the 1982 Population Census of the PRC*, p. 325.
59. J. Salaff, 'Youth, Family, and Political Control in Communist China', Ph.D. thesis (Department of Sociology, University of California, Berkeley, 1972).
60. Chen Pi-Chao, *Rural Health and Birth Planning in China* (North Carolina: International Fertility Research Program, 1981).
61. Han Suyin, 'Population and Family Planning in the People's Republic of China', in *Family Planning in China* (Population Crisis Committee, Spring 1971).
62. Zhang Zeyu, 'Population Policy for Minorities', *Beijing Review*, 29 (48), 15–18 (1 Dec. 1986).
63. Li Jiepin and Qi Yiju, 'Shanghaishi jihuashengyu qingkuang fenxi (Analysis of the Family-Planning Programme in Shanghai)', *Renkou Kexue Congkan (Population Science)*, No. 1 (Sept. 1981).
64. These contraceptive prevalence rates may be inflated. See e.g. R. Freedman *et al.*, 'Local Area Variations in Reproductive Behaviour in the People's Republic of China: 1973–1982', paper presented at the annual meeting of the Population Association of America, San Francisco, Apr. 1986. However, this should not seriously affect our regional comparison.

65. D. L. Poston, 'Patterns of Contraceptive Use in China', *Studies in Family Planning*, 17 (5), 217–27 (1986).
66. Ibid.
67. See e.g. *People's Daily*, 13 Sept. 1980.
68. D. Davin, 'The Single-Child Family in the Countryside', in E. Croll *et al.* (eds.), *China's One-Child Family Policy* (London: Macmillan, 1985), 37–82.
69. Chen Quangen, 'Population Policies and Fertility Decline in China', M.Sc. diss. (University College, University of Wales, 1986).
70. 'China: Our Arduous Task', *People*, 11 (4), 1984.
71. S. Greenhalgh, 'Shifts in China's Population Policy', *Population and Development Review*, 12 (3), 491–516 (1986).
72. Central Committee of the Chinese Communist Party, Document No. 7 (1984). See *Handbook of Chinese Population Information, 1987*, 3–5.
73. Qian Xinzhong, 'China's Population Policy: Theory and Methods', *Studies in Family Planning*, 14 (12), 302–17 (Dec. 1983).
74. The measure in 1979 and 1980 may overestimate the outcome of the campaign. For example, the higher percentage of one-child certificates may result from real achievement, but also may be due simply to selection bias, since couples who already had two or more children were excluded from the calculation of the index.
75. S. E. Fraser, *China: Population Education and People* (Melbourne: School of Education, La Trobe University, 1987).
76. Wu Naitao, 'Dealing with the "Spoiled Brat" ', *Beijing Review*, 29 (19), 26–8 (12 May 1986).
77. See e.g. S. Greenhalgh and J. Bongaarts, 'Fertility Policy in China: Future Options', The Population Council Working Papers, No. 127 (Oct. 1986).
78. *People's Daily*, 21 Jan. 1988.
79. 'No Slackening in Family Planning', *Beijing Review*, 29 (10), 6 (10 Mar. 1986).
80. It should be noted that there is no standard criterion for late marriage in 1979, although it is commonly higher than 23 years.
81. Wang Wei, 'Guanyu jihua shengyu gongzhou qingkuang de jianghua (A Speech on Family Planning)'. See *Handbook of Chinese Population Information, 1987*, 13–19.
82. *People's Daily (Overseas edition)*, 14 May 1988.
83. Information on age-specific rate of contraceptive is collected by China's 1982 Fertility Survey, and tabulated results can be seen in *Handbook of Chinese Population Information, 1987*.
84. Wang Wei, 'On Family-Planning Work', *Handbook of Chinese Population Information, 1986*, cited in n. 35, above.
85. M. K. Whyte and S. Z. Gu, 'Popular Response to China's Fertility Transition', *Population and Development Review*, 13 (3), 471–93 (1987).
86. E.g. *Beijing Wan Bao*, 25 Nov. 1987; *Beijing Review*, 29 (22), 18–26 (2 June 1986).
87. *Beijing Review*, 31 (27), 25–6 (4–10 July 1988).

3

Determinants of China's Fertility Transition

WE have reviewed the development of China's family-planning programmes over the last four decades. Coale in 1973 summarized the three pre-conditions of the fertility transition: (1) fertility must be within the calculus of conscious choice; (2) effective techniques of fertility reduction must be known and available; and (3) reduced fertility must be perceived to be advantageous.[1] In this chapter, we shall investigate how far these conditions were met and examine the main determinants of the regional differentials in China's fertility transition.

Fertility determinants can be roughly grouped into proximate determinants and ultimate determinants as summarized by Freedman.[2] Quantifying the effects of the proximate determinants on fertility is one of the most important achievements in fertility research.[3] Unfortunately, available data do not allow us to analyse the proximate determinants in detail, although one of these variables, nuptiality, will be examined in Chapter 4. Rather, consideration is given to the link between the ultimate variables (such as socio-economic and institutional factors) and fertility transition.

I. Family-Planning Programmes

The importance of the family-planning programme on fertility transition is a subject of controversy. While Mauldin argued that family-planning programmes had a significant, independent effect on fertility,[4] Handwerker claimed that family-planning services could not initiate fertility transition.[5] Both views are partly true.

There is no doubt that the very successful family-planning programme is one of the major factors responsible for the rapid fertility decline in China. Since the early 1960s, control of population growth has been strongly advocated by the Chinese leadership, no matter who has been in power. With the shift of the Party's priority from political struggle to economic construction, more and more efforts have been made to bring down the birth-rate and modernize reproduction. The regional differentials in the timing and pace of the transition are to a great extent a result of the differentials in the implementation of the local family-planning programme.

We have shown that the first two family-planning campaigns in China were largely urban-orientated and left the dominant rural areas almost untouched. Furthermore, although large-scale propaganda was conducted to disseminate the knowledge of birth control, the supplies of effective contraceptives were far from being sufficient to meet the needs of China's immense reproductive population in the 1950s, and this state probably persisted into the 1960s. In other words, even if Chinese couples accepted the new idea of birth control at that time, technical obstacles prevented further progress, unless major changes in nuptiality and breastfeeding took place. In China's rural areas contraceptives became easily accessible only after the establishment of the rural co-operative health system during the Cultural Revolution period. This is one of the major causes of the earlier transition in China's urban areas.

We will show in later chapters that the initial fertility decline in urban areas started within a very short period of time in almost all provinces soon after the launch of the second family-planning campaign in the early 1960s. Although the onset of the transition in Shanghai emerged before that date, the propaganda for birth control in the 1950s played an important role in disseminating contraceptive knowledge. Spontaneous fertility limitation is believed to have been practised in some areas among certain social strata before the government-sponsored family-planning programme. The overall fertility decline, however, was brought about, or at least speeded up, by these programmes.

The timing of the onset of the fertility transition in China's rural areas varied considerably between provinces. Nevertheless, the rural fertility transition did not commence earlier than the programmes in any of the provinces. Generally speaking, family-planning programmes were carried out earlier and more efficiently in the eastern provinces, whereas the programmes were enforced later and less rigidly in the most western provinces. This by and large coincides with the provincial patterns of China's fertility transition.

The uneven progress of local family-planning programmes and the differentials in fertility transition are often attributed to the leadership provided by local administrators. Besides the major municipalities, Jiangsu and Sichuan have frequently been cited as model areas in family-planning work. By contrast, the poor record of population control in Guangdong province has been viewed as a result of lack of effective efforts on birth-control campaigns. The inferior record of the family-planning programme in provinces with a large proportion of ethnic minorities is due in part to the overall policy towards minority populations.

China is a multi-ethnic country. Minority populations account for about 7 per cent of the national total. Most of these minority populations reside in the western part of China. The percentage of the population which is of minority origin ranges from 26 in Guizhou to 60 in Xinjiang.[6] This area is also the one with the highest fertility level within China. In the past China's family-planning programme was vigorously implemented in the vast majority of Han areas. Population policies adopted in the minority areas were very flexible, and some were in fact pronatalist.[7] This is certainly responsible for the high fertility in those areas.

The one-child policy may be one of the most ambitious family-planning programmes in the world. The policy linked control over population growth with economic modernization. The Chinese government has been firmly committed to limit population growth and has played a prominent role in the implementation of the programme. Education is assigned a high priority in China's family planning. Meanwhile, complicated packages of incentives and disincentives have been adopted throughout the country. Although coercion has been continually opposed by the state, coercive measures were sometimes taken by local cadres when persuasion failed. This has attracted criticism, especially from abroad. One scholar described the Chinese programme as 'the world's first national compulsory family planning programme'.[8]

It is true that there have been weaknesses in China's population policy and modifications have been made frequently in order to make the policy more acceptable. China's birth control is carried out in a country with one billion population. Negligence and mistakes are inevitable. Nonetheless, it is hard to imagine that China could bring down the population growth rapidly just by coercion.[9] In addition, confronted with its immense population and enormous childbearing potential, China, has every reason to carry out a strict population policy. As the Chinese government puts it, China's socio-economic development requires a planned control of its population growth, which is also conducive to the prosperity and stability of the world.[10]

It is ideal for couples to bear the number of children they think appropriate at a time suitable to them.[11] The focus of population control lies not in the execution of administrative mandates and economic sanctions, but rather in how to broaden the people's cultural knowledge and change their traditional attitudes towards child-bearing.[12] However, few rural communities in China, not even the most developed, approach the development level prevailing at the time of the fertility transition in most European countries. In addition, Chinese culture has strongly stressed family and kinship instead of the individual, as did Western civilization. This has made the fertility transition in China more difficult.

Moreover, historically, when economic and political conditions have improved, China's population has tended to increase even at the expense of progressive deterioration in the national standard of living.[13] Individual desire in many cases is in conflict with national and societal interests. Hence the view is taken that, although such intensive family-planning affects personal freedom of action and frequently generates dissatisfaction, in the long run a smaller population will benefit the entire nation.[14] In other words, the sacrifices made today will hopefully win time for succeeding generations.[15]

However, the impact of the family-planning programme on fertility transition should not be overstated. As pointed out by Gille, family-planning provision is unlikely to bring about a fertility reduction, unless accompanied by structural changes.[16] The success of this government-sponsored programme is to a great extent reliant on China's distinctive social and value system, and facilitated greatly by many other reforms which have been carried out in all aspects of social life since 1949. The Chinese revolution created a very favourable network of social organizations for the implementation of the family-planning programme.[17]

For example, the achievement of the birth-control campaign in the 1970s most likely resulted from combining family-planning efforts with organizational reforms and rural re-emphasis during the Cultural Revolution period.[18] The integration of the family-planning network with the health-care system has made China's contraceptive delivery system the largest community-based system in the world.[19] In addition, all the networks of the Party and other major mass organizations have been mobilized to promote family planning. The major responsibility for family planning lies with the Party. The health and educational networks assist in whatever ways they can. In the cities, contraceptive services are widely available, and people have been under double pressures from organizations in both their workplace and residence (i.e. Neighbourhood committees) to practise family limitation. In rural areas, one of the primary tasks of barefoot doctors, who were the backbone of the community collective medical-care system, has been to disseminate and distribute birth-control knowledge and services. Hence, ideological work has been supplemented by a well-built family-planning network to implement birth control with effective contraceptives, something that was not available in the previous campaigns in China and probably not in most of developing countries either. Therefore, the achievements of the family-planning programme have been to a great extent associated with the efficiency of these organizations. This in turn affects the process of the fertility transition. In 1981 about 70 per cent of provincial differences in the total fertility rate could be explained by differences in contraceptive prevalence between provinces.[20]

II. Fertility Differentials among Different Social Strata

Socio-economic differentials in fertility are a fundamental source of evidence on the underlying determinants of fertility.[21] It is worth noting, however, that none of these socio-economic variables can affect fertility directly. They must operate through 'proximate determinants' (termed as 'intermediate variables' for many years), such as marriage and contraceptive use. Bongaarts and Hobcraft and Little have made important advances in empirical analysis of the effects of proximate determinants on fertility.[22] In this section, we examine the fertility differentials in different social strata distinguished by education, occupation, and place of residence.

Data and Methodology

Data on the number of children ever born to women with different educational levels and occupations were collected separately in China's 1982 National Fertility Survey for each of China's 28 provinces, separating the rural from the urban population. Those data are further tabulated in a cross-classified format for women aged 35, 40, 45, 50, 55, 60, and 67 at the time of the survey. This information gives us the opportunity to examine how fertility behaviour was related to these variables during the process of China's fertility transition. Due to the structure of the data, some attention needs to be given to analytical methodology. The major objective of this study is to analyse how fertility is related to different socio-economic variables. However, variables which refer to criteria for the cross-classification are not independent among themselves, making the assessment of their relative effects on mean parities difficult. Proper controls should be introduced in order to avoid over- or underestimating the impacts which we are searching for. In addition, although the number of respondents in each subgroup is known, the distribution of the variable and the variance within the cells is not.[23]

The log-linear additive model has been used for analysis of WFS data, which have similar features to the data used here. This procedure is employed in this study by using the computer program GLIM. Poisson error distribution is chosen for the model. The general idea behind fitting models is to distinguish significant features from insignificant details, which makes interpretation much easier and more explicit.[24] A major assumption of the model is that the ratio of the estimated parities for two levels of one factor, with the levels of the other factors fixed, is the same for all levels of the other factors.[25] This enables us to estimate the difference in mean parities between any two levels of one variable, with other variables controlled.

Women aged 35 at the time of the survey, 1982, were born in and around 1947, and they reached reproductive age in about the mid-1960s. Their fertility behaviour was greatly affected by the government's birth-control efforts which started in the early 1960s and were carried out vigorously in the 1970s. In contrast, the family-planning programmes had little, or no, direct influence on women aged 50 and over. By analysing the differential fertility for these different age cohorts, we can examine how the effects of socio-economic variables on fertility change under different conditions. Theoretically speaking, women who are younger than 50 years old have not completed their reproductive cycles. It is, therefore, not plausible to compare mean parities directly for women in different age groups. Thus, models are fitted for each age group and the results are then compared. Differences between cohorts can also be viewed as evidence for time trends. To simplify the presentation, and considering the small number of respondents, women aged 50 and over are combined into a single age group.

China's fertility transition is a process of diffusion. We will return to this point later. There are marked rural–urban and provincial differences in the timing and pace of the transition. To examine how those socio-economic variables operate differently in different places, type of residence, and province location are the two main influences to be tested in the models.

Type of residence refers to rural–urban differences. All provinces are classified into six groups based roughly on geographical location and similarity in fertility transition. The first consists of three major municipalities: Beijing, Tianjin, and Shanghai. Five eastern coastal provinces: Zhejiang, Jiangsu, Shandong, Hebei, and Liaoning, comprise the second. The northern group is composed of Heilongjiang, Jilin, Nei Monggol, Shaanxi, Shanxi, and Henan provinces. The southern group includes Sichuan, Hubei, Hunan, Fujian, Guangdong, and Anhui. The northwest group contains four northwest provinces, Xinjiang, Qinghai, Ningxia, and Gansu; and the southwest includes Guizhou, Yunnan, Guangxi, and Jiangxi—which is located in southeast China but has a pattern of fertility transition that is similar to those in the southwest. It should be said that the classification is not very strict, but it is representative.

Effects of Education on Mean Parity

Mass education is often regarded as the primary determinant of fertility transition.[26] The effects of education on mean parity in China are examined by fitting log-linear additive models. These models contain three variables: educational level, type of residence, and province location. There are four levels of education in the model: illiteracy, primary schooling, junior middle school, and higher schooling (including higher middle school and university). Models are fitted for four age cohorts separately. The principle of model fitting is to find as parsimonious a model as possible.[27] This is to say, the criterion of model selection is not only the closeness of fit but also simplicity. Chi-squared tests of the absolute fit are carried out. These tests indicate that, except for the model for the cohort 50+, a model with the main effects of three variables provides a satisfactory fit. Thus, interactive effects are omitted and the three main effects model is chosen.[28] The model for the 50+ group does not fit satisfactorily, which is thought to be mainly caused by large variations between and within each province. Nevertheless, the model is consistent with those of the other age groups, and the result is used for further comparison.

The results of those models are summarized in Table 3.1. Fitted values of the mean parity of women in each category are compared with the reference and ratios are presented.

The effect of education on mean parity is clear: the number of children ever born to women in all four age groups declines constantly with increasing education. These models show that the highest mean parity is always for women with no education, while women with high school or higher education bear the smallest number of children. Differences between illiterate women and those who received primary education are small, and in all cases less than 10 per cent. The gap widens as education rises.

TABLE 3.1. *Ratios of mean parities for women with different education, type of residence, and province location to reference* (based on log-linear three effects models)

Variables	Age groups			
	35	40	45	50+
Education: Illiterate as reference				
Primary school	0.95	0.93	0.91	0.92
Junior middle school	0.87	0.84	0.80	0.80
Higher	0.71	0.72	0.64	0.62
Type of Residence: Rural as reference				
Urban	0.70	0.72	0.75	0.84
Province Location: Municipalities as reference				
East coast	1.17	1.14	1.10	1.02
South	1.44	1.37	1.28	1.12
North	1.46	1.42	1.32	1.11
Southwest	1.65	1.53	1.44	1.13
Northwest	1.71	1.48	1.40	1.03

Some suggest that education's impact on fertility may increase over time.[29] However, Table 3.1 shows an opposite trend. After controlling for residence and provincial location, the relative differences between different educational groups diminish as women become younger, although the change is not very significant. It can be seen that mean parities of women who received junior middle school education are estimated to be 20 per cent lower than those for illiterate ones for the 45 age group. The difference between illiterate women and women in the higher education category is 36 per cent. But these differences reduce to 13 and 29 per cent respectively for the 35 age group. A similar trend can be found in other groups. This phenomenon may result from the fact that the younger the women are, the less complete their reproductive cycle is. However, a more plausible explanation is that this tendency is caused by the progress of family-planning programmes in China. Support for this argument comes from a cross-national study done by the United Nations, which showed that educational differentials tend to be smaller in places with an effective family-planning programme, because the programme brings birth control to lower educational strata where it might otherwise have come more slowly.[30]

The number of children born to urban women is consistently lower than that for their rural counterparts. Urban women aged 35 are estimated to have 30 per cent fewer children than those living in the rural areas, even after controlling for education and province location. The time trend, however, is different from that for education. The difference between the urban and rural categories widens as women became younger: from 16 per cent for the 50+ age group to above 30 per cent for the 35 age group. Furthermore, the impact of rural–urban difference on fertility seems stronger compared with the effects of education, for the younger age groups.

Another salient finding concerns regional diversities. Women's fertility behaviour is not only affected by their educational level and place of residence, but also by the province in which they live. Table 3.1 shows that with the same education and place of residence, women in the three large municipalities tend to have the smallest family size. They are followed by women in eastern coastal provinces. On the other hand, highest mean parities are found in the two western groups. The situation for women in the north and south of China is estimated to be in-between. The classification of provinces may seem arbitrary, but such regional differences are observed to persist and widen over time. The difference for women aged 50+ is minor, and the largest difference of 13 per cent is estimated to be between the municipalities and southern provinces. Then the regional gaps in general become bigger as women's age decreases. The mean parity of women in northwestern provinces for the 35 age group is about 70 per cent higher than that of women in municipal areas.

The time trend of those changes, which refers to differences between age cohorts, is further illustrated in Figure 3.1. To summarize, education is an important determinant of fertility behaviour, but the effect is reduced with the passing of time. By contrast, the rural–urban and regional differences have not just been sustained, but have become more prominent.

Effects of Occupation

The effects of occupation can be analysed in a similar way. Type of residence and province location remain as the two main variables. Four occupational groups are used: peasant, worker, cadre, and housewife.[31] The association between occupation and type of residence is certainly closer than that with education. Almost all peasant women live in rural areas, while women with other occupations could be living in either rural or urban areas. Nevertheless, the effects of all three variables are established by the chi-squared tests of relative fit. In addition, the chi-squared tests of absolute fit indicate that the three main effects log-

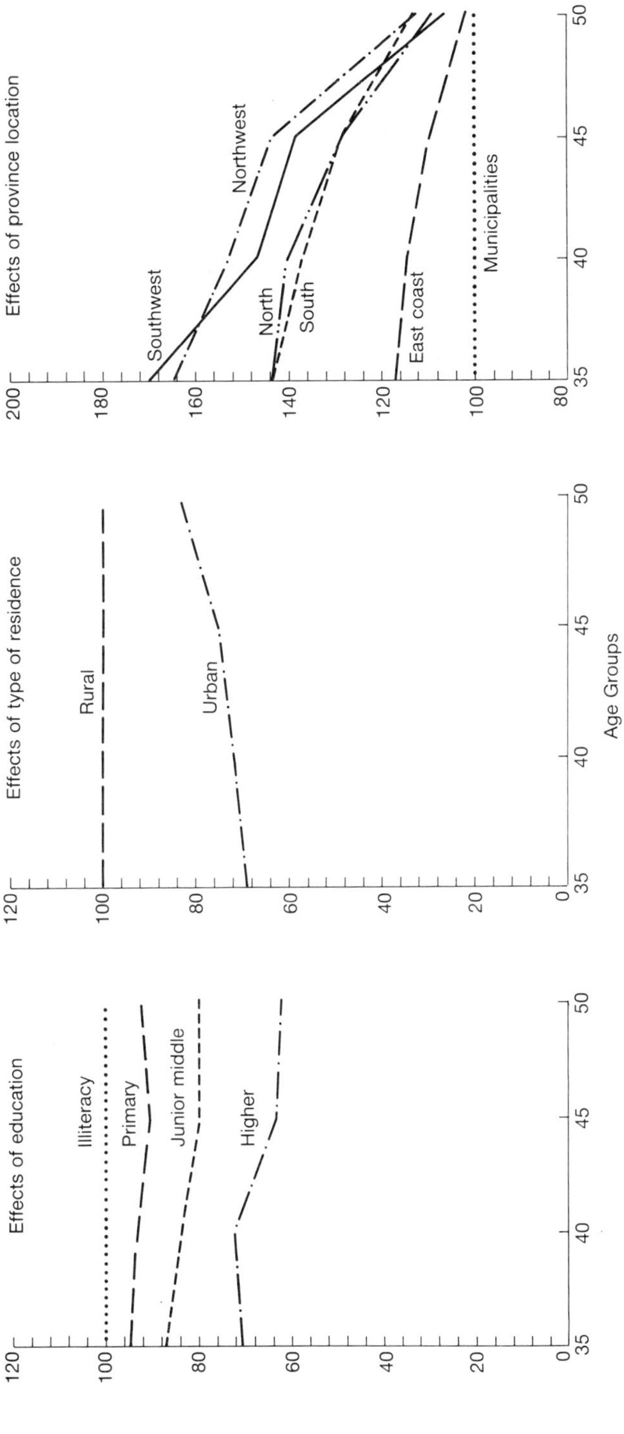

Fig. 3.1 Effects of education, type of residence, and province location on mean parity

linear models are satisfactorily fitted at 5-per-cent level, except for the 50+ groups.[32] Thus, the three main effects models are selected and results are presented in Table 3.2.

The occupational differentials are clear. It seems obvious that Chinese peasants have invariably had more children than the rest of the population. The fertility behaviour of housewives is to some extent similar to that of peasants, and the differences between them are less than 5 per cent for all ages. The mean parities of workers are about 10 per cent less than those for peasants. Chinese women classified as cadres are the social group with smallest family size. When residence and provincial location are controlled, cadres are estimated to have 26, 28, and 38 per cent less children ever born, compared with peasants, for the 35, 40, and 45 age groups respectively.

In view of the time trends it is noteworthy that cadre women are estimated to have 37 per cent less children than peasant women for the 45 age group, but with the gap reduced to 26 per cent for the 35 age group. On the other hand, differences between workers, housewives, and peasants are more or less constant between cohorts.

Rural–urban and regional differences estimated by the occupation models are consistent with those we discovered in education models. With the same occupation and type of residence, women in municipal

TABLE 3.2. *Ratios of mean parities for women with different occupation, type of residence, and province location to reference* (based on log-linear three effects models)

Variables	Age groups			
	35	40	45	50+
Occupation: Peasant as reference				
Worker	0.89	0.88	0.86	0.89
Cadre	0.74	0.72	0.63	0.67
Housewife	1.03	0.96	1.00	0.98
Type of Place: Rural as reference				
Urban	0.71	0.76	0.80	0.84
Province Location: Municipalities as reference				
East coast	1.21	1.14	1.13	1.03
South	1.48	1.37	1.32	1.13
North	1.48	1.40	1.35	1.12
Southwest	1.71	1.54	1.50	1.14
Northwest	1.78	1.49	1.45	1.04

areas and in east coast provinces produce less children than those in the other parts of China. The situation in the north and south is somewhat similar. Women in the two western groups are always estimated to have more children than the others. After controlling for occupation and province location, urban women always bear fewer children. The time trend of the residential and locational effect on mean parity in the occupation models is similar to the one we have found in the education models (see Figure 3.2). While the occupational differences diminish, the rural–urban and provincial differences increase over time.

Impact of Changing Population Composition on Overall Fertility

Great efforts have been made to promote China's mass education during the last several decades. It is also significant that more and more women are participating in economic activities. Chinese women's educational and occupational compositions are estimated for the four age cohorts by province. It can be seen from Table 3.3 that while about 88 per cent of women in the 50+ cohort were reportedly illiterate, the figure for the 35 cohort was only 39 per cent. On the other hand, the percentage of women who received primary-school education increased from 9.5 for the 50+ group to 43.6 for the 35 cohort. This is certainly a great achievement. Changes in occupational distribution are not so remarkable. The percentage of housewives declined from 8.5 for the 50+ group to 1.2 for the 35 age group. All other occupations increased their shares. Peasants remained as the largest occupational group, which accounted for more than 80 per cent of the total female population. The question here is what are the impacts of these compositional changes on the overall fertility.

An index of overall fertility (F_i) is created. This is:

$$F_i = D_{ij} \times R_{ij}$$

Where i = Age cohort

j = Educational or occupational categories (as used in Log-linear models above)

D_{ij} = percentage distribution of cohort i category j

R_{ij} = Ratio of mean parity for cohort i category j to reference (see Tables 3.1 and 3.2).

By using the index, overall fertility levels of the different age cohorts can be compared directly. By assuming that the educational (and occupational) differentials in mean parity remain unchanged between

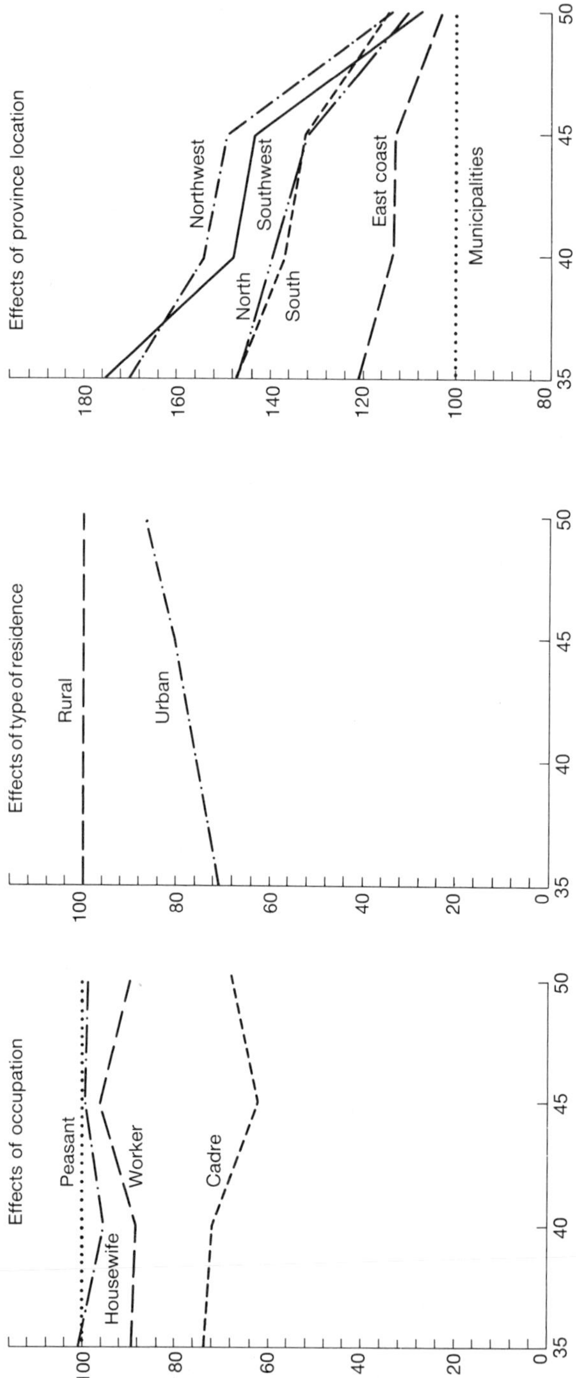

Fig. 3.2 Effects of occupation, type of residence, and province location on mean parity

TABLE 3.3. *Changes in population composition and their impacts on average parity for selected cohorts*

1. Population composition

	Age cohorts			
	35	40	45	50+
Educational:				
Illiteracy	39.2	54.5	71.2	87.9
Primary school	43.6	30.1	21.4	9.5
Junior mid-school	12.9	10.1	4.3	1.5
Higher	4.3	5.3	3.1	1.1
TOTAL	100.0	100.0	100.0	100.0
Occupational:				
Peasant	83.0	80.0	78.2	80.3
Worker	12.1	12.7	14.0	9.4
Cadre	3.7	5.2	4.2	1.8
Housewife	1.2	2.1	3.6	8.5
TOTAL	100.0	100.0	100.0	100.0

2. Impacts on average parity (in %)

	Educational			Occupational		
	35	40	45	35	40	45
Municipalities	12.4	13.2	7.9	3.4	5.8	4.3
East coast	6.3	5.4	2.0	1.2	1.2	1.3
South	5.1	3.6	1.5	0.3	0.6	0.3
North	7.6	7.3	3.6	0.9	2.7	2.7
Southwest	4.4	3.0	0.5	0.7	0.7	0.4
Northwest	7.8	7.1	2.3	4.9	4.8	2.5
CHINA TOTAL	7.3	6.6	3.0	1.6	2.3	1.8

Note: the 50+ cohort is taken as the 'standard'.

Source: Population compositions are calculated from data in China's 1982 Fertility Survey.

cohorts, the influence of changing educational (occupational) distribution on overall fertility can be assessed by employing the standardization method. Here, the ratios for the 50+ cohort have been chosen as the 'standard' schedule and the educational (occupational) distributions are multiplied by that 'standard'. The resulting F_i's are then compared with that of the 50+ cohort. Differences between F_i's for the 50+ cohort and standardized F_i's for the other age cohorts are estimated for six province groups respectively, which can be regarded as the net impact of distributional changes on overall fertility.

In Table 3.3 overall fertility for the 50+ cohort has been regarded as the reference. Other things being equal, changes in educational distribution for China as a whole can reduce the overall fertility by 7.3 per cent for the 35 cohort, 6.6 and 3.0 per cent for the 40 and 45 cohorts respectively. These figures are relatively small compared with the dramatic fertility decline that has occurred. Although Chinese women's education level did improve greatly, most of the improvement was in primary schooling. As was analysed earlier, the difference in mean parity between women who received primary education and those who were illiterate is small, so that the impact of this improvement alone is not very significant.

In view of the regional differences, one can see that the impact of distributional change in municipalities is the greatest, where improvement of education alone could bring down the overall fertility by 12 per cent, other things being equal. By contrast, educational improvement in the southwest region could result in total fertility declining by only 4 per cent. The effects of educational achievements on fertility in the north and northwest parts of China were relatively greater than those in southern China.

Table 3.3 also suggests that changing occupational distribution has little influence on reducing overall fertility. This may result from the fact that occupational distribution in China is very stable due to strict government control.

In summary, one can say that educational and occupational differences in fertility are important in understanding fertility behaviour. But their impact on reducing the overall fertility is moderate. It is unlikely that China's remarkable fertility decline mainly resulted from mass education or occupational mobility. Rather it came from changes affecting the whole population and overall socio-economic structures.

Possible Causes of Differential Fertility among Social Strata

The effects of education on fertility have been thoroughly studied.[33] The inverse relationship between fertility and education is consistently confirmed by numerous empirical studies. Schooling delays marriage, weakens the traditional family authority, and disseminates new ideas. More educated couples tend to have more interests unconnected with family life, and are engaged in more roles outside family, such as professional careers. Education for women increases the opportunity cost of having children. Those with higher education might have access to more information on birth control and might be more efficient family planners.[34] These speculations are commonly valid in the case of China.

In China people's education is closely associated with their occupation and place of residence. China's 1982 census shows that among all occupations, the agricultural labour force has the lowest schooling attainment and highest illiteracy rate. At the same time, peasants have the highest average parity. In contrast, the average educational level is the highest for people working as professionals, such as those classified as cadres: small families are more common among them.[35] The overall educational level of the urban population is also much higher than that of the rural population, which is due in part to the inequality of educational opportunities between rural and urban areas. Furthermore, for a long time, high education has been one of the surest ways for the rural youngsters to move into urban areas. Different educational composition, therefore, may be one of the major causes of the differentials in occupational fertility.

Differences in educational and occupational fertility may also be attributed to the differences in organization and control. Chinese society is well organized and controlled by various administrative and social organs. In urban areas, people are organized in their workplace as well as in their residence. Since they work and reside in the same location, members of the rural population are controlled basically in their production teams. During the third family-planning programme, population quotas were assigned to these grass-roots units. Therefore, couples in the cities were exposed to double pressures (one, from where they worked; the other, from where they lived) to pledge birth control. Both their career and wage promotion would be affected if they did not fulfil the requirements. Furthermore, it was very difficult to live in the cities without rations for food, clothing, and other supplies and services in the 1960s and 1970s. By contrast, control in rural areas was far looser. This was particularly true when the working target of the local family-planning personnel was his relatives.

However, some other factors are also responsible for higher fertility in rural areas and among peasants. It is necessary to consider the reasons for having children (especially amongst peasants) in order to understand the differential fertility among different social strata.

Feudal Influence

Feudal influence is often cited as one of the most important factors responsible for high fertility among peasants.[36] Values supporting early marriage and large family are deeply ingrained in Chinese culture, and closely linked to traditional concepts of family roles and to ideas about self-fulfilment, filial piety, fortune, and fate.[37] In a culture with strong ancestor cults and patrilineal tradition, it was considered not only a sign of 'blessing' but also of 'good moral conduct' to have many sons. Having only a few children, and especially no son, was viewed as a punishment for evil doings.[38] Ancestor worship was practised as a central rite of Chinese family life for thousands of years. Although the government has taken a firm stand to shift the loyalty from the family to the State since 1949, the importance of patrilineal descendants continues to affect thinking about the ideal family size and composition, especially among peasants.[39] Another traditional motive which has not disappeared entirely is the desire to have a son who will get on in the world and bring wealth and honour to the family.[40] These feudal vestiges are much stronger in rural areas and among those who have attained less education. However, a peasant's desire for more children is by no means only a product of ignorance or superstition. There is more to it than this.

Costs and Benefits of Childbearing

Demand theory is often used as a framework to explain the reproductive behaviour of households.[41] Analyses of the costs and benefits of childbearing have been made by the Chinese government and by scholars.[42] It has been estimated that the cost of bringing up a child to working age is about 7,000 *Yuan* in the large, economically and culturally developed cities, whereas it costs two-thirds of that figure in less developed small- and medium-sized cities, and only one-quarter of that cost (about 1,600 *Yuan*) in the rural areas. A large part of these differences can be attributed to government expenditures on public services such as schooling and health care. Nevertheless, the differences in the parent's direct costs are substantial (4,689 *Yuan* in cities and 1,193 *Yuan* in the countryside). Moreover, the cost of a child in rural areas with low living standards is perceived as even lower based on the belief that it is 'as easy to handle a flock of sheep as just one'.

By contrast, bringing up children involves more economic difficulties for couples in the cities with universally low wages.[43] It is hard to imagine having a child without lowering living standards. In addition, urban young couples tended to spend much of their time, energy, and earnings in educating their children. This is particularly true for those who came back from the countryside. Their education and career had often been ruined by the Cultural Revolution, and they put their hopes on their children. This may also be a consequence of the family-planning policy. The policy stressed fewer but better children. Small family size made high spending on children possible.

Children in rural areas make themselves useful very early. Although collectivization had reduced the importance of the family as an economic unit, the size of the labour force remained the deciding factor conditioning a family's income in China's rural areas. This became more crucial as the economic reforms in China's rural areas progressed after the late 1970s. Even in collectives, small children made contributions to a family's welfare by weeding, or tending pigs and chickens, and looking after babies. In addition, for decades many local regulations, such as those governing the allocation of grain rations and private plots, also made children a source of family well-being. Since each family's allotment was based on the number of family members rather than the work contributed by the family, an extra child could bring in more land and rations. In many cases, grain allocated to households with many children was enough for them throughout the year, but families with few children often ran out of grain and had to purchase at high prices in the market. This naturally stimulates more births. As a Chinese proverb says: 'the more sons the more happiness'. The economic benefits of bringing up a child in the rural areas was probably in excess of the cost.

In contrast, children in urban areas are net consumers until they graduate from school. They can not provide much help to the family when they are small. In the early 1980s about 93 per cent of school-age children under the age of 15 in the urban areas were studying in school, while only 78 per cent of children did so in rural areas.[44] The difference in higher education has been much greater. Furthermore, rural children reaching the minimum working age (usually 16) would automatically enter the labour force of their production teams and start to earn income if they worked there. In urban areas, youngsters have to wait for a while after their graduation in order to find a job. There were few means of income generation outside wage employment in the 1960s and 1970s. A large number of urban youths were sent to the countryside—a process which reached its climax during the Cultural Revolution period. It was reported that during the period 1966–76 about 14 million urban youths were sent to the countryside to accept so-called 're-education'. When working in the poor rural areas, these urban youngsters had to rely on their parents for financial support in addition to the small amount of government subsidy.[45] Those who remained in the cities and towns after leaving school without being assigned jobs had to depend on their parents for a living. The cohorts born in the 1950s and 1960s, together with those returned from the countryside, encountered somewhat severe unemployment problems in the cities. By the end of 1984 the urban population classified as 'people waiting for job' amounted to about 3.4 million.[46] Thus children in the urban areas are more an economic liability than an asset.

Old-age Security

More important is the concern about old age. The old-age security motive for fertility is commonly strong in less developed countries.[47] A survey conducted in the rural area of Hubei province in 1982 shows that while 21 per cent of interviewees wanted many children mainly in order to increase the household labour force, 25 per cent were concerned with continuance of the ancestral line, and more than one-half wanted to produce sons to support them in their old age.[48] Another survey carried out in the outskirts of Shanghai reported that out of 198 interviewees, 108 wished to have sons to ensure financial support for old age, and 80 said the motivation was to increase family labour force and income.[49] More evidence can easily be found in Chinese literature.

Although tremendous progress has been made since 1949, China's social welfare system is not yet well developed. There is no universal retirement scheme to give everyone some sort of old-age pension. In 1982 there were about 80 million people aged 60 and over in China. Only about one-eighth were in receipt of pensions, and another 3 million obtained the provision of 'the five guarantees' (of food, clothing, medical care, housing, and burial expenses). Among 60 million old people in China's rural areas, only 0.9 million received some kind of old-age security.[50] Most elderly people have to turn to their adult children for financial support in old age as in traditional China. Furthermore, supporting aged parents is a child's legal responsibility, according to the Chinese Constitution and marriage law.[51]

There are great rural–urban differences. On the one hand, a majority of the labour force in non-agricultural sectors are employed by State or locally owned enterprises. When they reach the limits of working ages (usually 60 for men and 55 for women) they may retire with pensions to support them through their remaining years. The regulations for labour insurance have been revised several times. The percentage of the urban labour force that is eligible for the pension scheme has increased, benefits have been improved and the minimum requirements reduced.[52] Moreover, all retired people continue to receive free medical care and other social benefits. One economic rationale for having several children has been greatly minimized for this section of the Chinese population.

On the other hand, despite the establishment of old people's homes and the provision of 'the five guarantees' for the childless, the majority of peasants have to depend on their savings and, more importantly, their adult children to support them when they are unable to earn a living. Locally funded retirement schemes have been implemented in some wealthy villages,[53] but nation-wide diffusion is not very promising in the current economic situation. Furthermore, the living standards of those who receive 'the five guarantees' are in general lower than those who are supported by their offspring.[54] This is particularly true in poor areas, since the standard is based on local economic conditions, which vary enormously. The old fears of loneliness, dependency, or hardship in old age remain a very strong factor in the childbearing decision. Thus, 'having sons to look after you when you are old' is not only a traditional attitude, but also reflects a practical problem. Combined with China's strong patrilineal tradition, a minimum of one son to take care of his parents and to carry on the family name is generally accepted among peasants. Many studies have suggested that the family-planning programme was more easily and efficiently implemented in places where financial support for the elderly was provided.[55]

This seems to confirm the validity of the wealth-flows theory proposed by Caldwell.[56] The net flow of wealth from children to parents is in general probably positive in China's rural areas. Therefore, bearing more children is economically rational. By contrast, the intergenerational wealth flow is by and large negative in China's urban areas, and parents continue to have children but only in small numbers and for non-economic reasons.

Decline in Infant Mortality

Before 1949 China's mortality level, especially infant mortality, was very high. It was estimated that life expectancy for a Chinese farmer in the 1930s was only between 20 and 25 years.[57] Estimates of infant mortality before 1950 were about 200 per 1,000 live births.[58]

Since 1949, mainly as the result of the improvement of living standards and development of health and medical services, China's mortality rate has fallen substantially. China, as suggested by Banister and Preston, has probably gained on average over 1.5 years of life expectancy for each calendar year since 1949. This is unprecedented among the world's populous developing countries.[59] By 1957 average life expectancy had risen to 57 years, and by 1975 to 68.2 years. Infant mortality rate has also shown a sharp decline. By 1981 China's officially reported infant mortality rate stood at 35 per 1,000 live births.[60] This great achievement is largely attributable to the Chinese government's effort in strengthening its maternity and child-care services.

The decline of mortality may not be a pre-condition of fertility transition. Nevertheless, this rapid reduction in infant mortality should reduce the demand for surviving children. It is probably not necessary now to have many children, as it was previously, to assure the continuity of the family line and old-age security. The decline in infant mortality has been a factor in the acceptance of family planning.[61]

Although many measures have been adopted by the government to improve the health service in China's rural areas, such as the introduction of barefoot doctors, there are still marked rural–urban differences in medical care, and mortality level as well. This may be one of the causes of the higher fertility amongst Chinese peasants.

Housing Problems

For the urban population, a shortage of housing stock becomes one of the main considerations associated with reproductive decisions. The rapid improvement of mortality and longer lifespan, higher fertility in the early years of the People's Republic, and lack of investment in urban infrastructure contributed to the crowded housing conditions in urban areas.[62] In fact, the average living space per head of urban inhabitants declined from 4.5 square metres in 1952 to 3.6 square metres in 1978.[63] A survey conducted in 216 cities in late 1979 revealed that about one-third of all urban households did not have sufficient living space.[64] Housing pressure in the cities has been gradually reduced in the 1980s, and the per capita living space increased to 4.89 square metres by 1984.[65] However, it is not easy to solve the problem within a short period. The situation in the older and larger cities, such as Shanghai, has been even worse. The very high age at first marriage in those cities is partly attributed to the difficulty in obtaining flats. The majority of China's urban residents relied on the local authority to allocate housing. It was said that it was easier to find a wife than to secure accommodation. Even among those who had registered for marriage, shortage of housing prevented them from living together,[66] and affected their reproduction. Lack of privacy in overcrowded cities may also strengthen cultural constraints on pre-marital sex and often inhibits post-marital sexual relations. The shortage of living space may lead to the popularity of the nuclear family. However, this limited accommodation may also hinder the development of the modern nuclear family, which may be a possible cause of the relatively greater proportion of large families in Shanghai.[67]

Female Labour Participation

It is worth mentioning another factor relevant to the rural–urban differentials in fertility: female labour participation. This is linked with the improvement of women's position in China. Since the 1950s, women's societal role has been transformed and the saying 'women hold up half the sky' has been taken seriously. All four Constitutions formulated since the founding of the new China have stipulations which demand women's equal rights with men in political, economic, cultural, educational, and other spheres of social life.[68] More and more women have participated in economic activities.[69] Women workers and employees accounted for about 18.8 per cent of all workers and employees in 1959. By the end of 1982 this figure had increased to about 36.3 per cent.[70]

The relationship between women's work and their fertility is a controversial topic.[71] None the less, this increased participation did offer women much more freedom of choice and the right to speak in family and childbearing matters. It has also become easier for working women to discuss and improve their knowledge of birth control. Meanwhile, they were exposed to the group pressure to accept the family-planning programme. Women workers' free time was to a certain extent occupied by frequent political meetings and involvement in other social activities in the past.

Although both work and motherhood are considered important roles for Chinese women, popular attitudes tend to favour the motherhood role as the primary one.[72] Heavy housework is another burden to bear, in part because of the lack of service facilities for the public. Surveys reveal considerable variations in the time actually spent on household chores.[73] But one thing is certain: that most of the housework was done by women, in what has traditionally been regarded as their role. In the rural areas, women were usually offered lower-paid part-time jobs, and the working arrangement was much more flexible. In contrast, working women in the cities worked the same as their male counterparts. They contributed six days a week, eight hours a day, spent one or two hours on daily commuting, plus about three hours on household chores per day. Although husbands may help in sharing these chores, life for working couples is tiring and exhausting, and is all the more so if a couple has more children.[74] This certainly affects their desire for children.

Summary

The effects of education and occupation on mean parities are quantified by fitting log-linear models. The results are consistent and convincing. Education and occupation are important determinants of Chinese women's fertility behaviour. Women who have received higher education tend to have smaller family sizes than those having less education. Peasant women are estimated to have more children than workers or cadres, and are similar to housewives. Women who work as cadres in general have less children than any other group.

The mean parity of rural women is consistently higher than that of their urban counterparts. It is of great interest that for the same educational level, same occupation, and same rural–urban identity, fertility levels vary substantially among provinces, especially between the eastern and western parts of China. Women in western provinces usually have more births than those in eastern China.

The time trends of the differentials are prominent. The effects of education and occupation on fertility have diminished over time, although they are still significant. By contrast, the effects of type of residence and province location increase over time. China can be roughly divided into three regions according to the findings from these models. The eastern part includes three large municipalities and five east coastal provinces. Mean parities in this part of China are usually low, and the fertility decline is earlier and faster. The western region contains eight provinces, and the mean parities for women in this part are estimated to be the highest in China, no matter what their education level and occupation. The middle part covers a large area from the north to the south of China. Here women's fertility behaviour shows some similarity to, and fertility levels and paces of transition are close to, the national average.

This seems to support our initial conclusion concerning the diffusive pattern of China's fertility transition. China's urban population took the lead in fertility decline, with the rural population well behind. Transition started among women who received high education and diffused to less educated women. Women classified as cadres reduced their family size first, then other occupations followed. Fertility regulation commenced earliest in large municipalities, followed by the eastern coastal provinces, and thereafter the interior regions. As time passed, the pace of fertility transition in eastern China accelerated, resulting in a widening gap between provinces.

Comparison of the effects of education and occupation on mean parity is not straightforward. Rural–urban differences, controlling for other factors, are consistently larger in the education models than in the occupation models. The strong association between occupation and type of residence may account for some of these differences. The regional differences, on the other hand, are estimated to be larger in the occupation models. In China, educational level is closely related to type of occupation. Generally speaking, the labour force engaged in agricultural activities has the lowest educational level, whilst cadres are usually those who have received better education.

The gradual increase in regional, and decrease in educational and occupational, differentials are the combined product of local government's efforts on birth control and people's responses to the programme. Although the policy initiative began centrally, the outcome of the family-planning programme to a large extent relied on local efforts. At the early stage of the transition, certain social groups, such as the better-educated and cadres, were more willing to use, and had better access to, birth-control services. In addition, urban intellectuals and cadres were the main target of the early family-planning programmes. With the progress of the programme, knowledge and provision of contraceptives became widely available to everyone in particular areas. Therefore, the pace of fertility transition was largely determined by local commitment to the programme. As a result, fertility differentials between social strata shrank, while regional differences widened.

This confirms the view that the fundamental forces of change operate at the societal level.[75] The micro-level processes seem to be largely determined by changes in macro-level conditions. It is plain to see that although individual differentials are important, Chinese women's reproduction is more likely to be affected by community or macro factors, especially with the implementation of the family-planning programme. The consistent and remarkable regional differentials in China's fertility transition lead us to look for possible determinants at macro-level.

III. Regional Fertility Variations and Socio-Economic Development

Several investigations have sought to examine the socio-economic determinants of China's regional fertility differentials.[76] However, these analyses are cross-sectional and focus on a certain time point, and none embraces different periods of China's fertility transition. In this section we try to link cross-sectional study with different phases of China's fertility transition, to shed light on the general mechanism of fertility transition, and the way in which roles played by socio-economic factors change over time.

Data for Study

The provincial administrative unit is the basic policy-making organ for the family-planning programme in China. Levels of socio-economic development vary greatly between provinces. The hypothesis to be examined in the following section, therefore, is that socio-economic factors are largely responsible for provincial differentials in fertility levels.

There are no systematic time–series data for any of China's provinces. But fragmentary information is available or can be estimated for most of China's provinces for the selected years: 1957, 1965, and 1978. These years are chosen mainly because of data availability. Nevertheless, these dates also represent important phases of China's population growth. As was mentioned earlier, there was no official birth-control policy in the 1950s, even though the issue was discussed in some circles. Thus 1957 represents a time when there was little impact of birth control on fertility. Family planning was first earnestly carried out, at least in urban areas, in the early 1960s. The data for 1965 show the socio-economic conditions in the early stage of the urban fertility transition. Finally, dramatic fertility decline has been achieved since the early 1970s. Accordingly, data for 1978 should reflect this period. Since the early 1980s abundant information is available. Because the main object of this study is to find out the possible determinants of the fertility transition which has taken place, our focus here is on the information for the past rather than for the most recent period. However, the relationships between socio-economic variables and provincial fertility in the early 1980s are treated separately.

Eleven sets of data have been collected, and they represent various social and economic conditions in China's provinces over time. Gross Product Value of Industry and Agriculture (GPVIA) is an index used by the Chinese government to reflect the general levels of economic development in a region. Per capita GPVIA is estimated for provinces, where sufficient data are available. Population density is calculated on the basis of current administrative boundaries. The urban proportion is derived from China's first two censuses. Because of the strict control of rural–urban migration, there was little change in the urban proportion between the mid-1960s and the 1970s. Therefore, the figure derived from the 1964 census is assumed to be valid until the end of the 1970s. The numbers of doctors and hospital beds per 10,000 population are estimated for most provinces and viewed as general indicators of each province's health-care conditions. Since an overwhelming majority of China's population are rural residents, the annual net income, and consumer expenditure, per person for China's rural population are estimated in order to examine relationships between income, expenditure, and fertility level. Several sets of data are used to show the general educational condition in provinces. They are collected from different sources and include the number of students enrolled in primary and middle school per 10,000 population; the proportion of illiterate and semi-illiterate among the total population aged 12 years and over; and the proportion of female illiterates. Finally, data on newspaper circulation per 10,000 population are used to examine the impact of the media on fertility.

The means and standard deviations for these variables are presented in Table 3.4. These figures represent the unweighted provincial average, not the national values.

Socio-economic conditions indicated by these variables vary substantially between provinces. More significant is the fact that for almost all variables, provincial differences increase over time. This indicates the uneven process of development. Taking per capita gross product value of industry and agriculture as an example, in 1957 the highest (1,215 *Yuan* in Shanghai) is about 11.4 times higher than the lowest (107 *Yuan* in Qinghai). The difference jumps to 18.8 times (2,374 *Yuan* in Shanghai, 126 *Yuan* in Guangxi) in 1965 and further rises to 20 times (5,153 *Yuan* in Shanghai and 257 *Yuan* in Guizhou) in 1978.

Correlation Coefficient Analysis

Our study begins with an analysis of the correlation coefficient. Negative relationships between total fertility rate and these variables, except illiteracy, are expected. All values of the correlation coefficients are presented in Table 3.5.

Some important features are revealed in the table. All values of the coefficients for 1957 are relatively small, and consistently have positive signs, except for illiteracy. This suggests a tenuous and positive relationship beteen TFR and these selected variables, which is contrary to our earlier expectation. In other words, more developed provinces tended to have a higher TFR in the mid-1950s. It can be seen that the GPVIA has the highest correlation with the total fertility rate ($r = 0.367$), while the density variable ($r = 0.107$) is least associated.

This picture has been totally reversed in subsequent years. The coefficients reach their highest values in 1965, but all the signs are reversed. Furthermore, all coefficients are close to 1. Even the smallest coefficient ($r = 0.646$), which is between the peasant annual consumer cost and the TFR, is much higher than the highest one ($r = 0.367$) in 1957. Thus, very close and, more importantly, negative relationships are established according to these figures. The total fertility rates in these more advanced provinces were relatively lower, which is the relationship that we anticipated. Newspaper circulation and GPVIA

TABLE 3.4. *Means and standard deviations for selected socio-economic variables*

Variables	1957		1965		1978	
	Mean	St.d	Mean	St.d.	Mean	St.d
1. Total fertility rate (TFR)	6.265(28)	0.763	5.904(28)	0.994	2.915(28)	1.001
2. Per capita gross product value of industry and agriculture (GPVIA) (Yuan)	260.7(23)	266.2	396.0(21)	501.0	831.0(23)	1040.0
3. Population density (Person/km^2)	202.0(28)	303.4	233.5(28)	333.5	281.0(28)	338.4
4. Percentage urban	18.68(28)	16.88	22.32(28)	15.68		
5. Doctors per 10,000 population	20.21(22)	9.16	25.80(20)	10.52	32.55(22)	15.50
6. Hospital beds per 10,000 population	8.57(23)	7.32	15.54(22)	8.46	22.44(24)	7.61
7. Peasant annual net income per head (Yuan)	90.47(22)	35.80	111.33(23)	25.30	144.08(23)	45.92
8. Peasant annual consumer cost per head (Yuan)	78.91(21)	18.93	101.57(16)	26.42	122.03(20)	28.61
9. Students enrolled per 10,000 population	1108.5(27)	210.4	1756.8(27)	271.0	2206.0(28)	318.5
10. Percentage illiterate and Semi-illiterate			35.98(24)	8.51		
11. Female illiteracy rate (%)	86.50(28)	10.47	68.25(28)	17.82	43.79(28)	18.02
12. Newspaper copies per 100,000 population	7.16(11)	9.16	6.65(12)	6.85	11.49(12)	15.07

Note: Figures in parentheses refer to cases available.

Source: 2, 5, 6, 12. From relevant provincial Statistical Yearbooks, Economic Handbooks, Statistical Abstracts.

3, 4, 10. Hu Huanyong and Zhang Shanyu, *Population Geography of China* (1986, in Chinese).

7, 8. Collected from *Collection of Data on Peasants' Income and Consumption for Provinces, Autonomous Regions and Major Cities* (Beijing, 1985, in Chinese), 207, 304.

9. Calculated from *Educational Yearbook of China, 1984* (Beijing).

11. Derived from China's 1982 Fertility Survey. Figure for 1957 estimated from women aged 50, 55, 60, and 67; figures for 1965 refer to women aged 45, and the average of the 35 and 40 age groups for 1978.

TABLE 3.5. *Correlation coefficients between TFR and socio-economic variables in selected years, China*[a]

Variables	Total fertility rate			
	1957	1965	1978	1982[b]
GPVIA	0.367(23)	–0.915(21)	–0.524(23)	–0.580(28)[c]
Density	0.107(28)	0.821(28)	–0.567(28)	–0.544(28)
Proportion urban	0.331(28)	–0.800(28)	–0.556(28)	–0.586(28)
Peasant income	0.333(22)	–0.622(23)	–0.526(23)	
Peasant consumption	0.291(21)	–0.646(16)	–0.131(20)	–0.555(28)
Doctors	0.268(22)	–0.848(20)	–0.539(22)	–0.478(28)
Hospital beds	0.183(23)	–0.735(22)	–0.374(24)	–0.365(28)
Students	0.149(27)	–0.719(27)	–0.068(28)	
Illiteracy (total)	*	0.650(24)	*	0.631(28)[d]
Illiteracy (women)	–0.271(28)	0.805(28)	0.519(28)	0.600(28)[d]
Newspaper	0.194(11)	–0.923(12)	–0.487(12)	–0.486(28)[e]

[a] Figures in parentheses refer to cases available.
[b] Quoted from Dudley L. Poston and Baochang Gu, 'Socioeconomic Development, Family Planning, and Fertility in China', in *Demography*, 24 (4), 1987.
[c] Refers to per capita industrial output only.
[d] In Poston and Gu's paper, the index of percentage of literate was used.
[e] Author's estimation.

Source: Cited in Table 3.4 and note b.

are the two variables which have the highest negative correlations with the TFR.

In 1978 the absolute values of all coefficients drop to around 0.5, but the negative signs remain. This seems to suggest that the relationship between socio-economic factors and fertility weakened over time. The proportion of students enrolled is almost totally unrelated to TFR, which is indicated by the very low value of the correlation coefficient between them (r = 0.068). This may be caused by the fact that the index is to a large extent affected by the population age composition.

Nineteen eighty-two follows a similar pattern although some variables are slightly different from those used for the other years. The relative effects of the variables representing illiteracy, proportion urban, and per capita output are among the highest, while the effect of health care is relatively small.

The correlation coefficient for per capita gross product value of industry and agriculture is consistently among the highest in the former three selected years. Therefore, the relationship between total fertility rate and per capita GPVIA is examined in more detail in Figure 3.3.

It is interesting to observe the changes in these curves. In the 1950s

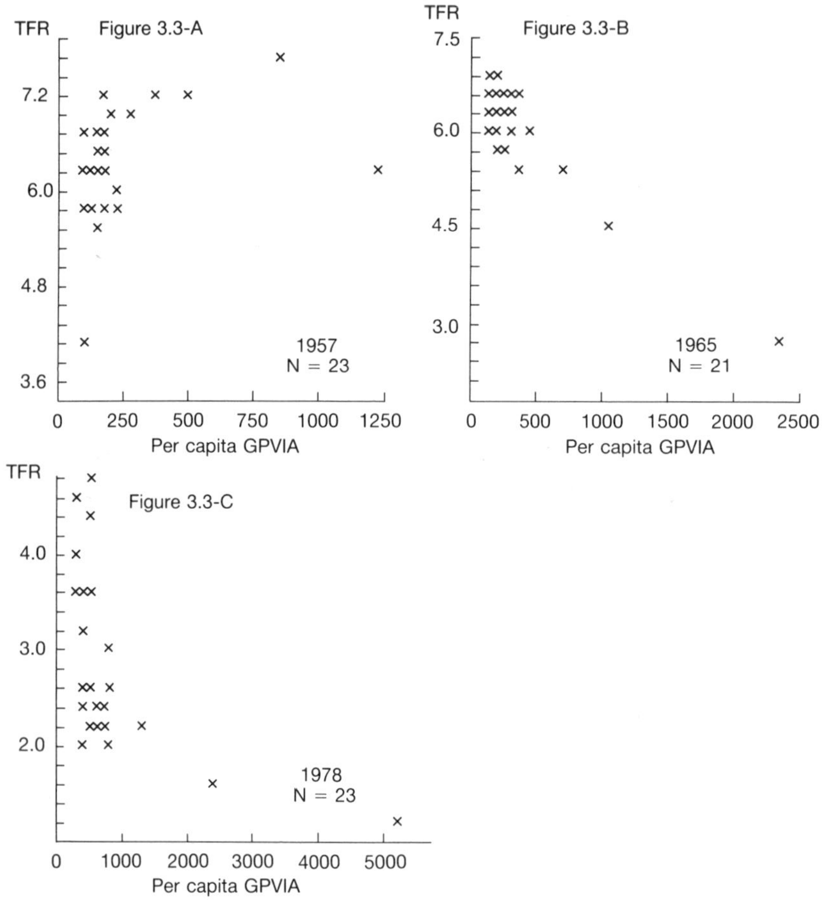

Fig. 3.3 Relationship between total fertility rate and per capita gross product value of industry and agriculture

panel A of Figure 3.3 shows that the relation between the TFR and per capita GPVIA was positive. The TFR was generally low for provinces with low per capita GPVIA. With the increase of per capita GPVIA, the TFR also became higher. However, the TFR for the province with the highest per capita GPVIA was lower, although not the lowest. This relationship is different in 1965. Panel B of Figure 3.3 suggests that the higher the provincial per capita GPVIA, the lower its TFR: These two indices, TFR and per capita GPVIA, are closely associated. In the later 1970s, although provinces with lower TFR are still those with higher per capita GPVIA, the negative relationship has become less clear and far from linear (see panel C of Figure 3.3). The curves in Figure 3.3 are largely determined by several extreme values. The general relationship becomes less close but remains valid, after the two extreme values (for Shanghai and Tianjin) are left out.

Some concluding points can be made. The positive, but tenuous, linkage between the total fertility rate and indices of development in 1957 suggests that in the pre-transition period, when birth-control measures were little in evidence, the effects of socio-economic structures on fertility were mostly positive. The fertility level in provinces with higher GPVIA, higher income, more health service, lower illiteracy rate, higher urban proportion, and higher population density was commonly higher than elsewhere. As we have noted, China experienced a steady increase in fertility level during the early 1950s. This to a large extent matches the pattern of the onset of demographic transition which was described by Dyson and Murphy.[77] Modernization might be the main cause of this early increase in fertility. However, the weak relationship between the TFR and socio-economic indices suggests that many other institutional factors, such as local social customs, cultural traditions, etc. may also be responsible for regional fertility differentials.

At the early stage of the transition and with fewer compulsory measures, there are close and negative relationships between fertility and socio-economic conditions. It can be said that if the transition were a spontaneous process, the influences of socio-economic conditions would be very important. The population in more advanced provinces was more willing to accept the new attitude to birth control, and better socio-economic conditions made the birth-control programme easier to implement.

These relationships tend to become tenuous again with the progress of the family-planning programme. Since knowledge of family planning and services had been widely propagated and became easily available, the early advantage of advanced socio-economic structure diminished over time. Resistance to fertility transition was deeply rooted in local institutional factors. During this period administrative efforts played a more important role in facilitating the transition.

Multiple Regression Analysis

The bi-variate relationships between the total fertility rate and selected socio-economic variables have been examined in the preceding section. Many of these variables, however, are closely related to each other (correlation matrix not shown). We therefore should further select indicators for carrying out a multiple regression analysis.

The variables of peasant annual income and consumer expenditure are closely associated (r = 0.95, 0.98, and 0.93 for 1957, 1965, and 1978 respectively). Only the income variable is chosen for the regression. Similarly, the high correlation coefficients between the number of doctors and hospital beds per 100,000 population (r = 0.87, 0.91, and 0.87 respectively) lead us to exclude hospital beds as an independent variable in the analysis. There are three sets of data on education. The proportions of illiterates and semi-illiterates for the total population aged 12 and over are only available for 1964. On the other hand, female illiteracy rates derived from the survey are for the different age cohorts rather than for the selected years. Moreover, they tend to be overstated and are exposed to the risk of sampling errors. Therefore, the number of students enrolled in primary and middle school has been chosen as the educational indicator, although this index is affected by the population age composition. Information on newspaper circulation is only available for 12 provinces, so this variable is left out. Now, we have one dependent variable (TFR) and six independent variables (per capita GPVIA, peasant annual income, number of doctors, percentage urban, population density, and students). We have regressed the total fertility rate on the six selected socio-economic variables for the years of 1957, 1965, and 1978. All values of these variables are available for 17 out of 28 provinces. Thus the regression is based on the situation in these 17 provinces, and the results are shown in Table 3.6.

TABLE 3.6. *Multiple regression analysis of socio-economic factors on TFR for selected years*

Independent variables	Dependent variables TFR n = 17		
	1957	1965	1978
Constant	5.994(0.765)*	8.771(1.031)*	3.869(0.3921)*
Income	0.024(0.008)*	0.004(0.004)	
GPVIA	0.006(0.002)*	–0.00003(0.0009)	0.0010(0.0007)
Student	–0.002(0.001)*	–0.0012(0.0005)*	
Doctor	0.051(0.029)	–0.0331(0.025)	
Urban	–0.099(0.037)*	0.0081(0.020)	–0.0461(0.0257)
Density	–0.002(0.001)*	–0.0017(0.0007)*	–0.0029(0.0013)*
Multiple Coeffficient of Determinants (R-squared adjusted)	64.30	93.50	34.10
Standard error	0.3291	0.2495	0.7730
F-ratio	5.807	39.581	4.786

Note: An asterisk indicates that the coefficient is significant at 5% level.
Figures in parentheses refer to standard deviation.

The general relationship between socio-economic factors and total fertility rate among China's provinces can be assessed. Table 3.6 shows that the R-squared values for both the 1957 and 1965 equations are significantly different from zero at a fairly high significance level, say, 0.01. About 65 per cent of regional diversity in fertility in 1957 may be explained by these six socio-economic variables, and 93 per cent in 1965. It is difficult to assess what the importance of each individual variable is in the overall equation. All factors except the number of doctors are statistically significant at the 0.05 level in the regression equation for 1957. However, even though the R-squared value is very high and significant, most of the parameter estimates in the 1965 equation are not. Clearly, this occurrence is associated with the problem of multicollinearity. The regression for 1978 is not satisfactory. The R-squared value of the regression with six independent variables is as low as 2.3 per cent. The best regression result is obtained from using three independent variables: the proportion urban, population density, and per capita GPVIA. In this regression equation, about 34 per cent of the variance in fertility can be explained by these variables. The equation is significant at the 0.05 level. Grouping or indexing variables may lead to better results.

The index of province location, which has been used in our micro-analysis, is introduced again into the regression. Now, the values of R-squared rise to 71.1, 93.7, and 61.8 for 1957, 1965, and 1978 respectively. This variable has little explanatory power for total fertility rate in the regressions for 1957 and 1965, but is significantly important in 1978. This finding leads to the suggestion that China's regional fertility patterns in the later 1970s are more clustered than before.

A path analysis has been conducted by Poston and Gu using most recent (1982) information on socio-economic development and family planning for China's 28 provinces.[78] Results of their study demonstrated very strong negative direct effects of structural development on fertility. Furthermore, indirect negative effects of development on fertility through family planning were also established.

While there was less regional fertility diversity in the pre-transitional period, China's fertility pattern has become more and more regionally clustered. The question to be asked is how this is associated with regional differentials regarding socio-economic structures.

Regional Differences

Available provincial data are combined and averaged according to province location. Results are recorded in Table 3.7. This procedure

TABLE 3.7. *Selected socio-economic variables for China's province groups*

Province location	TFR	Income	GPVIA	Student	Doctor	Urban	Density
1957							
Municipal	6.699	152.33	1033.1	1382	35.69	0.624	768
East coast	6.466	87.99	245.9	1240	24.06	0.154	273
South	6.251	87.78	161.6	1058	16.62	0.119	165
North	6.504	86.23	233.1	1184	18.72	0.165	98
Southwest	6.161	63.33	127.6	982	16.23	0.088	87
Northwest	5.387	69.80	115.1	897	11.52	0.131	17
1965							
Municipal	3.478	165.40	1706.2	2369	45.84	0.604	929
East coast	5.737	108.28	329.6	1874	22.12	0.190	305
South	6.294	113.02	206.2	1726	20.68	0.153	180
North	6.069	104.30	311.1	1801	25.73	0.240	114
Southwest	6.709	106.11	145.5	1593	18.04	0.117	99
Northwest	6.295	85.30	241.7	1447	29.45	0.166	18
1978							
Municipal	1.448	222.90	3756.8	2102	64.79	0.604	970
East coast	2.172	144.76	760.8	2215	29.33	0.190	381
South	2.902	137.40	446.1	2222	25.18	0.153	244
North	2.653	136.50	575.1	2296	30.77	0.242	152
Southwest	4.209	119.95	302.3	2037	20.13	0.117	142
Northwest	4.061	100.50	593.0	2282	31.64	0.166	27

Correlation coefficients between TFR and socio-economic variables

	1957	1965	1978
Income	0.635	−0.912	−0.867
GPVIA	0.583	−0.985	−0.720
Student	0.884	−0.935	−0.018
Doctor	0.779	−0.919	−0.722
Urban	0.515	−0.982	−0.764
Density	0.652	−0.974	−0.833

Note and Source: Cited in Table 3.4.

conceals the variance within province groups but highlights differences between them.

There do exist marked regional differences in socio-economic conditions. All selected socio-economic variables in the municipal region are well ahead of the rest, followed by the east-coast region. The western regions are generally less developed compared with the others. This pattern persists over time, and coincides with the overall pattern of regional fertility differentials. The high values of correlation coefficients between TFR and socio-economic variables provide further evidence of the close relationship between fertility transition and its socio-economic context.

But compared with fertility differentials, regional differences in the selected socio-economic variables are small. This may suggest that Chinese women's fertility behaviour is very sensitive to surrounding social conditions. On the other hand, it may also indicate that many other non-socio-economic factors are at work, such as policy issues and regional traditions.

Summary

On the whole, the findings of our study parallel the results of several other studies. We share with others the opinion that the government's programme, although important, has not operated in a vacuum.[79] Socio-economic structures are closely associated with the fertility transition, but their impact differs over time. In general, socio-economic factors seem to be more relevant to China's regional fertility differentials in the pre- and early period of the fertility transition, but less so at the later stage, at least in terms of a linear relationship. The direct role played by socio-economic factors in bringing about China's rapid fertility decline may be minor, as some analysts have suggested.[80] Nevertheless, these developments brought about fundamental changes in society and paved the way for the family-planning programme.

As already mentioned, decentralized policy implementation is one of the major features of China's family-planning programme. Although the fundamental principles of policy are the same, the detailed regulations vary widely among provinces. Furthermore, acceptance of, or resistance to birth control are closely associated with local conditions. The kinship system, the traditional value of children, etc. are quite different between regions. Other things being equal, populations with similar cultures and environments tend to have a similar response of fertility to socio-economic and other changes.[81] The analysis of socio-economic determinants of fertility should not be separated from that of such institutional factors.

IV. Institutional Determinants

The regional differentials in China's fertility transition are to a great extent attributable to the uneven progress of the family-planning programme among localities. In addition, population programmes appear to have been more influential where economic circumstances are better, but less so where socio-economic change has lagged.[82] However, a large part of the fertility decline cannot be explained by these factors.

Let us take Guangdong as an example. The family-planning programme in this province was carried out very actively in the 1960s and the 1970s. The development level in this province is also one of the highest nationally. Peasants in Guangdong are richer than in many other parts of China.[83] Moreover, Guangdong is one of the provinces in which western influence is relatively strong owing in part to its geographic location. However, the resistance to fertility change in the rural areas of Guangdong has been very strong. While many other less developed provinces, such as Sichuan, experienced rapid fertility decline during the 1970s, the transition in Guangdong was very slow and the fertility level in the rural areas of Guangdong consistently remained relatively high.

Government intervention and modernization fail to explain this phenomenon. An alternative explanation lies in the institutional approach.[84] On the basis of their study of Guangdong, Parish and Whyte argue that the implementation of these programmes depends to a great extent on the concrete features of village life, features which support some changes and obstruct others.[85]

The institutional settings in Guangdong province are in many ways distinctive. Its special political history, the strength of kinship and family lineages, the strong linkage with overseas Chinese, and so on made Guangdong differ from other provinces. The mechanism through which those unique institutional factors affect the fertility transition is far from being adequately studied.

Guangdong is not the only province with peculiar local characteristics. China is such a large and heterogeneous country that various local 'little traditions' exist.[86] They each play their part in determining the regional differentials in the fertility transition. While there were conspicuous and long-enduring patterns of nuptiality and fertility that followed linguistic and cultural lines in the European fertility transition,[87] the regional patterns in China are less clear. Much more work on the linkage between the local tradition and the regional differences in fertility and marriage behaviour, is needed in order to understand fully the features of China's fertility transition.

The content of 'institutional factors' in many cases remains undefined or unspecified. In the following sections, we shall briefly examine several important factors which affect an individual's demographic decision-making. These factors may be viewed as 'objective' institutional environments, as termed by McNicoll.[88]

Sex Preference

Sex preference is common in many societies throughout the world.[89] Rooted deeply in the feudal tradition, preference for sons over daughters can be found almost everywhere in China, especially in the rural areas.[90] Fragmentary information indicates the regional differentials in the effects of son preference on fertility.[91]

There is clear evidence of boys receiving more favourable treatment in Anhui, Guangdong, and some western provinces. It is reported that in Anhui province 78.5 per cent of boys of school age enrolled in schools, while only 58.7 per cent of girls did so. The figures in Guangdong were 88.1 and 66.4 per cent respectively. In contrast, sex differences in attendance at school were minor in many other provinces.[92]

Traditionally, Anhui has been a province in which the sex ratio has consistently been above the national average. It was reported that its sex ratio for children under the age of 5 was as high as 126.62 in 1934.[93] The areas with a high sex ratio for children were concentrated along the middle and lower Huai River Valley.[94] Female infanticide is closely related to this phenomenon. Although the incidence fell sharply after 1949, female infanticide still occurs, and in some areas very widely. In 1981 the reported sex ratio at birth for Anhui as a whole was 112.45, but higher than 130 in some rural counties. In Quanjiao county, infanticides (most of them, of female babies) accounted for nearly 5 per cent of all births.[95] This cruel practice has been severely criticized by the Chinese government and many measures have been adopted to curb such barbarity.[96]

Apart from Anhui, the sex ratios for infant children in 1981 were 110.69, 110.47, and 110.32 for Guangxi, Guangdong, and Henan respectively. It was reported that the sex ratio at birth exceeded 144 in 9 counties in Hunan province in 1982.[97] In addition, a 1984 survey reveals that the sex ratios for children under the age of 15 in Anhui, Fujian, Shanxi, and Nei Monggol were all above 111, while the national figure was 107.4.[98] Since couples can not influence the sex of their children, the only way they manifest sex preference in their fertility decision is in their choice to have another child,[99] and in their different treatment towards boy and girl. These high sex ratios may result from high mortality for infant girls and clearly indicate the strong son-preference in these provinces. There is also evidence that during the one-child campaign, Guangdong was the first province officially to allow rural couples to have a second child, if their first one was a girl.[100]

It is not surprising that the fertility level in all these provinces was above the national average.

Modern Shanxi[101] provides a good example for examining the relationships between socio-economic conditions, son preference, and reproductive behaviour. Traditionally, women in Shanxi province were rarely involved in economic activities and male-domination and son preference were strongly in evidence in this province. Female infanticide was common. As a result, the sex ratio in modern Shanxi was very high and some men could not get married because of the imbalance in the marriage market. Consequently, marriage tended to take place very early, due in part to fears of failing to find a partner.[102] Early marriage in turn results in early childbearing. Social reform and economic development have brought about changes in Shanxi's marriage customs. Nevertheless, old traditions can not disappear in a very short period, and they remain important factors to take into account. It is likely that some other northwest provinces follow the same pattern.

It has been suggested by Feeney and Yu that eliminating son preference for China as a whole might reduce completed family size by about 9 per cent.[103] It is believed that the effects of eliminating son preference in the provinces mentioned above would be much larger.

Family and Kinship

In addition to feudal influences and the economic rationale already referred to, son preference and fertility level are also associated with structures of the local community and kinship system. In Guangdong province, one of the main reasons for seeking an extra son is to obtain clan superiority in communities.[104] This is less important in Hunan and Anhui,[105] and is not relevant at all in many other provinces.

Mainly owing to diversities in cultural, social, political, ecological, and economic conditions, strong family lineages were traditionally more prevalent in the central and southern parts of China than in the north.[106] Many studies show that some villages in southeastern China, especially in Guangdong and Fujian, are inhabited almost exclusively by the members of one clan. In most places, several clans live side by side, each one occupying a distinct section of the village.[107] By contrast, most of the villages in central and north China are not clan villages.[108] Similarly, higher proportions of extended families are found in the coastal south, the red basin (part of Sichuan province), and some parts of the northern region. By contrast, nuclear families are more prevalent in the southeastern and lower Yangzi river areas.[109]

The Chinese family structure has undergone a profound transformation since the Chinese revolution in 1949. However, it has been often observed by sociologists that changes in family mores tend to lag behind other social changes. In any given society present-day family patterns and values are continuous with the patterns and values of its past.[110] China's regional differences in family systems have by and large remained. Data from the 1982 census show that the proportion of families with three or more generations is commonly high in southern coastal provinces and in loess plateau areas around Shaanxi province. By contrast, families in the eastern and the northeastern provinces are relatively small.[111]

The importance of these primary groups in determining marriage and fertility patterns diminished with the development of a new form of political authority or polity in China. However, they are still active forces, not only competing with political organizations and authorities for control of marriage patterns but also active in the competition between the generations and organizations.[112]

It is easy to understand the difficulties faced by the family-planning personnel when working in an environment which has strong lineal traditions, especially when the working targets are members of their own clan. The obstacle raised by this institutional factor to fertility regulation is insignificant or does not exist at all in the northern provinces, but may be one of the decisive causes of the poor performance of the birth-control campaign in several southern provinces, such as Guangdong and Fujian.

Youngsters in China's rural areas are still to a great extent dependent economically on their parents for marriage expenses, such as dowries and bride wealth. The need to obey their parents' wishes on marriage and childbearing considerably reduces their freedom of choice.[113] Reproductive behaviour of young couples living with their parents is often affected by older generations.[114] In contrast, young couples who make their own decisions more easily and willingly accept and practise fertility limitation. With a few exceptions, there is a very close relationship between the provincial fertility level and the proportion of large families there.[115]

The linkage with overseas Chinese is particularly strong in Guangdong and Fujian provinces. It is estimated that in the 1950s, 68 per cent of about 12 million overseas Chinese were originally from Guangdong, and 25 per cent from Fujian.[116] In 1982 one-quarter of the population in Fujian province had relatives abroad.[117] The availability of large-scale overseas remittances provides the necessary condition for co-residence of large extended family groups.[118] On the whole, the impact of this linkage on the fertility transition is negative. On the one hand, the family-planning programme towards this part of the population was less rigid and they have enjoyed certain privileges in childbearing.[119] On the other hand, their reproductive behaviour was largely determined by their relatives, especially their husbands abroad. The stronger traditional mentality, better economic well-being, and relative lack of exposure to the pressure of birth control made their desire for children much higher than the government's requirement. Consequently, the implementation of family-planning programmes was more difficult, and fertility levels were relatively higher in those regions with a large proportion of overseas relatives.[120]

The impacts of institutional settings on regional fertility differentials are very complicated. Often, several counter-balancing sets of factors work together. Much more work is needed on this subject.

V. Some Tentative Conclusions

In this chapter, we have tried to examine the determinants of China's fertility transition and its regional diversities. Factors touched on in the foregoing sections include the family-planning programme, socio-economic conditions, and institutional changes. It seems clear that much more research should be done in order to formulate a general theory of the determinants of the fertility transition in China. Nevertheless, by way of summary a few tentative conclusions may be drawn.

China's fertility transition seems to provide an exception to the classical theory of demographic transition. Although there has been great improvement in living standards, health care, and education since the 1950s, China has not modernized enough to reach a level at which people might be motivated to limit family size spontaneously. Nevertheless, China has attempted and obviously succeeded in beginning to change public attitudes towards marriage and childbearing, and to bring down population growth.

The effective family-planning programme is undoubtedly one of the main causes of the rapid fertility decline in China. This programme has been endorsed by officials at the highest level of the Chinese leadership, and supervised and managed through all levels of the Communist Party and the government administrative apparatus. The programme matched the political education with social and economic policies; combined the contraceptive delivery system with the well-established health-care network. Mass organizations and local communities were all mobilized to promote birth control and family limitation. There has been societal awareness of the urgency of population control. The Chinese experience suggests that initial fertility transition can occur in a society at a relatively low level of modernization, as long as there is strong government commitment and an effective family-planning programme.

The success of the Chinese family-planning programme owes much to China's unique social structure which was established by the Chinese revolution, but which was also partly a heritage of the Chinese culture. The organizational behaviour of the Chinese people, the mass participation, and effective government control allowed the programme to be carried out relatively more easily.

Since 1949 China has undergone some fundamental social and economic changes. The process of socialization and collectivization has considerably weakened the traditional importance of family and kinship on economic production, child care, education, and all aspects of individual life. Traditional values supporting large families are being eroded. Women have been greatly emancipated and are involved in every activity of socio-political affairs now. Considerable progress has been made in reducing not only infant and maternal but also general mortality. (This is a very important determinant of fertility, but one which it has not been possible to consider in detail owing to the lack of systematic data.) These changes provide a very good environment for the Chinese programme.

The regional differentials in fertility transition are mainly determined by the commitment of the local government to the population issue and socio-economic development of the local community. In carrying out the programme, local government is responsible for providing birth-control services, setting population targets, and formulating family-planning regulations. At the start of the transition, the fertility differentials amongst social strata and localities were the combined products of birth-control diffusion and development factors. As the transition has progressed and birth-control services become easily accessible, the reproductive decision has clearly been determined by social factors other than the availability of birth-control methods. In this stage, the government intervention has played an important role in determining the pattern of the transition.

However, the role of development and culture is more fundamental in long-term fertility transition. China is such a large country that different regional cultural backgrounds have strong impacts on fertility transition. The effect of culture, in general, operates through socio-economic development. However, they may also directly influence reproductive behaviour through sex roles, family structure, and kinship system. The economic development will ultimately change people's attitude towards family and childbearing.

While the government-sponsored family-planning programme has succeeded in changing the fertility behaviour of Chinese women in a very dramatic way for a while, further fertility declines, and the completion of the fertility transition as well, are likely to occur more gradually and in line with socio-economic development. It seems certain that the regional differentials in fertility will exist in the near future, and probably follow some sort of cultural pattern. This deserves more systematic study.

NOTES

1. A. J. Coale, 'The Demographic Transition', in *Proceedings of the International Population Conference 1973* (Liege: IUSSP, 1973), 53–72.
2. R. Freedman, 'Fertility Determinants', in J. Cleland and C. Scott (eds.), *The World Fertility Survey: An Assessment* (London: Oxford University Press, 1987), 773–95.
3. Ibid.
4. W. P. Mauldin, 'Population Trends and Prospects', *Science*, 209 (1980), 148–58; also id., 'The Determinants of Fertility Decline in Developing Countries: An Overview of the Available Empirical Evidence', *International Family Planning Perspectives*, 8 (1982), 119–27.
5. W. P. Handwerker, 'Culture and Reproduction: Exploring Micro/Macro Linkages', in W. P. Handwerker (ed.), *Culture and Reproduction: An Anthropological Critique of Demographic Transition Theory* (Boulder: Westview Press, A Westview Special Study, 1986), 1–29.
6. In Xizhang (Tibet) Autonomous Region, Tibet nationalities account for about 95% of the total population. We leave out Xizhang from our general analysis because relevant demographic data are not available to the author.
7. Zhang Zeyu, 'Population Policy for Minorities', *Beijing Review*, 29 (48), 15–18 (1 Dec. 1986).
8. J. Banister, *China's Changing Population* (Stanford, Calif.: Stanford University Press, 1987), 195.
9. Wu Cangping, 'Family Planning Meets Social Progress', *Beijing Review*, 28 (45), 15–17 (11 Nov. 1985).
10. *Beijing Review*, 28 (40), 7–8 (7 Oct. 1985).
11. Banister, *China's Changing Population*, p. 216.
12. See *Beijing Review*, 29 (22), 18–26 (2 June 1986).
13. Ho Ping-ti, *Studies on the Population of China, 1368–1953* (Cambridge, Mass: Harvard University Press, 1959).
14. C. Pannell and Laurence Ma, *China: The Geography of Development and Modernization* (London: Edward Arnold, 1983), 109.
15. Song Jian, 'Population Development—Goals and Plans', in Liu Zheng *et al.*, *China's Population: Problems & Prospects* (Beijing: New World Press, 1981), 25–31.

16. H. Gille, 'Policy Implications', in J. Cleland and J. Hobcraft (eds.), *Reproductive Change in Developing Countries* (Oxford: Oxford University Press, 1985), 273–95.
17. Wu Cangping, 'Theoretical Explanations of China's Rapid Fertility Decline', *Population Research*, No. 1 (1986) (in Chinese).
18. J. Kaufman, *A Billion and Counting: Family Planning Campaigns and Policies in the People's Republic of China* (San Francisco: San Francisco Press, 1983), 36.
19. Chen Pi-Chao, 'Birth Control Methods and Organization in China', in E. Croll *et al.* (eds.), *China's One-Child Family Policy* (London: Macmillan, 1985), 135–48.
20. Peng Xizhe, 'China's Regional Fertility Differences and Related Socioeconomic Factors', M.Sc. diss. (London School of Economics, 1984).
21. I. Alam and J. B. Casterline, 'Socio-Economic Differentials in Recent Fertility', *WFS Comparative Studies*, No. 33 (1984).
22. J. Bongaarts, 'A Framework for Analysing the Proximate Determinant of Fertility', *Population and Development Review*, 4 (1), 105–32 (1978); J. Hobcraft and R. Little, 'Fertility Exposure Analysis: A New Method for Assessing the Contribution of Proximate Determinants to Fertility Differentials', *Population Studies*, 38 (1), 21–45 (1984).
23. This is a result of the tabulation process. It is possible now to use original tape of the survey with approval of Chinese authorities.
24. Technical details of the procedure can be found in *WFS Technical Bulletins*, No.5/ Tech. 834, Oct. 1978.
25. Ibid. 16.
26. See e.g. J. C. Caldwell, *Theory of Fertility Decline* (London: Academic Press, 1982), 301.
27. *WFS Technical Bulletins*, No. 5, p. 4.
28. The chi-squared values for all but the 50+ model, with the main effects of three variables, are not significant at the 5% level, which indicates satisfactory fits. See *WFS Technical Bulletins*, No. 5, p. 36. Details of models can be found in the Appendix of this book.
29. See e.g. S. H. Cochrane, 'Effects of Education and Urbanization on Fertility', in R. A. Bulatao and R. D. Lee (eds.), *Determinants of Fertility in Developing Countries* (New York: Academic Press, 1983), ii. 609.
30. United Nations Department of International Economic and Social Affairs, *Relationships between Fertility and Education: A Comparative Analysis of World Fertility Survey Data for Twenty-two Developing Countries*, ST/ESA/SER.R/48.
31. Roughly speaking, 'Worker' mainly includes those working in a factory, shop, or other service involving physical labour; 'Cadre' refers to government employees, such as officials, teachers, doctors, managers, etc.; 'Housewife' refers to women with no formal work outside the home.
32. For details of the models see the Appendix.
33. e.g. Cochrane (1983); Caldwell (1982).
34. R. Andorka, *Determinants of Fertility in Advanced Society* (London: Methuen, 1978), 259.
35. State Statistical Bureau of PRC, *10 Percent Sampling Tabulation of the 1982 Population Census of the PRC* (Beijing, 1983), 380–91, 444–5.
36. e.g. Tian Xueyuan, *Xinshiqi renkoulun (Population Theory in the New Era)* (Haerbin: Heilongjiang People's Press, 1982), 31–2.
37. J. S. Aird, 'Fertility Decline in China', in Nick Eberstadt (ed.), *Fertility Decline in the Less Developed Countries* (New York: Praeger, 1981), 119–227.
38. Ibid.

39. D. Davis-Friedmann, 'Old Age Security and One-Child Campaign', in Croll *et al.*, (eds.) *China's One-Child Family Policy*, pp. 149–61.
40. I. W. Mabbett, *Modern China: The Mirage of Modernity* (New York: St. Martin's Press, 1985).
41. e.g. T. P. Schultz, *Economics of Population* (Reading, Mass.: Addison-Wesley, 1982).
42. See e.g. Chen Muhua, 'To Realize the Four Modernizations it is Necessary to Control Population Growth', in *People's Daily*, 11 Aug. 1979; Tian Xueyuan, 'A Survey of Population Growth since 1949', in Liu Zheng *et al.*, *China's Population: Problems & Prospects* (Beijing: New World Press, 1981), 32–54.
43. For decades the government policy stressed universal employment, but low and equal wages. See Xue Muqiao, 'Guanyu gongzi wenti de tanhua (Talk on the Problem of Wage)', *Woguo dangqian de jingji wenti (Current Economic Problems in our Country)* (Beijing: People's Press, 1980), 122–38.
44. China Population Information Centre, *Handbook of Chinese Population Information, 1985* (Beijing, 1985), 384.
45. Author's personal experience.
46. *Handbook of Chinese Population Information, 1985*, p. 97.
47. J. B. Nugent, 'The Old-Age Security Motive for having Children', *Population and Development Review*, 11 (1), 75–98 (1985).
48. Cheng Du, 'Hubei sheng nongcun shengyuli diaocha (Fertility Survey in the Rural Areas of Hubei Province)', *Renkou Yanjiu (Population Research)*, No. 5 (1982).
49. *Beijing Review*, 26 (28), 1983.
50. In 1984, 660,000 rural old people were provided with pensions, another 240,000 were living in Jin Lao Yuan (Old People's Home). See Zhu Chuanyi, 'It is an Urgent Task to Establish a Social-Security System for the Rural Elders', *Laonian wenti Yanjiu Ziliao (Research Information on Problem of Ageing)*, No. 54 (Nov. 1985).
51. 'China's Marriage Law', *Beijing Review*, 24 (11), 24–7 (16 Mar. 1981).
52. Davis-Friedmann, 'Old Age Security and the One-Child Campaign', cited in n. 39, above.
53. 'Peasants Enjoy Pensions', *Beijing Review*, 25 (40), 8 (4 Oct. 1982).
54. e.g. Yang Jishun, 'Laoyou suoyang zai nongcun jihua shengyu gongzuo zhong de diwei he zuoyong (The Importance of Old-Age Security on Rural Family-Planning Works)', *Shandong Renkou (Shandong Population)*, No. 3 (1983).
55. e.g. Liu Junzhe, 'The Impact of Old Age Security on Family Planning', in *Xibei Renkou (Northwest Population),* No. 1 (1984).
56. Caldwell, *Theory of Fertility Decline*, cited in n. 26, above.
57. J. Banister and S. H. Preston, 'Mortality in China', *Population and Development Review*, 7 (1), 98–110 (1981).
58. Wu Cangping, 'Theoretical Explanations', cited in n. 17 above.
59. Banister and Preston, 'Mortality in China'.
60. Wu Cangping, 'Theoretical Explanations'.
61. P. Kane, *The Second Billion: Population and Family Planning in China* (London: Penguin Books, 1987), 173.
62. Su Wenming (ed.), *Population and Other Problems* (Beijing: *Beijing Review* Special Feature Series, 1981), 35–57.
63. *Beijing Review*, No. 48, 1979.
64. See Editorial Committee, *Zhongguo baike nianjian (Encyclopaedia of China) 1981* (Beijing: Encyclopaedia Publish House, 1981), 540–1.

65. State Statistical Bureau of PRC, *China Urban Statistics, 1985* (London: Longman, 1985), 456.
66. In a survey carried out at Luwan district in Shanghai in 1981, about one-third of all newly married couples could not live together owing to the shortage of accommodation.
67. The 1982 census shows that in Shanghai about 21% of families have three or more generations living together, which made Shanghai among the highest third nationally. *10 Percent Sampling Tabulation of the 1982 Population Census of the PRC.*
68. *Beijing Review*, 27 (42), 27–8 (15 Oct. 1984).
69. This refers to women who are employed to work for a wage in institutions outside their home. As argued by Ware, almost all women work, irrespective of the proportion of women who are included in the official definition of the labour force. See H. Ware, *Women, Demography and Development* (Canberra: The Australian National University Press, 1981).
70. *Statistical Yearbook of China, 1983*, p. 145.
71. See e.g. S. Kupinsky, *The Fertility of Working Women* (New York: Praeger, 1977).
72. J. C. Robinson, 'Of Women and Washing Machines: Employment, Housework, and the Reproduction of Motherhood in Socialist China', *The China Quarterly*, No. 101 (Mar. 1985), 32–57.
73. See 'Nuzhigong shijian fenpei zhuangkuang qianxi (Primary Analysis of Female Worker's Time Arrangement', *Zhongguo Funu (Women of China)*, No. 8 (1987); *Xinhua*, 21 May 1983; E. J. Croll, 'The Chinese Household and its Economy: Urban and Rural Survey Data', *Contemporary China Centre Resource Paper* (Oxford: Queen Elizabeth House, 1980).
74. Qiao Xinjian, 'Possible Obstacles to the Realisation of the One-Child Family', extended essay, David Owen Centre for Population Growth Studies, July 1982.
75. J. Cleland and C. Wilson, 'Demand Theories of the Fertility Transition: An Iconoclastic View', *Population Studies*, 41 (1), 5–30 (1986).
76. See e.g. Tien H. Yuan, 'Induced Fertility Transition: Impact of Population Planning and Socio-Economic Change in the People's Republic of China', *Population Studies*, 38 (3), 385–400 (1984); Peng Xizhe, M.Sc. Dissertation, 1984; D. L. Poston and Baochang Gu, 'Socioeconomic Development, Family Planning, and Fertility in China', *Demography*, 24 (4), 531–51 (1987).
77. T. Dyson and M. Murphy, 'The Onset of Fertility Transition', *Population and Development Review*, 11 (3), 399–440 (1985).
78. Poston and Boachang Gu, 'Socioeconomic Development'.
79. See N. Birdsall and D. T. Jamison, 'Income and Other Factors Influencing Fertility in China', *Population and Development Review*, 9 (4), 651–75 (1983); Poston and Baochang Gu, 'Socioeconomic Development'; Tien H. Yuan, 'Induced Fertility Transition'.
80. J. Bongaarts and S. Greenhalgh, 'An Alternative to the One-Child Policy in China', *Population and Development Review*, 11 (4), 585–618 (1985).
81. Dyson and Murphy, 'Onset of Fertility Transition', p. 431.
82. Tien H. Yuan, 'Provincial Fertility Trends and Patterns', in E. Croll *et al.* (eds.), *China's One-Child Family Policy*.
83. e.g. the per capita net income for Guangdong's peasants is 193 Yuan in 1978 and 396 in 1983. The figures are 111 and 299 yuan for Guangdong's north neighbouring province Hubei, 143 and 316 for Hunan. Source is as cited in Table 3.5
84. G. McNicoll, 'Institutional Determinants of Fertility Change', in C. Hohn and

R. Mackensen, *Determinants of Fertility Trends: Theories Re-examined* (Liege: Ordina Editions, 1982), 147–69.
85. W. L. Parish and M. K. Whyte, *Village and Family in Contemporary China* (London: University of Chicago Press, 1978), 199.
86. L. Moser, *The Chinese Mosaic: The Peoples and Provinces of China* (Boulder: Westview Press, 1985).
87. A. J. Coale and S. C. Watkins (eds.), *The Decline of Fertility in Europe* (Princeton, NJ: Princeton University Press, 1986).
88. G. McNicoll, 'The Nature of Institutional and Community Effects on Demographic Behaviour: A Discussion', in J. Casterline (ed.), *The Collection and Analysis of Community Data* (Voorbury, Netherlands: International Statistical Institute, 1985), 177–84.
89. R. Repetto, 'Son Preference and Fertility Behaviour in Developing Countries', *Studies in Family Planning*, 3 (4), 70–6 (1972).
90. F. Arnold and Liu Zhaoxiang, 'Sex Preference, Fertility, and Family Planning in China', *Population and Development Review*, 12 (2), 221–46 (1986).
91. Arnold and Liu did provide a regional pattern of the extent of son preference. However, their results should be interpreted with great caution because of the regional differences in family-planning achievements.
92. China Population Information Centre, *Handbook of Chinese Population Information, 1985* (Beijing, 1985), 378–94.
93. Hu Huanyong and Zhang Shanyu, *Zhongguo renkou dili (Population Geography of China)* (Shanghai: Eastern Normal University Press, 1986), 140.
94. Cheng Fenggao, 'Anhui renkou xianzhuang de chubu fenxi (Preliminary Analysis of Current Situation of Anhui's Population)', in *Renkou (Population)*, No. 1 (1985).
95. Zhang Wansong *et al.*, 'Nongcun yinger xingbili shitiao yao yinqi gaodu zhongshi (Attention Should be Paid to Unbalance of Infant Sex Ratio in the Countryside)', *Anhui Renkou (Anhui Population)*, No. 1 (1983).
96. *Beijing Review*, 26 (5), Jan. 1983.
97. Deng Yan, 'Dui wosheng renkou xingbiebi de fenxi (On the Sex Ratio of our Province)', *Renkou Tansuo (Exploration on Population)*, Supplementary Issue (1984).
98. *Handbook of Chinese Population Information, 1985*, pp. 378–94.
99. Arnold and Liu, 'Sex Preference', cited in n. 90, above.
100. *Jihuashengyu tongxun (Newsletter of Family-Planning Work)*, No. 1 (1985), 43; *Handbook of Chinese Population Information, 1985*, p. 38.
101. Refers to the early 20th century.
102. See Xing Long, 'Shanxi jindai renkou gao xingbili jiqi Houguo (High Sex Ratio and its Consequences in Modern Shanxi Province)', *Renkou Yanjiu (Population Research)*, No. 5 (1986).
103. G. Feeney and Yu Jingyuan, 'The Effect of Son Preference on Fertility in China', paper presented at the 1986 annual meetings of the Population Association of America, San Francisco, Apr. 1986.
104. Office of Population Census of Guangdong Province, *Guangdong renkou zhuangkuang fenxi yu yuce (Analysis and Projection of Population Situation in Guangdong Province)* (Guangzhou: Zhongshan University Press, 1985).
105. Yang Xiuyu, 'Yingxiang nongcun zhisheng yitai de yinsu fenxi (Factors Affecting Single-Child Policy in the Rural Areas)', *Renkou Tansuo (Exploration on Population)*, Supplementary Issue (1984); Cheng Fenggao, op. cit., in n. 94 above.

106. J. M. Potter, 'Land and Lineage in Traditional China' in M. Freedman (ed.), *Family and Kinship in Chinese Society* (Stanford, Calif. Stanford University Press, 1970), 121–38.
107. See e.g. M. Freedman, *Lineage Organization in Southeastern China* (London School of Economics Monographs on Social Anthropology, No. 18; London: Athlone, 1970).
108. O. Lang, *Chinese Family and Society* (New York: Archon Books, 1968).
109. I. Taeuber, 'The Families of Chinese Farmers', in Freedman (ed.), *Family and Kinship in Chinese Society*, pp. 63–85.
110. F. R. Elliot, *The Family: Change or Continuity?* (London: Macmillan Education, 1986).
111. See State Statistical Bureau, *10 Percent Sampling Tabulation of the 1982 Population Census of the PRC* (Beijing, 1983), 401.
112. E. Croll, 'A Conflict for Control of Marriage Patterns: Primary Groups versus Political Organizations', in S. L. Greenblatt *et al.* (eds.), *Organizational Behavior in Chinese Society* (New York: Praeger Publishers, 1981), 231–55.
113. A survey conducted in 10 rural communes of Anhui province showed that out of 1,952 marriages that took place in 1979–82, only 61 (less than 13%) were marriages of free choice, because of the economic dependency. See *Shehui Kexue (Social Sciences)*, No. 1 (1984).
114. Five Cities Family Research Project Group, *Zhongguo chengshi jiating—wuchengshi jiating diaocha ziliao huibian (Family in China's Urban Areas: Collection of Data and Reports on a Family Survey in 5 Cities)* (Jinan: Shandong People's Press, 1985).
115. The correlation coefficient for the total fertility rate and the proportion of families with three or more generations in 1981 is 0.726 for 24 provinces. Shanghai, Guangxi, Ningxia, and Xinjiang are excluded from the comparison by virtue of their special status.
116. Hu Huanyong and Zhang Shanyu, *Population Geography of China*, p. 342.
117. Yie Wenzhen, 'Silun qiaoqu dui renkou kongzhi de libi (On the Advantage and Disadvantage of Population Control in Areas Where a Large Proportion of Families have Overseas Relatives)', *Fujian Renkou (Fujian Population)*, 1983.
118. E. S. H. Yu, 'Overseas Remittances in South-Eastern China', *The China Quarterly*, No. 78 (June 1979), 339–50.
119. For instance, the second child is commonly allowed for those couples where both or one spouse is an overseas Chinese in almost all provinces in the 1980s.
120. Yie Wenzhen, op. cit., in n. 117, above.

4

National Trends in Fertility and Nuptiality

FROM this chapter, our focus turns to a detailed demographic analysis of China's fertility transition. China's rapid fertility change at the national level has been widely studied by demographers both in and out of China.[1] However, this does not mean that the subject has been exhausted. The main aim of this study is to analyse the provincial patterns. However, it is advantageous to begin with an analysis of national trends in fertility and nuptiality, in order to provide a general picture for the past several decades. This also serves as an important reference point for understanding fertility transition at the provincial level.

I. General Fertility Trends

Estimates of the Total Fertility Rate

Age-specific and total fertility rates are derived from data collected in China's 1982 One-Per-Thousand Fertility Survey. The upper-age limit of the survey was set at 67, which means that women aged 67 at the time of survey were 25 years old in 1940, 35 in 1950, and so forth. As a result, the information required for direct calculation of complete sets of age-specific fertility rates are only available from 1964 onward. For the period prior to 1964, we only have truncated fertility rates for younger ages. These incomplete sets of fertility rates are valuable and can be examined extensively by using analytical techniques developed by the World Fertility Survey.[2] Nevertheless, since the total fertility rate is one of the best summary measures for the description of fertility trends, it is worthwhile to fill in the missing age-specific fertility rates prior to 1964 and complete the sequences of the total fertility rates in the 1950s, at least at the national level.

Several efforts have been made. A curve-extrapolation method was employed by Chinese demographers on the basis of normal relations between two sets of age-specific fertility rates of different years.[3] This approach provides a complete set of age-specific fertility rates by single years of age from 15 to 49 over the period 1940 to 1979. However, those estimated rates prior to 1964 were subject to the risk of distortion by single-year fluctuation, either from sampling error or real variation.

More recently, Coale and Chen reconstructed total fertility rates by age, and total marital fertility rates by duration, for the whole period between 1945 and 1981. They estimated the total fertility rate for 1945–63 from duration-specific fertility rates (recorded and estimated) and total first-marriage rates.[4] Yearly and single-age fluctuations were smoothed. The basic assumptions of the above two mentioned methods are similar. But the total fertility rates estimated by Coale and Chen are lower in the early years and higher in the later years, compared with the estimates made by Chinese demographers. Coale and Chen's approach seems to underestimate slightly the fertility rates before 1964.[5] On the other hand, the Chinese estimates are closer to the real situation.

In this chapter, estimates of TFR between 1949 and 1963 given by Chinese demographers are accepted with caution of single-year fluctuation. Rates from 1964 onward are derived directly from the survey.

National Trend

Table 4.1 and the accompanying graphs in Figure 4.1 contain the total fertility rates over the past 34 years from 1949 to 1982 for China as a whole and for the rural and urban population separately.

The fertility level before the founding of the People's Republic is not so clear. However, a TFR of around 5.4 was estimated for the 1940s using China's 1982 Fertility Survey data. This is close to that estimated by George Barclay and others for the Chinese rural population in the 1930s.[6] In the mid-1950s China's national total fertility rate (TFR) was around 6 and remained so until the end of the 1960s. Since the early 1970s, fertility transition has accelerated. The national TFR declined from 5.8 in 1970 to 3.6 in 1975, and further to 2.31 in 1980. In other words, China's fertility decreased by more than 50 per cent in only one decade. In 1985 the TFR was reported by a national sample survey on population change to be 1.996.[7] More recently, China's fertility rose slightly, but remains at a low level.

Before proceeding to more detailed analysis, let us first divide China's fertility transition into periods or stages according to the level of the TFR. The criteria for such divisions may be subjective, but the dates when marked fertility changes occurred are informative, especially

TABLE 4.1. *China's total fertility rates, 1949–1982*

Year	Nation	Urban	Rural	Year	Nation	Urban	Rural
1950	5.81	5.00	5.96	1967	5.31	2.91	5.85
1951	5.70	4.72	5.90	1968	6.45	3.87	7.03
1952	6.47	5.52	6.67	1969	5.72	3.30	6.26
1953	6.05	5.40	6.18	1970	5.81	3.27	6.38
1954	6.28	5.72	6.39	1971	5.44	2.88	6.01
1955	6.26	5.67	6.39	1972	4.98	2.64	5.50
1956	5.85	5.33	5.97	1973	4.54	2.39	5.01
1957	6.40	5.94	6.50	1974	4.17	1.98	4.64
1958	5.68	5.25	5.77	1975	3.57	1.78	3.95
1959	4.30	4.17	4.32	1976	3.24	1.61	3.58
1960	4.02	4.06	4.00	1977	2.84	1.57	3.12
1961	3.29	2.98	3.35	1978	2.72	1.55	2.97
1962	6.02	4.79	6.30	1979	2.75	1.37	3.05
1963	7.50	6.21	7.78	1980	2.32	1.20	2.56
1964	6.18	4.40	6.57	1981	2.71	1.47	2.99
1965	6.08	3.75	6.60	1982	2.62	1.50	2.86
1966	6.26	3.10	6.96				

Note: Data prior to 1964 from *Population and Economy* (Special issue), 1983.

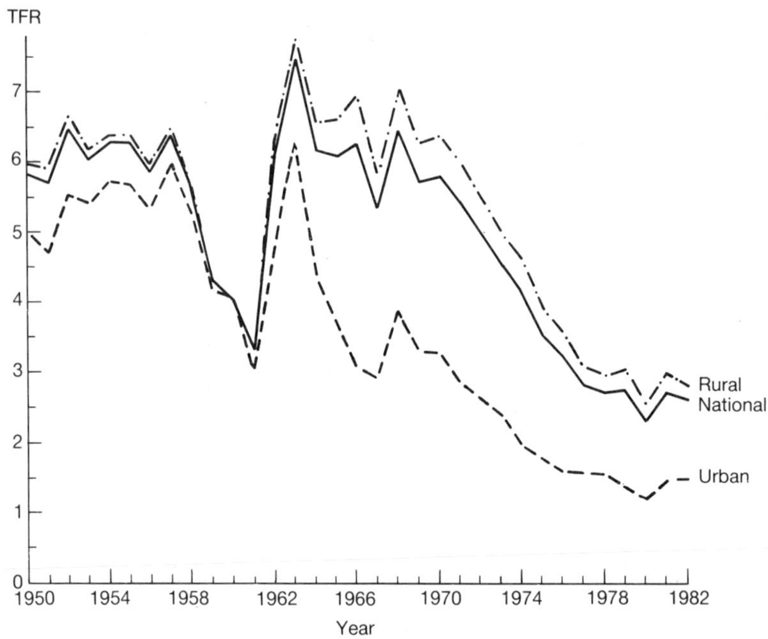

Fig. 4.1 Total fertility rates, China 1950–1982

when linked to other socio-economic factors and the efforts of the Chinese government to control population growth. Here, the emphasis is mainly on the fertility change since the founding of the People's Republic of China in 1949, the fertility situation before that year being excluded as being largely unrepresented by the survey.

China's fertility transition took place in roughly five stages.

First period: 1949–1957. China's fertility level during this period rose steadily to reach a peak in 1957. The total fertility rates maintained a fairly high level at around 6, with small fluctuations. Peaceful social conditions, better health care, and the modernization process are the major factors responsible for this early fertility increase.[8] Birth control was discussed at certain times, but no effective family-planning policy was implemented. Such an increase can also be attributed to several other policy factors, among which the blind following of the development strategy of the Soviet Union was important.[9] In fact, the government policy at this time was a pronatalist one. Bearing more children was even encouraged by the government and prolific mothers were widely honoured. The fertility level in this period can be viewed as the natural fertility level in China.

Second period: 1958–1963. This period was characterized by massive fertility fluctuations. In early 1958 the Great Leap Forward was launched by the Chinese leadership. The general line which guided the Leap was 'Going all out, aiming high and achieving greater, faster, better, and more economical results in building socialism'.[10] The entire country was mobilized to take part in the campaign for steel and iron, and the communization movement. The Great Leap Forward soon led to disaster and precipitated a nation-wide famine between 1959 and 1961. As a consequence, fertility dropped dramatically in 1959 and reached a trough in 1961. Thereafter, as the situation improved, the TFR rose to a peak value of 7.5 in 1963, the highest since 1949. On the whole, the net fertility deficit, which refers to total births lost during this period after taking fertility compensation into account, amounted to about one normal year's total births.[11]

Third period: 1964–1970. After the massive fluctuations of the previous period, the TFR returned to a relatively stable level. Although there were some variations associated with the Cultural Revolution, the average value of national TFR in this period was as high as that in the 1950s. Alarmed by the great famine and huge fertility compensation, the Chinese government started to carry out a birth-control programme in the early 1960s. This early programme focused on the urban population and no compulsory measures were adopted.

The response to the programme was very impressive and urban fertility experienced a sharp reduction in a few years. On the whole, fertility transition started in some large municipalities and some provinces located on the east coast, whereas the fertility in the rest of China remained very high till the early 1970s.

Fourth period: 1971–1979. This period is well-known for its marked fertility decline. The TFR reduced from 5.812 in 1970 to a very low value of 2.7 in the late 1970s, a decline of almost 60 per cent within ten years. Factors that brought about this substantial decline have been discussed in the earlier chapters. Simply speaking, it is generally agreed that the reduction was largely due to the success of China's family-planning programme. The nation-wide programme, known as 'Wan, Xi, Shao' (later marriage, longer birth intervals, and fewer children), went into effect in 1971. Contraceptive devices were for the first time widely available to everyone. A well-organized birth-control network played an especially important role in reducing fertility.

Fifth period: 1979–now. During this period, a more strict birth-control programme—single-child policy—has been implemented. More recently, there have been some modifications of the policy, especially at the local level. But the basic principle remains. The population target has been set at 1.2 billion by the year 2000. The population policy in this period has been very vigorous. However, it is of interest that the TFR shows a slight increase, although it is still well below half of the 1970 level. The estimated total fertility rates are 2.29 and 2.64 for 1986 and 1987 respectively.[12] The major factors responsible for such increase are a large marriage boom and relaxation of birth-control efforts, which is partly the by-product of the country's economic reform.[13]

Rural–Urban Difference

The fertility trend for rural population is virtually identical to that at the national level, as can be seen from Figure 4.1. This is unsurprising, since the majority of Chinese population live in the rural areas.

The urban fertility trends show some differences, though the broad trends are similar. Generally speaking, the urban TFRs were always lower than rural ones.

In the first period, the urban fertility level was as high as rural fertility with only minor differences. The high urban fertility level was certainly affected by rapid urban expansion in this period, as the overwhelming majority of the new immigrants to the cities were young adults who comprised the most fertile age group of the total female population.

In the second period, both the urban and rural fertility experienced major fluctuations. The urban TFR began to decline in 1959 and approached a trough in 1961, before recovering. This is a pattern similar to the rural one and indicates that both the rural and urban populations were affected by the Great Leap Forward and natural calamities at that time. However, the magnitude of this urban fluctuation was much smaller than the rural one. The rural–urban difference in TFR during this period was very small in 1960 and increased to a substantial 1.3 times in 1963. In addition, the timing of this fertility disturbance differed between rural and urban areas. It seems likely that the urban population suffered relatively less in the early period of the disturbance, but the rural population recovered much earlier and more rapidly.

The third period is very important for the analysis of fertility differentials. After the recovery from the massive fertility deficit, sustained fertility decline occurred in the urban areas, while the rural fertility remained at a high level until 1971. By 1965 the urban TFR was already roughly 40 per cent lower than that of the mid-1950s. By contrast, the rural TFR was even higher than that of a decade earlier. As a result, the absolute difference in TFR between urban and rural population grew from 0.04 in 1957 to 3.11 in 1970. In other words, urban TFR in 1970 was only about half of the corresponding rural figure. This is obviously associated with the early and better implementation of family-planning programmes in urban areas.

The urban fertility trend since the early 1970s has been similar to the rural one. During the 1970s the urban TFR declined by 58 per cent, from 3.267 in 1970 to 1.373 in 1979. Meanwhile, the rural TFR dropped from 6.371 in 1970 to 3.045 in 1979, a 52 per cent reduction. In 1970 the rural TFR was 1.95 times the urban TFR. The rural–urban difference increased to 2.23:1 in 1979. In the early 1980s TFR in both the urban and rural sectors experienced some increase.

Ethnic Difference

China is a multi-ethnic country: there are fifty-six different ethnic groups. Apart from the majority Han nationality which constitutes roughly 93 per cent of China's total population, the other fifty-five minorities with a total population of 67 million account for 7 per cent of the national total. The national identities of these minorities have been encouraged by the government and remain strong. 'Equality, unity, and mutual assistance' is the constitutional guideline for the relationship between China's races.[14] In the face of the great variety in life-style, religious practice, culture, custom, socio-economic development, etc. between ethnic groups, central policies implemented in the predominant Han areas were sometimes not enforced on minority populations, as was the case with birth control. Consequently, paces of fertility transition vary widely between ethnic populations.

In Table 4.2 ethnic differences in terms of the total fertility rate for the period 1964–81 are presented. For the sake of clarity, all fifty-five minority groups are combined in comparison with the Han population. Several points can be drawn from the table.

First, both Han and minority populations experienced fertility reduction, but the decline for the Han population was much sharper. During this 18-year period, the total fertility rate for the Han population dropped by more than 58 per cent, in contrast to 33 per cent for the minorities. As the transition progressed, the gap between Han and other minority populations became bigger than ever before, as can be seen from trends of those ratios in Table 4.2.

TABLE 4.2. *Ethnic differences in total fertility rate, 1964–1981*

Year	Total			Urban			Rural		
	Han	Minority	Ratio[a]	Han	Minority	Ratio[a]	Han	Minority	Ratio[a]
1964	6.031	6.717	1.11	4.404	3.989	0.91	6.412	6.876	1.07
1965	5.931	6.713	1.13	3.766	3.845	1.02	6.447	6.886	1.07
1966	6.111	6.988	1.14	3.098	2.472	0.80	6.826	7.243	1.06
1967	5.172	6.004	1.16	2.927	3.061	1.05	5.705	6.192	1.09
1968	6.281	7.024	1.12	3.834	3.178	0.83	6.861	7.246	1.06
1969	5.569	6.577	1.18	3.321	3.407	1.03	6.101	6.769	1.11
1970	5.649	6.491	1.15	3.268	2.929	0.90	6.219	6.708	1.08
1971	5.287	6.013	1.14	2.836	3.036	1.07	5.864	6.198	1.06
1972	4.782	5.854	1.22	2.575	2.938	1.14	5.296	6.042	1.14
1973	4.338	5.893	1.36	2.374	1.813	0.76	4.795	6.161	1.28
1974	3.936	6.012	1.52	1.924	2.466	1.28	4.392	6.249	1.42
1975	3.356	5.517	1.64	1.731	1.935	1.12	3.722	5.754	1.55
1976	3.030	5.138	1.69	1.565	1.677	1.07	3.356	5.371	1.60
1977	2.667	4.458	1.67	1.522	1.613	1.06	2.926	4.650	1.59
1978	2.575	4.148	1.61	1.519	1.520	1.00	2.818	4.326	1.54
1979	2.598	4.490	1.73	1.327	1.815	1.37	2.891	4.675	1.62
1980	2.121	4.007	1.89	1.118	1.656	1.48	2.358	4.164	1.77
1981	2.521	4.492	1.78	1.379	1.484	1.07	2.796	4.699	1.68
MEAN			1.40			1.05			1.32
ST.D.			0.28			0.19			0.27

[a] Ratio = $TFR_{Minority}/TFR_{Han}$

Secondly, while the ethnic differences in fertility for the rural are very close to those for the total population, the trend for the urban population is quite different. It can be seen that despite some fluctuations, the minority population living in the urban areas follow the same pattern of fertility decline as the Han population. This seems to suggest that the process of national integration in urban China is much faster than in rural areas. Although couples with minority status living in cities and towns enjoy some privileges in terms of childbearing, the fertility difference is minor. Minority population living in the urban areas are, in general, those with relatively high education, better occupational choice, and a high standard of living compared with those in the rural areas. They may also have better access to family-planning services. Therefore, development factors and a stronger birth-control programme overtake the ethnic identity and lead to similar fertility levels for the urban Han and minority populations.

To summarize, China's fertility experience since 1949 can be classified into five periods. The massive fertility fluctuation, which was caused mainly by the Great Leap and famine, was abnormal. Except for that, the TFR for the rural population stayed at a level of about 6 until the end of the 1960s. Since then rapid and sustained fertility decline has occurred. In urban areas, fertility declined much earlier, beginning immediately after the recovery from the famine. Because of this difference in timing in fertility transition, the rural–urban difference widened over time. While the urban residents, no matter what nationality they are, share the same fertility trend, the rural Han population experiences much faster transition than their minority counterparts.

II. General Nuptiality Trend

Nuptiality is an important determinant of fertility levels and trends. Marriage patterns, especially the age at marriage and the prevalence of marriage, are directly relevant to the study of fertility.[15]

Universality and Stability of Marriage

Marriage patterns are closely related to the diversities of socio-economic development, religion, and cultural traditions. Over the last several decades, a profound change in marriage pattern has occurred in China. Shortly after the founding of the People's Republic, a new marriage law was promulgated, which affected every aspect of Chinese marriage.[16] The importance of marriage control on population growth was soon realized and has been regarded as one of the major effective measures for family planning. However, there are several features, such as universality and stability of marriage continually present over time.

Universality is one of the major characteristics of the Chinese marriage pattern. In traditional Chinese society, particularly in the rural areas, the family and kinship circle were the most important units of organization to serve the individual's social and economic needs.[17] Since marriage was the first step in the creation of a family, it was regarded as one of the critical means to perpetuate the family lineage and to make the family the centre of loyalty. In addition to these tasks, marriage also provided protection and security to the family unit. Therefore, to get married was not only a matter of personal interest, but also a duty of the young to their families and to society.

Marriage for family lineage and loyalty is feudalistic in ideology and has been widely criticized since the founding of the People's Republic of China. Marriage was redefined and regarded as a measure for founding a new society resting on socialist principles. The marriage system was reformed to match socio-economic development.[18] However, getting married upon reaching a certain age is still accepted by the society as a moral obligation. The Chinese folk saying is that 'when a man (or girl) is old enough he (she) should get married' (Nanda danghun, nuda dangjia). Remaining unmarried by certain ages, say the late 20s, is still seen by the general public as abnormal. Spinsters and bachelors have never been encouraged by Chinese tradition. Public opinion and social pressure worked together to push youngsters into getting married. The recent trend in the increasing number of unmarried youngsters in their late 20s and over has been regarded by the Chinese masses as a social problem and a source of social unrest. Local agencies have been established by mass organizations (e.g. Women's Federation and Youth League) to provide information and opportunities to those in need. Every effort has been made to help these people to cope with the difficulty of finding suitable mates and eventually to get married.[19]

Although the occurrence of women remaining unmarried at the end of their childbearing ages, especially in urban areas and among professional women, has increased recently, virtually universal marriage persists. The proportion of women remaining single for every year of age has been estimated, using the 1982 survey data. The results are presented in Table 4.3 for China as a whole, and for the rural and urban population separately. Figures for women aged 50 and over are combined.

TABLE 4.3. *Proportion of women never married, China 1982* (%)

Age	Proportion			Age	Proportion		
	Nation	Urban	Rural		Nation	Urban	Rural
15	99.80	100.00	99.78	33	0.52	2.19	0.21
16	99.16	100.00	99.05	34	0.54	2.05	0.26
17	97.57	99.75	97.24	35	0.41	1.44	0.23
18	93.99	99.61	92.90	36	0.27	0.49	0.23
19	87.94	98.36	85.90	37	0.18	0.63	0.10
20	73.94	94.68	70.19	38	0.27	0.67	0.20
21	61.60	87.31	54.10	39	0.23	0.38	0.21
22	49.29	79.25	40.70	40	0.28	0.45	0.25
23	33.19	65.24	25.08	41	0.18	0.00	0.22
24	20.71	49.18	14.27	42	0.21	0.11	0.23
25	12.12	32.81	7.60	43	0.16	0.10	0.17
26	7.31	23.34	3.61	44	0.09	0.22	0.06
27	3.99	13.69	1.92	45	0.15	0.11	0.16
28	2.15	8.53	0.86	46	0.21	0.19	0.21
29	1.55	6.72	0.57	47	0.20	0.00	0.26
30	1.21	4.96	0.52	48	0.09	0.21	0.05
31	0.94	3.73	0.38	49	0.11	0.22	0.08
32	0.98	4.27	0.34	50+	0.26	0.47	0.21

It is apparent that the majority of Chinese women get married before the age of 25, and almost all women are married by their early 30s. Only 0.2 per cent of women aged 35 and over reported never being married in the survey. In other words, Chinese women achieved very close to 100 per cent entry into marriage.

This table also shows that Chinese women ultimately get married regardless of the place of residence. Although the proportion never married is higher for the urban women in general, the rural–urban difference here is negligible for the older ages and lies rather in the timing of the process. Generally speaking, Chinese women living in rural areas are more likely to get married earlier than those in urban areas. More than 60 per cent of rural females get married before they reach the age of 23, whereas, the percentage for urban females is less than 40. With increasing age, this difference diminishes. The timing factor in marriage will be studied in detail in the later section.

Another principal characteristic of Chinese marriage is its stability. Traditionally, there were rigid institutional restrictions on divorce so as to enforce family solidarity.[20] In principle the freedom of divorce is guaranteed in both 1950 and 1980 marriage laws. However, society and cultural tradition stress the stability of the family, and divorce is still looked down upon in Chinese society.

As has been widely observed,[21] most Chinese marriages are stable. Couples are expected to stay married for life. Both local kinship and government policies encourage such stability. When a marital dispute occurs, various attempts at mediation ensue, in order to get the couple back together. Only when such mediation fails, is the case sent to a local court. Divorce is to be avoided if at all possible.

The new marriage law, which went into effect on 1 January 1981, gives more freedom of divorce and places more emphasis on the emotional factor in ensuring happy marriages and preserving family life. Partly as a result of that, the number of divorces increased rapidly from 113,600 in 1979 to 427,000 in 1982.[22] But, if population increase is taken into account, the divorce level of 1982 was similar to the average for the years between 1950 and 1981.[23]

Data from China's 1982 Fertility Survey show that in 1982 the proportion of women aged 35–49 remaining in marital unions which were created by first marriage was 89.1 for all China, and 92.5 and 88.3 for urban and rural populations respectively. The higher proportion in the urban areas may reflect the fact that the life expectancy of the urban population is higher than that of the rural population. Among all ever married women aged 15–49, only 0.27 per cent were reportedly currently divorced at the national level, significantly higher (0.73 per cent) in the urban than in rural populations (0.189 per cent). The survey also reveals that 12.9 per cent of women aged 50 and over were remarried, 19 per cent were widowed, and only less than 0.5 per cent were currently divorced. These remarried women might be either previously divorced or widowed. Remarriage is not easily accepted by the public or tradition. Action by the younger generation to obstruct widowed or divorced parents from remarrying is one of the major issues in this subject and has attracted a lot of attention.[24] Nevertheless, the relatively high proportion of remarriages suggests that remarriage is common, and Chinese women are more likely to live in marriages rather than to stay single.

Table 4.4 shows the international comparison of crude divorce rates, which are defined as the number of final divorce decrees granted under civil law per 1,000 mid-year population, for selected countries in 1982. All these data indicate that marriage in China is stable.

Having considered two important features of contemporary Chinese marriage, universality and stability, our focus shifts to the trends of Chinese marriage pattern.

In China's 1982 Fertility Survey, women were asked about their

TABLE 4.4. *Crude divorce rate for selected countries, 1982*

Country	Rate (‰)	Country	Rate (‰)
US	5.08	Japan	1.38
Canada	2.86	Singapore	0.86
England	2.94	China	0.41

Source: Demographic Yearbook 1983, United Nations; Li Ning 1985.

current marital status as well as marital history, such as the date of the marriage and so on. The events of marriage were then classified by the year when the marriage occurred and the age of the bride at that time. Based on this age-period measurement, the mean age at first marriage and the age-specific first-marriage rate can be derived.

The Mean Age at First Marriage

In China, at least for the majority Han population, sexual activities outside marriage have been a cultural taboo. The phenomena of cohabitation and illegitimate births do exist, but are rare. An overwhelming majority of conceptions take place within marriage in line with Chinese customs. Hence, the age at marriage obviously signifies a milestone in the life course of youngsters and can be used with confidence as an indicator of the beginning of a woman's exposure to the risk of childbearing in the case of China, even though this may be misleading in many other developing countries.[25]

The mean age at first marriage (MAFM) in the 1940s was 18.46 for the country as a whole, and 19.16 and 18.32 for the urban and rural population respectively. This was roughly a year higher than the average (17.52) for the Chinese farm population in 1929–31.[26] Since the early 1950s (see Table 4.5 and Figure 4.2), the mean age at first marriage has increased continually. This increase was relatively slow before 1970 and accelerated during the subsequent decade. The national mean age at first marriage increased by 1.6 years over the 1950s and the 1960s, an annual increase of 0.08 year. The marriage age then rose rapidly during the decade beginning in 1970. In this ten-year period, the national value of mean age at first marriage increased from 20.19 in 1970 to 23.12 in 1979, an annual increase about 0.3 year. Since the early 1980s, the age at marriage has decreased slightly but is still at a level of 22.66 years in 1982 and 22.54 in 1986. In short, the mean age

TABLE 4.5. *Mean age at first marriage, China 1940–1982*

Year	Nation	Urban	Rural	Year	Nation	Urban	Rural
1940–9	18.46	19.16	18.32	1966	19.86	22.86	19.44
1949	18.57	19.16	18.44	1967	20.03	22.73	19.57
1950	18.68	19.41	18.52	1968	20.17	22.62	19.73
1951	18.69	19.43	18.54	1969	20.29	22.45	19.94
1952	18.49	19.75	18.76	1970	20.19	22.38	19.89
1953	18.94	19.85	18.71	1971	20.29	22.80	19.96
1954	19.00	20.12	18.72	1972	20.56	23.23	20.22
1955	19.07	20.28	18.81	1973	20.95	23.48	20.60
1956	19.19	20.51	18.87	1974	21.38	23.79	20.99
1957	19.23	20.40	18.90	1975	21.74	24.13	21.36
1958	19.15	20.77	18.78	1976	22.30	24.61	21.90
1959	19.35	20.81	19.01	1977	22.57	24.99	22.11
1960	19.57	21.25	19.24	1978	22.83	25.10	22.41
1961	19.70	21.46	19.40	1979	23.12	25.40	22.64
1962	19.61	21.49	19.27	1980	23.05	25.19	22.54
1963	19.58	21.49	19.25	1981	22.82	24.71	22.28
1964	19.55	22.04	19.17	1982	22.66	24.93	22.07
1965	19.74	22.57	19.30				

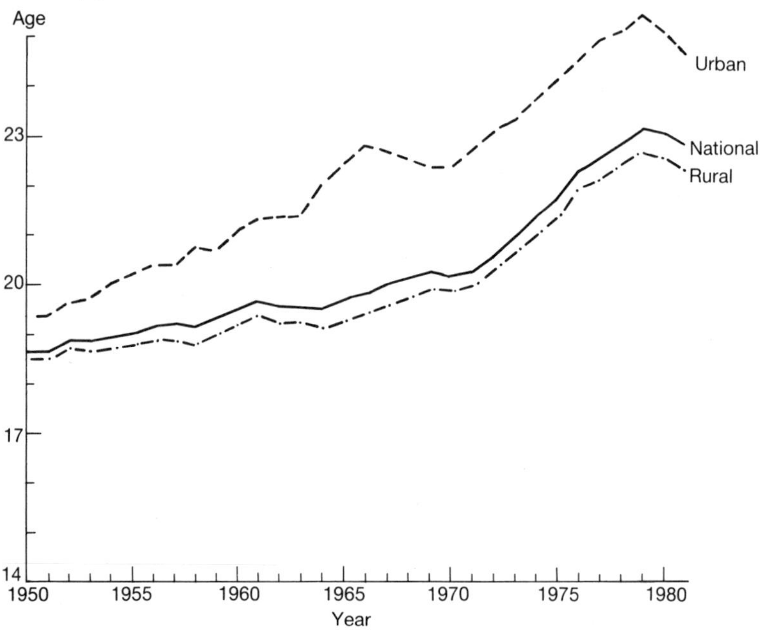

Fig. 4.2 Mean age at first marriage, China 1950–1981

at first marriage for China as a whole rose by about 4 years over the period 1950–82.

Nowadays, no matter where they live, women marry later than they did 30 years ago. But the tempo of this change in marriage ages has been different in the rural and the urban areas. In general, the mean age at marriage for urban females has been consistently higher than that of their rural counterparts. Before 1970 the increase of mean age at first marriage in urban areas was much quicker, especially in the early 1960s. This led to a wider gap between the rural and urban areas. The rural–urban difference in mean age at first marriage increased from 0.89 year in 1950, jumping to 2.01 years in 1960, and further to 2.49 in 1970. In 1966 the urban MAFM was 3.42 years higher than the rural MAFM. Since 1971 the increase of marriage age in both the rural and the urban areas has followed a similar momentum, and the gap has remained relatively constant around 2.5–3 years. In 1982 the mean age at first marriage was 24.9 for urban and 22.1 for the rural females, which were 5.77 and 3.63 years higher than those 32 years ago.

There are many factors associated with the increase of marriage age. Their relative importance varied in different periods. The legal minimum ages at marriage set by the 1950 marriage law were 18 and 20 years old for females and males respectively. More importantly, this marriage law formally abolished 'arranged marriage' and introduced greater freedom for young women to choose their husbands. The implementation of the law and the accompanying mass campaigns to inhibit very early marriage during the 1950s must have played the most important role in the postponement of marriage. The causal mechanisms by which social and economic changes affect age at marriage have not been satisfactorily studied. Nevertheless, it is certain that socio-economic circumstances at that time were also in favour of postponing marriage.[27] Encouragement of female employment, better educational opportunities for young girls, and so on all contributed to delaying marriage. The first marriage law was not an act to limit population growth. However, the rapidly diminished incidences of very early marriage no doubt had some impact on population growth. During this period, the government's efforts to postpone marriage were mainly restrained to persuasion rather than force.[28] The accompanying campaign was generally a gradual process of education among the masses.

For the whole period of the 1960s the mean age at marriage for rural females rose slowly but steadily. By contrast, the mean age at marriage in urban areas rose very fast in the first half of the 1960s, reaching a peak of 22.86 years in 1966, and fell afterwards in the second half of the

1960s. Two events must be responsible for this situation. In the early 1960s the Chinese government carried out its first effective family-planning programme. The rapid increase in marriage ages was no doubt a positive response of the urban population to the programme. The second is related to China's political condition. Nineteen sixty-six was the year in which the Cultural Revolution was launched. Family planning gave way to political activities and ceased to function. Schools were closed and the normal social order was broken. Earlier incentives for delaying marriage disappeared. Furthermore, as Edgar Snow commented, the behaviour of male and female Red Guards, plus a certain loosening of sexual taboos, stimulated earlier marriage.[29] Consequently, this chaotic movement led to the decline in mean age at first marriage till the restoration of order. The above data suggest that the marriage behaviour of urban females is more likely to be affected by China's political conditions.

The continuous and rapid increase in the mean age at first marriage in the 1970s largely resulted from the population policies implemented by the Chinese government. In 1971 the family-planning programme was resumed after the most chaotic period of the Cultural Revolution. A population programme known as 'Wan, Xi, Shao' (later marriage, longer birth interval, and fewer children) was being strictly pursued. Appropriate marriage age was set out, normally around 23–5 for females, by local authorities. Women were encouraged, in some circumstances forced, to postpone their marriages. In addition, a large number of urban youths, about 17 million in total, were sent to the countryside during the first half of the 1970s, which led to postponement of marriage among urban females.[30] This is also regarded as one of the main causes of the imbalance in the urban marriage market.

Since 1979 the mean age at first marriage has continuously declined from 23.12 years in 1979 to 22.66 in 1982, and 22.54 in 1986. Losing control on late marriage is certainly responsible for this downward trend. As we have shown earlier, the controlling age at marriage in the later 1970s was not the legal age for marriage, but rather the recommended age set by local authorities which was usually 23 years old for females. Hence, the high level of mean age at first marriage in the later 1970s is a combined product of a secular trend of delaying marriage and some forced late marriages. In the 1980s the previous recommended age for marriage has ceased to be effective and the only controlling age is the legal marriage age, say 20 years old for female, set by China's 1980 marriage law. Although late marriage is still strongly encouraged by family-planning programmes, it is no longer a compulsory obligation of youngsters. Therefore, it can be said, on top of other causes, the current mean age at marriage is more likely to reflect the secular trend of marriage pattern.

First Marriage Rates

China's annual total first marriage rates betwen 1950 and 1981 are calculated on the basis of the age-specific first-marriage rates. The marriage data collected in China's 1982 Survey were tabulated on an age-period basis. Some adjustment was undertaken to transfer the age-period marriage rates to age-cohort ones in order to match the proportion of ever married for each age cohort. The tabulated data are not detailed enough to enable us to reallocate the marriage events directly. A simple but reasonable method of adjustment is employed here. Ratios of the number of women ever married at each age in mid-1982 to the number of marriages cumulated from the tabulated age-period marriage events for the corresponding cohort are calculated. It is reasonable to use women's marital status at the time of survey as a basis for the adjustment. Assuming that the difference between the age-period marriage events and the age-cohort ones are the same as the ratio through the relevant diagram, we transfer the marriage data into a kind of age-cohort format. The age-specific first-marriage rates are then calculated, as are the total first-marriage rate (TMR). China's total first-marriage rates for both rural and urban population, are presented in Table 4.6 and illustrated in Figure 4.3.

TABLE 4.6. Total first marriage rate, China 1950–1981

Year	Nation	Urban	Rural	Year	Nation	Urban	Rural
1950	1.016	0.957	1.036	1966	0.728	0.605	0.744
1951	0.883	0.805	0.910	1967	0.824	0.831	0.818
1952	0.920	0.893	0.933	1968	0.998	1.064	0.985
1953	0.878	0.901	0.878	1969	0.994	1.003	0.996
1954	0.887	0.905	0.887	1970	0.829	0.740	0.850
1955	0.885	0.798	0.909	1971	0.715	0.610	0.740
1956	0.918	0.902	0.918	1972	0.675	0.581	0.698
1957	0.894	0.958	0.876	1973	0.641	0.568	0.665
1958	0.878	0.804	0.890	1974	0.665	0.652	0.676
1959	0.738	0.721	0.735	1975	0.675	0.650	0.690
1960	0.889	0.780	0.910	1976	0.741	0.741	0.752
1961	0.988	0.788	1.023	1977	0.749	0.761	0.755
1962	1.189	1.039	1.201	1978	0.819	0.772	0.842
1963	1.007	0.896	1.016	1979	0.922	0.931	0.941
1964	0.786	0.651	0.801	1980	1.137	1.193	1.141
1965	0.707	0.618	0.717	1981	1.303	1.507	1.267

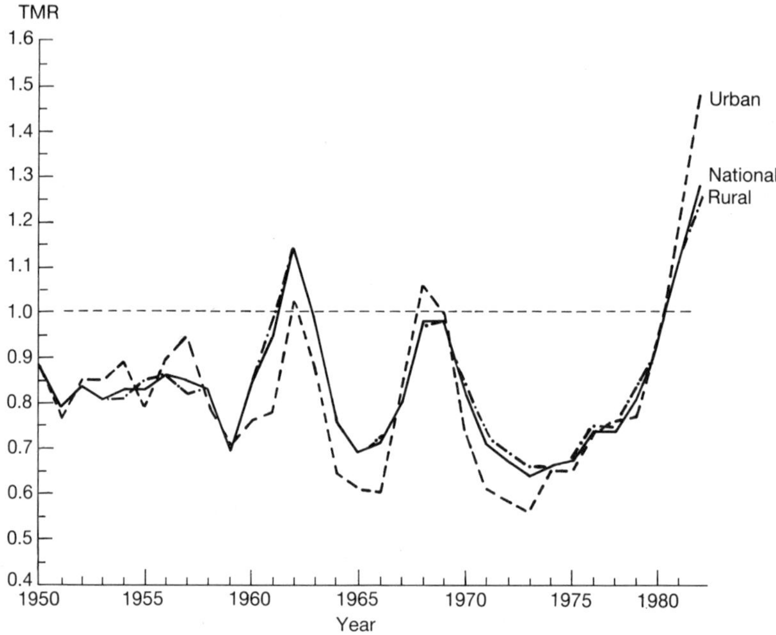

Fig. 4.3 Total first-marriage rates, China 1950–1981

During the early 1950s the TMRs stayed at a level of 0.9, and reached an initial trough in 1959, when the value fell to 0.74. The TMR then increased to a peak of 1.19 in 1962. The TMR afterward fell again down to 0.71 and 0.73 in 1965 and 1966, and rose to a point very close to unity in 1968 and 1969. The lowest TMR, 0.64 was recorded in 1973. Since then, the TMR has increased continually and reached a peak of 1.30 in 1981, which is the highest value for the whole period from the late 1940s to 1981.

The Chinese marriage pattern is characterized by its universality. However, the annual total female first-marriage rates (TMR) differed from unity in most years during the period concerned and experienced several large fluctuations. Coale gives two possible explanations for difference from unity in the annual TMR even when every cohort achieved very close to 100 per cent entry into marriage: the first is temporary deficit and excess in the number of marriages, and the second is continual increase in mean age at first marriage.[31] His explanations are shared by this study. On the whole, the case of China fits the formula which was suggested by Norman Ryder very well. Over the last four decades, mean age at first marriage for China as a whole increased by 4.9 years. The average TMR for the same period should be 0.874, using Norman Ryder's formula, which is very close to the real situation.[32]

The time trend of the total marriage rate is closely associated with socio-political conditions in China. The 1959 trough is clearly a consequence of the Great Leap Forward and the massive famine. Subsequently, the 1962 peak reflects the recovery from the disaster. This large marriage boom was also partly responsible for the marriage deficit in the following years.

The impact of the Cultural Revolution on TMR is twofold. During the early and most militant period, youngsters were heavily involved in the movement. Personal affairs were subjugated to the revolution and youths were too busy to get married. Shortly after that, political fanaticism cooled. Young people caught up with getting married. Building their small family was also regarded as a way of avoiding meaningless political conflicts. This might have been responsible for the increase in the total marriage rate in the late 1960s. Of course, it is dangerous to oversimplify the matter. The varied impact of the Cultural Revolution on people's daily lives are more complicated, and this is by no means a complete explanation.

The earnest implementation of the family-planning programme in the early 1970s, which led to a rapid rise in the mean age at first marriage, was certainly associated with the 1973 trough. The recent surge of the TMR is believed to be the product of another marriage boom, mainly caused by a relaxation of control.

The marriage boom, which followed the disturbance in the early 1960s, was smaller in the cities. This may suggest that urban life was less severely interrupted by the massive famine. The marriage fluctuation in the second half of the 1960s was much greater for the urban population, compared with their rural counterparts and indicates that it was more active in the political movement. The deep trough of urban TMR in the early 1970s was clearly related to the movement of sending urban youths to China's countryside. Nineteen eighty-one is the year in which the new marriage law went into effect, setting the legal age of marriage well below the official requirement prevailing in the previous period. On the whole, it can be summarized that marriage behaviour of China's urban women was more strongly influenced by the country's social and political conditions.

Composition of Marriage Events

Figure 4.4 shows the composition of marriage events for all China from 1950 to 1982. Here three-year age groups are used and the marriages

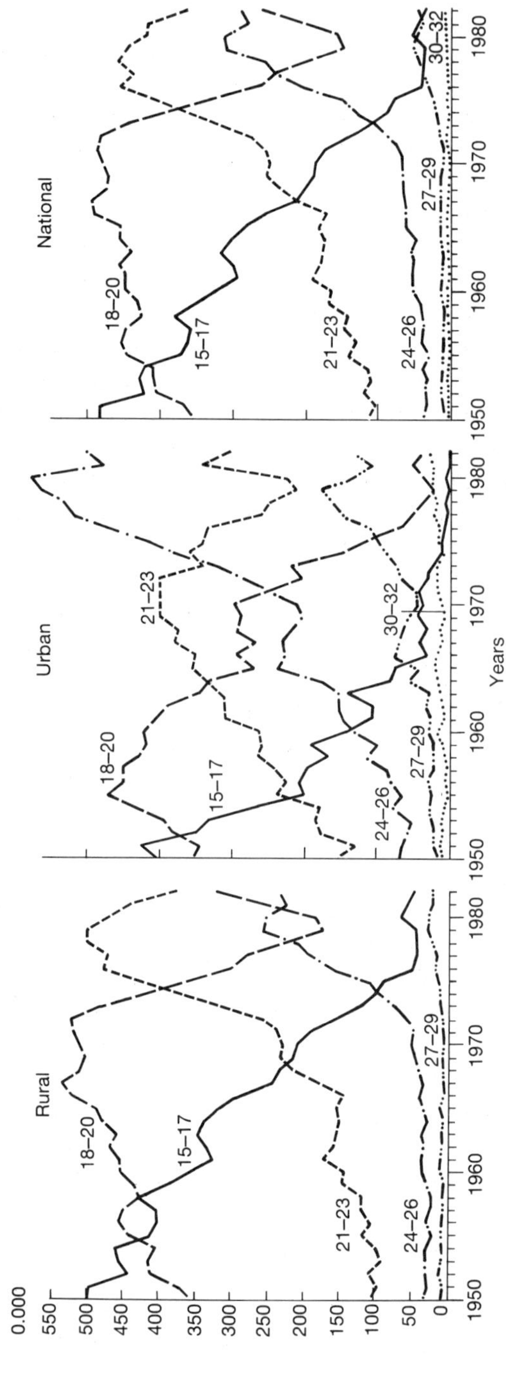

Fig. 4.4 Contributions to total marriage by age group, China 1950–1982

involving women aged 33 and over are left out for clarity. As mentioned above, almost all Chinese women get married before 30 and this simplification will not therefore affect the result.

We consider the national pattern first. The contribution of the 15–17 age group to total marriages has been declining sharply and continuously since 1950. In 1950 marriages occurring in this age group accounted for almost 50 per cent of total yearly marriages. This figure decreased to about 30 per cent in the middle 1960s and to less than 4 per cent in the later 1970s. On the one hand, this change was brought about by the implementation of the 1950 marriage law which set the minimum age at marriage at 18 years. On the other hand, changes were in part due to developmental factors, such as universal education and women's emancipation. Reducing incidence of very early marriage was obviously the main cause of the increase in mean age at marriage, at least in the 1950s.

As far as the 18–20 age group is concerned, its contribution to total annual marriages increased rapidly in the 1950s and then remained relatively constant until 1973. This may be because of the corresponding decline in very early marriage. During the period 1960–72, about half of Chinese women married in their later teens and early 20s. Since the early 1970s, this situation has changed sharply. By 1979 married women in this age group accounted for only about 15 per cent of annual total marriages. The turning-point coincided with the launch of 'Wan, Xi, Shao' campaign, and undoubtedly indicates the success of this aspect of the family-planning programme. After the promulgation of the new marriage law in the early 1980s, there was a tendency for Chinese women to get married younger than before, and the percentage contributions for the 18–20 age group increased again. In the first half of 1982, about 26 per cent of marriages belonged to this age group.

Figures also reveal that the contribution of the 21–3 age group increased gradually before 1967, and has risen quite sharply since then. In 1950 only 11 per cent of women married when they were 21–3 years old. The percentage increased to 18 in 1965 and up to 46 per cent in 1978. Since 1979 the contribution of this age group has decreased at the expense of an increased contribution by the 18–20 age group.

The trend of the 24–6 age group shows a similarity to that of the 21–3 group, with the difference being in the beginning time of sharp increase. For this group matches that of the 21–3 group, except that its sharp increase began 5 years later in 1972. This is certainly associated with the adoption of an official target for age at marriage, which was usually 23 for the rural women and 25 for their urban counterparts.

Changes in percentage contributions for the two older age groups, the 27–9 and the 30–2 were very small over time. This suggests that notwithstanding the strict implementation of the late-marriage policy, a majority of Chinese women get married before their late 20s.

On the whole, this figure demonstrates the process of China's marriage transition: considerable postponement of marriage over the last three decades and a setback in recent years.

Moving from early to late marriage took place in both rural and urban areas. But the process occurred much earlier and faster in urban areas. For the urban population, the incidence of very early marriage (i.e. women married 15–17 years old) was always lower than that for the rural. By 1966 very early marriage had already fallen below 5 per cent of total urban marriages, whilst rural population reached this point ten years later in 1976.

While about 50 per cent of all rural marriages affected women aged 18–20 till 1972, only 20 per cent fell within this category amongst the urban population. In the urban areas, the share of the 18–20 age group reached its peak of 47 per cent in 1955 and then decreased consistently. In 1982 less than 4 per cent urban females married under the age 21, while the figure for the rural areas was still as high as 32 per cent.

The contribution of the 21–3 age group for the urban population increased continually during the 1950s and the 1960s. During the later 1960s to early 1970s, this age group was the once which accounted for the highest percentage of total marriages. Since 1972 its position has been assumed by the 24–6 age group. On the other hand, the 21–3 age group of the rural population has superseded the 18–20 group—a situation which has persisted until the present day.

In the early 1980s about half of the urban marriages involved women aged 24–6, whereas the figure for the rural areas was around 25 per cent. In urban areas, about 15 per cent of women married in their later 20s in the 1980s, but the proportion for rural women was insignificant.

The analysis of time trends for China's marriage composition gives us a clear picture about the movement from very early marriage to late marriage over the past several decades. The logical conclusion is that nuptiality transition occurred earlier in China's urban section. Among relevant factors, rigid control of marriage age in urban areas has been particularly important. This also reflects the fact that the urban population responded to family planning quicker and more positively. Although there has been a recent setback in terms of late marriage, it seems unlikely that the general trend of China's marriage pattern will be significantly reversed.

III. The Age Pattern of Fertility Trends

Data collected in China's 1982 Fertility Survey make an analysis of changes in the age patterns of fertility possible. While the trends in the TFR tell us the general direction of China's fertility transition, or the quantum changes, examination of the trends in age patterns yields more detailed information on when and in which age groups the entire movement started. The focus on tempo changes may help us to understand the cause and process of the quantum changes. We begin by looking at the trends of the age-specific fertility rates.

Age-Specific Fertility Rates

Table 4.7 contains the average values of the Age-Specific Fertility Rate (ASFR) over the past 30 years for all China, and for the rural and urban population separately. Changes in ASFR are also presented in the table.

Closely connected with the postponement of marriage is the consistent decline in the age-specific fertility rate for the 15–19 age group. By the early 1980s the ASFR for the 15–19 age group was only 0.01, in contrast to 0.1 three decades ago.

The ASFRs for the 20–4, 25–9, and 30–4 age groups remained more or less constant for China as a whole, and for the rural population as well, over the first two decades. Sustained fertility decline for these age groups occurred during the 1970s, but the reduction of the ASFRs for the urban population can be traced back to the mid-1960s.

Data for the older age groups are not complete. However, it can be seen that the turning-point of fertility decline for the 35–49 age groups was earlier than for the 20–34 age groups. It seems likely that this sustained fertility decline for the three oldest age groups started in the late 1960s for China as a whole, and for the rural population. The decline in urban areas is likely to have been earlier. In the late 1970s there were almost no births that occurred to urban women in their forties, and the incidence for the rural population was also greatly diminished.

Over the last three decades, the ASFR of the 15–19 age group declined substantially by 85 per cent for the rural population, and even more for the urban population. Changes in ASFRs for the three oldest age groups are as great as that for the 15–19 group. In contrast, the decline for women in their twenties and early thirties is modest. The rural–urban difference is clear. Compared with the early 1950s, the

TABLE 4.7. *Age-specific fertility rates for selected periods*

Age group	1952–4	1955–7	1958–60	1961–3	1964–6	1967–9	1970–2	1973–5	1976–8	1979–81
National										
15–19	0.099	0.084	0.054	0.057	0.062	0.047	0.039	0.024	0.014	0.013
20–4	0.287	0.289	0.214	0.267	0.294	0.279	0.265	0.214	0.164	0.161
25–9	0.291	0.297	0.233	0.291	0.314	0.314	0.300	0.253	0.217	0.207
30–4	0.251	0.251	0.199	0.246	0.261	0.250	0.234	0.168	0.105	0.077
35–9	—	0.194	0.152	0.178	0.198	0.180	0.162	0.106	0.057	0.033
40–4	—	—	—	0.073	0.094	0.086	0.075	0.048	0.025	0.014
45–9	—	—	—	—	0.011	0.009	0.008	0.006	0.004	0.002
Rural										
15–19	0.104	0.091	0.057	0.061	0.068	0.054	0.044	0.028	0.017	0.016
20–4	0.294	0.294	0.212	0.276	0.314	0.298	0.287	0.239	0.186	0.189
25–9	0.293	0.297	0.229	0.296	0.334	0.330	0.314	0.265	0.225	0.216
30–4	0.254	0.254	0.200	0.255	0.288	0.279	0.260	0.184	0.114	0.083
35–9	—	0.199	0.154	0.187	0.220	0.206	0.190	0.126	0.068	0.039
40–4	—	—	—	0.078	0.104	0.098	0.088	0.058	0.031	0.017
45–9	—	—	—	—	0.012	0.010	0.009	0.007	0.005	0.003
Urban										
15–19	0.079	0.059	0.040	0.037	0.025	0.012	0.010	0.004	0.002	0.002
20–4	0.256	0.268	0.222	0.230	0.195	0.175	0.149	0.088	0.057	0.043
25–9	0.281	0.301	0.246	0.268	0.236	0.248	0.226	0.188	0.178	0.163
30–4	0.233	0.237	0.193	0.209	0.150	0.139	0.129	0.094	0.061	0.045
35–9	—	0.169	0.138	0.133	0.096	0.067	0.053	0.027	0.013	0.006
40–4	—	—	—	0.052	0.042	0.027	0.018	0.007	0.003	0.001
45–9	—	—	—	—	0.006	0.003	0.002	0.001	0.001	0.000

Changes in age-specific fertility rate (%)[a]

	15–19	20–4	25–9	30–4	35–9	40–4	45–9
National	−87	−44	−29	−70	−83	−85	−82
Rural	−85	−36	−26	−67	−82	−84	−75
Urban	−97	−83	−42	−80	−94	−98	−100

[a] Changes for the 15–19, 20–4, 25–9, 30–4 age groups refer to period 1952–4/1979–81, changes for the other age groups refer to 1964–6/1979–81.

ASFRs for the 20–4 and 30–4 age groups declined by 80 per cent for the urban population, but only 36 and 67 per cent for the rural population. This indicates that fertility transition among the urban population was more dramatic and births are more likely to be concentrated in a relatively shortened age span.

The Percentage Contribution

National Pattern

In Figure 4.5, the percentage contributions of each five-year age group to overall fertility over the past 30 years are illustrated. The denominators used for these calculations prior to 1964 are the TFRs estimated by Chinese demographers. It can be seen that China's fertility composition has changed substantially over time.

The percentage contribution of the 15–19 age group has been continuously falling since the founding of the People's Republic. The average percentage value was around 7 in the 1950s, 4.8 in the 1960s, and less than 3 in the 1970s, with the lowest value being 2.1 in 1977. Such a trend is closely related to the tendency to delay marriage over the last 30 and more years. Those figures also show that even in the early 1950s, when the mean age at first marriage was about 17 years, the contribution of this age group to the TFR was only about 7 per cent.

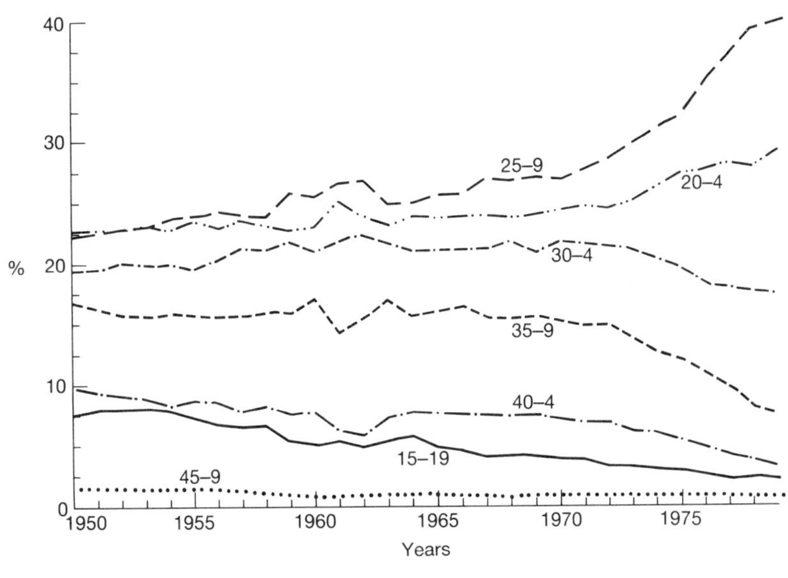

Fig. 4.5 Contribution of ASFR to TFR, national 1950–1979

This indicates that the importance of fertility reduction of the 15–19 age group on overall fertility may be small, even though the decline itself is significant.

The 20–4 age group contributed about 22 per cent of total fertility in the 1950s, 23 in the 1960s. From the early 1970s its share began to increase, reaching its highest level of 34.6 per cent in 1981.

The trend of the percentage contribution for the 25–9 age group shows a similarity to that for the 20–4 age group, although the increase was more rapid. In the 1950s this age group shared on average 23 per cent of total fertility, and 26 per cent in the 1960s. Since 1971 the increase has accelerated and reached its highest value of more than 40 per cent in the early 1980s. In other words, in the early 1980s, more than 40 per cent of all annual births occurred to mothers aged 25–9.

Meanwhile the contribution of the 30–4 age group remained constant at a level of around 20 per cent throughout the 1950s and 1960s. Thereafter, the percentage contribution of this age group started to decline and fell to 14 in 1981.

The contribution of the 35–9 age group has constantly declined, slowly in the 1950s and 1960s but speedily since the beginning of the 1970s. Its share to the TFR dropped from 17 per cent in the early 1950s to about 6 per cent in the first two years of the 1980s.

The contribution of the 40–9 age groups prior to 1964 is calculated according to the age-specific fertility rates estimated by Chinese demographers. The 40–4 age group produced about 10 per cent of total annual births in the early 1950s, but only 2.4 per cent in 1981, a similar trend to the 15–19 age group. The 45–9 age group was never an important one in terms of its contribution to TFR, ranging from a high of 1.6 per cent in 1960 to a low of 0.4 in 1981.

From the above discussion, some important features of the age pattern of China's fertility change can be discerned. Nineteen seventy-one can be viewed as a turning-point. Before 1971 the contributions to the TFR of the very young and the older age groups fell slightly but continuously. On the other hand, the age groups in-between increased their contributions. These different changes offset each other. Since 1971 this pattern has shifted substantially. The reduction of contributions by the 15–19 and 35–49 age groups has accelerated, giving way to more and more births in the age groups in between. In 1981, the three age groups between 20–34, within the period of peak human fecundity, accounted for 90 per cent of the TFR, compared with 64.4 per cent in 1950.

It is interesting to note that changes in age group contribution to TFR did not necessarily lead to changes in total fertility rate. Although the age group composition of the TFR did change, the national fertility level remained more or less constant over the first two decades of the People's Republic. This mainly resulted from an increase in fertility for the 20–34 age groups.

Figures in Table 4.7 for 1958–60 and 1961–3 may be affected by the massive fertility fluctuation during the famine and the recovery period. Comparing the period 1964–6 with the 1950s, it is clear that although the TFRs of these two periods were similar at around 6.2, the age patterns were a little different. The ASFR for the 15–19, and for the three older age groups as well, fell during this period. By contrast, fertility of the age groups 20–34 was higher in the mid-1960s.

The lower ASFR of the 15–19 age group in the 1960s was related to marriage, as has been discussed above. The increased ASFRs of the 20–34 age groups in the same period may also be partly due to the postponement of marriage. Several studies have shown that women who get married late may give more births in the first few years of their marriage. In other words, delaying marriage from a very early age had the effect of increasing the ASFR of the next few age groups.[33] Therefore, the reduction of the ASFR of the 15–19 age group became one of the main reasons for the increase in ASFRs of the later age groups. When there was no effective birth-control programme, fertility decline in the very young ages was offset by the increased ASFRs of the 20–34 age groups, and resulted in a near constant TFR at the end of the 1960s.

In conclusion, over the last 30 years, childbearing in China has shifted heavily towards women in their twenties. Meanwhile, fertility in both the youngest and older age groups has declined. Moreover, since the change in the contribution of the 15–19 age group to TFR was relatively small compared with the older age groups, especially the 35–44 groups, it can be said that the reduction of China's overall fertility has mainly come from changes in the older age groups. The relative importance of delaying marriage and reducing ultimate family size will be discussed in a later section.

Rural–Urban Difference

Now let us turn to the rural–urban differentials in trends of percentage contribution. Here, the concepts and measurements are the same as those discussed earlier, except that the three oldest age groups, 35–9, 40–4, and 45–9, are combined. As was mentioned above, the percentage contribution of the 40–4 and 45–9 groups has been small, especially for the latter age group, during the past 30 years, so that this simplification will not significantly affect the present analysis.

The time trend for the rural population in terms of distribution is identical to that at the national level. During the past 30 years, the percentage contribution for rural females aged 15–19 fell continuously from 7.3 in 1950 to 2.6 in 1979. The contributions of the other age groups remained more or less constant before 1970 with only small annual changes. Nineteen seventy-one was the year in which this stability was broken. Since then, the two age groups in the twenties have increased their shares of the TFR, and the shares of the older age groups have declined. However, even in 1979, the fertility of the 35–49 age group still accounted for one-eighth of the total births. Births to women at such ages are normally higher order births, and this phenomenon indicates that higher order births were still common in the rural areas. Nevertheless, women in their twenties contributed 70 per cent of the total births in 1979.

The time trends for the urban population show a different picture. Before 1964 the shares of different age groups to the TFR were relatively constant, with fluctuations only occurring around the famine period. At that time the contribution of the 15–19 age group declined continuously, just as for the rural population. Meanwhile, the percentages for the 20–4 and 25–9 age groups rose slightly and moved away from the older age groups. Since 1964 a marked change has occurred. The contribution of the 15–19 group was already very small and left little room for further reduction. The shares of the 30–4 age group were relatively constant. The most striking changes occurred for the other three groups. The 35–49 group began to experience a decline in its share of the TFR in 1964, from 21 per cent in that year to 12 in 1970 and further down to less than 5 per cent in the late 1970s. The 25–9 age group moved in the opposite direction. Its contribution rose consistently from 30 per cent in 1964 to about 60 per cent by the end of the 1970s. In other words, in 1979, a remarkable 60 per cent of annual urban births occurred to mothers aged 25–9. The 20–4 age group stood at its previous level until 1970, then began to decline and reached its lowest value of 12.5 per cent in 1979.

A few observations can be made with respect to the rural–urban differences. First, the change of fertility composition occurred much earlier in urban than rural areas. The turning-point for urban areas is around 1964, and 1971 for rural.

Secondly, as far as the age groups are concerned, the direction of movement for the 25–9 age groups is the same for both rural and urban. And so are the ones for 35–49 age groups. However, the behaviour of the other two groups deserve the greater attention. While the share of 20–4 age group began to decline in 1970 for the urban population, it increased in rural areas. As for the 30–4 group, it remained constant in the urban, but fell in the rural sector. There are at least two factors responsible for this urban–rural contrast: the differences in marriage age and in family size. Since rural girls got married earlier than their urban counterparts, they also gave birth to their first or second child earlier, usually in their early or middle twenties. Owing to the strict control of higher order births, they tended to stop their reproductive activities then. On the other hand, as a result of delayed marriage, urban women postponed their first childbearing to 25–9 years old and then stopped their fertility activities as a positive response to the family-planning programme.

Cumulated Period Fertility

By setting the period TFR as unity and making the cumulated fertility rates up to certain age a percentage of the corresponding TFR, it is possible to describe the age patterns of family formation. Comparison of such patterns is likely to highlight the tempo changes, net of the absolute TFR levels.

Our analysis shows that China's family formation pattern evolved gradually, moving from a pattern of starting at an early age and continuing to very old age, to that of starting late and finishing early. It means that family formation in China became more and more concentrated in a shortened period, particularly during the recent past.

To make the picture clearer, an index called the 80-per-cent interval (A_{80}) is used. The index indicates the age intervals between the ages when the cumulated fertility rate reached 10 and 90 per cent of the TFR respectively. In other words, it identifies women's most active age span in childbearing during which more than 80 per cent of children are born at a given time point. We have:

$$A_{80} = A_{90} - A_{10}$$

Where:

A_{10} refers to the age by which 10 per cent of the TFR is completed and A_{90} as the 90 per cent.

Table 4.8 contains indices of A_{10}, A_{90}, and A_{80} for eight selected years for China as a whole, and for rural and urban areas. From these figures, it is clear that no matter where the place of residence is, Chinese women now spend less time in forming their families than earlier cohorts. For the country as a whole, and for rural areas, there are signs of a gradual compression of the childbearing range up to the mid-1970s, but with the main reduction taking place in the second half

TABLE 4.8. *80-per-cent intervals for selected years*

	1951	1955	1959	1963	1967	1971	1975	1979	1981
National									
A_{10}	20	20	20	21	21	21	22	22	21
A_{90}	40	39	39	38	39	38	38	35	34
A_{80}	20	19	19	17	18	17	16	13	13
Rural									
A_{10}	20	20	20	21	21	21	21	22	21
A_{90}	40	39	39	38	39	39	38	35	34
A_{80}	20	19	19	17	18	18	17	13	13
Urban									
A_{10}	20	20	21	21	22	22	23	24	23
A_{90}	39	39	39	37	36	36	34	32	30
A_{80}	19	19	18	16	14	14	11	8	7

of the 1970s. During this 5-year period, the value of the index of 80-per-cent interval fell from 17 years to 13 years, an average decline of 0.8 years per annum. For the period 1950–79 as a whole, the A_{80} interval fell six years, the A_{10} delayed two years, and A_{90} was four years earlier. These changes reflect the impact of postponement of marriage and reduction in ultimate family size.

The A_{80} values for the urban population are usually smaller than those for rural females. The direction of the change in the index for the urban population is the same as for the rural, but the speed of change is much quicker. Consequently, the difference in A_{80} values between the urban and rural populations increased as time passed. During the 1950s the rural–urban difference was one year. The gap became larger after the second half of the 1960s. By 1981 this difference had increased to six years. Both the A_{10} and A_{90} contributed to this change. For instance, in 1981, the difference in A_{10} and A_{90} between urban and rural areas is two years and four years respectively, which indicates that urban females began their family formation later and completed their fertility much earlier than rural females.

In urban areas, the family formation was largely concentrated in a mere 8-year period in 1979. It reached its 10 per cent point at the age 24, and reached the 90 point by age 32. This confirms our early conclusion that women living in urban areas were more likely to delay their marriage and accept a small family.

The conclusion is that during the past three or four decades the time intervals for forming a family became shorter in both rural and urban areas. Family formation tended to become more and more concentrated in a shorter period. The most important contributors to the TFR in the urban areas were women in their later twenties, while women in their early twenties and early thirties in the rural areas were still very active in terms of childbearing. This clearly reflects the rural–urban differences in the marriage age and the ultimate family size.

Birth Order

Closely associated with age pattern of fertility change are changes in birth order. To reduce births of higher order was one of the major programme objectives of China's family planning, particularly the 'One-child policy'. Therefore, analysis of changes in birth orders can help us to understand the mechanism of China's fertility transition, and the success story of the family-planning programme as well.

Table 4.9 and Figure 4.6 show the contribution of each birth order to total yearly births for 1970, 1977, 1981, and 1984 respectively. These dates are chosen solely because of data availability.

From Table 4.9 we see that, since 1970, the contribution of the first birth to total births has increased consistently. By contrast, the share of the higher order births, which refers to births of the third and higher orders, has declined. The contribution of second order births has remained more or less constant for China as a whole as well as for the rural population, but has declined for the urban population.

Before the nation-wide implementation of the effective family-planning programme, the figures show that more than 60 per cent of total births were the third or higher orders. The first births accounted for only 21 per cent of the total births.

This situation reversed as time passed. In 1984 births of the first order contributed 68 per cent of total births for China as a whole, and only 10 per cent of total births were higher orders. This is unequivocal evidence of the success of China's one-child policy.

The rural–urban difference emerges clearly. The occurrences of births of higher orders are always lower in the urban areas for the period concerned. In 1970 while 64 in every 100 births were higher orders in the rural areas, the equivalent figure for the urban population was 46 per cent. By 1977 the proportion of higher order births was already below 20 per cent in the urban areas, but remained as high as 50 per cent in the rural areas. Five years after the implementation of the 'one-child policy', the occurrence of second and higher order births in the urban areas fell to 16 per cent (1984). But there were still 37 per cent of rural births in this category. It is evident that the one-child

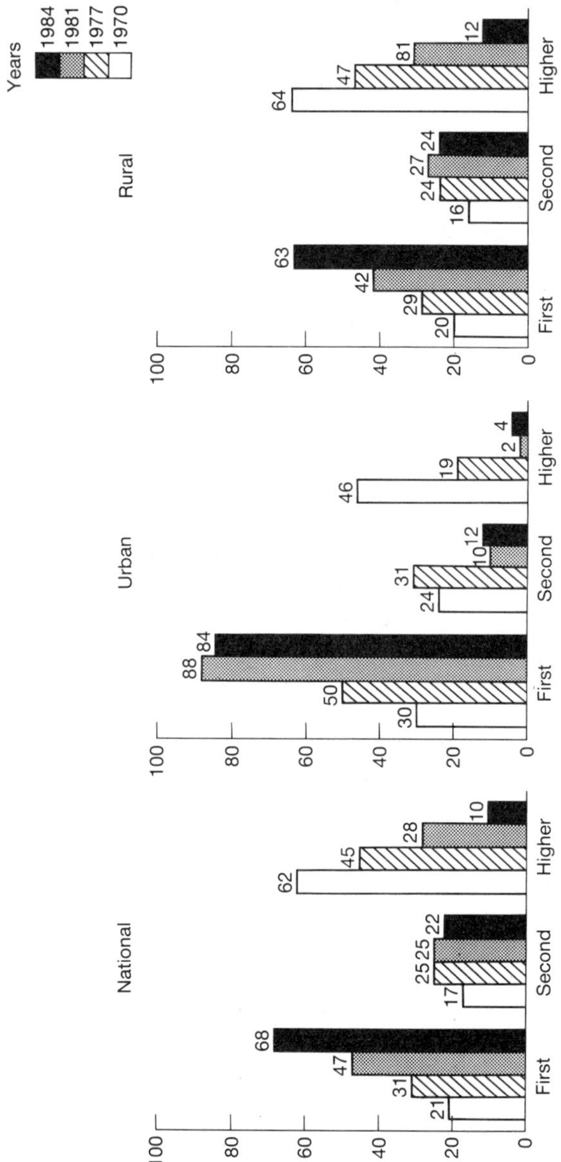

Fig. 4.6 Contribution of total births by birth order, China

TABLE 4.9. Contribution to total births by birth order (%)

Year	First			Second			Higher		
	National	Urban	Rural	National	Urban	Rural	National	Urban	Rural
1970	21	30	20	17	24	16	62	46	64
1977	31	50	29	25	31	24	45	19	47
1981	47	88	42	25	10	27	28	2	31
1984	68	84	63	22	12	24	10	4	12

Sources: Data for 1970, 1977, and 1981 from China's 1982 Fertility Survey, data for 1984 from China's Population Information Centre, *Handbook of Chinese Population Information, 1985*.

policy was more likely to be accepted by the urban population than their rural counterparts.

Cohort Fertility

Above analyses are all based on period measures. What is the situation of cohort fertility? Although most of the women interviewed in China's 1982 Fertility Survey have still not completed their reproductive life, the comparison of cumulated cohort fertility rates up to certain ages for the past three decades can show us the trend of cohort fertility. Estimates of cumulated cohort fertility (age cohort) are presented in Table 4.10. Here, the three-year average is used which smoothes the single-year fluctuation, especially for the period 1958–63. The focus here is on the general trend of cohort fertility trend.

The broad trend of cohort fertility is similar to that of the period fertility. However, compared with the period measures, the change in cohort fertility is modest and the time point for this change is later. We consider the national pattern first.

The cohort fertility up to age 19 has been declining continuously and dramatically. In the early 1950s women aged 19 on the average had 0.5 children, as against less than 0.065 in the early 1980s. This largely resulted from the postponement of marriage.

However, delaying marriage did not simultaneously bring about falls in the number of children born to a woman by the age of 24, as might have been expected. As a matter of fact, women who married later lost no time in childbearing in their early married life and caught up quickly. This can be seen from the trend of the first-birth interval (Table 4.11). The median interval between the first marriage and the first birth declined steadily through successive marriage cohorts. The first-birth interval was 2.5 years for the 1957 marriage cohort, was compressed to less than 2 years for the 1970 cohort; and fell further to 1.7 years for the 1980 cohort. In other words, the efforts expended in raising marriage age were not fully rewarded by later childbearing as had been assumed by China's family-planning programme.

As suggested by W. Lavely, the birth-control programme itself and the pre-marital pregnancy may be responsible for this tendency.[34] It may also be related to biological factors such as teenage subfecundity. Consequently, the cumulative cohort fertility up to age 24 did not change until the first half of the 1970s. By the early 1980s the average number of children ever borne for women aged 24 had halved, compared with 30 years ago.

So far as the rural–urban comparison is concerned, it is clear that the

TABLE 4.10. *Cumulated cohort fertility rate up to the end of age group*

Age group	1952–4	1955–7	1958–60	1961–3	1964–6	1967–9	1970–2	1973–5	1976–8	1979–81
National										
15–19	0.496	0.453	0.324	0.261	0.326	0.247	0.211	0.133	0.077	0.065
20–4	1.764	1.855	1.839	1.562	1.665	1.800	1.692	1.492	1.190	0.932
25–9	—	3.147	3.191	3.112	3.195	3.158	3.277	3.174	2.872	2.408
30–4	—	—	—	4.236	4.394	4.464	4.436	4.255	3.979	3.556
35–9	—	—	—	—	5.115	5.283	5.267	5.184	4.853	4.428
40–4	—	—	—	—	—	—	5.618	5.679	5.497	5.190
45–9	—	—	—	—	—	—	—	—	5.691	5.638
Rural										
15–19	0.514	0.485	0.348	0.277	0.358	0.281	0.241	0.156	0.091	0.079
20–4	1.797	1.898	1.877	1.597	1.744	1.919	1.824	1.655	1.337	1.082
25–9	—	3.195	3.221	3.157	3.277	3.296	3.456	3.355	3.066	2.606
30–4	—	—	—	4.290	4.501	4.649	4.689	4.530	4.219	3.771
35–9	—	—	—	—	5.237	5.458	5.534	5.537	5.200	4.735
40–4	—	—	—	—	—	—	5.828	5.940	5.843	5.576
45–9	—	—	—	—	—	—	—	—	5.910	5.940
Urban										
15–19	0.425	0.332	0.231	0.179	0.147	0.064	0.059	0.024	0.012	0.007
20–4	1.617	1.671	1.698	1.430	1.323	1.181	0.947	0.655	0.424	0.256
25–9	—	2.931	3.059	2.927	2.885	2.625	2.460	2.178	1.809	1.387
30–4	—	—	—	3.984	3.930	3.747	3.456	3.179	2.788	2.355
35–9	—	—	—	—	4.554	4.494	4.120	3.876	3.504	3.128
40–4	—	—	—	—	—	—	4.652	4.517	4.074	3.741
45–9	—	—	—	—	—	—	—	—	4.661	4.332

TABLE 4.11. *Median first-birth intervals and the mean age at first marriage for selected marriage cohorts* (in years)

Marriage cohort	National		Urban		Rural	
	Interval	MAFM	Interval	MAFM	Interval	MAFM
1957	2.455	19.23	1.907	20.40	2.655	18.90
1964	2.173	19.55	1.740	22.04	2.264	19.17
1970	1.906	20.19	1.679	23.38	1.945	19.89
1977	1.708	22.57	1.573	24.99	1.739	22.11
1980	1.679	23.05	1.651	25.19	1.687	22.54

decline in cohort fertility started much earlier in urban areas. The age pattern of cohort fertility for China's rural population as a whole in 1979–81 was similar to that of the urban population in 1967–9, a time-lag of more than one decade. Changes in cohort fertility in urban areas took place smoothly throughout the 1960s and the 1970s, while changes for the rural population occurred sharply in the 1970s.

It was not until the second half of the 1970s that the cohort fertility rate for women aged 29 began to decline. Despite the vigorous implementation of the 'one-child policy', by the age of 30, women had already had 2.4 children on average in the early 1980s.

Changes affecting older age groups are even smaller. This is not surprising since there was no strict birth control for the most of their reproductive life. They were affected by the 'Wan, Xi, Shao', programme. Longer birth interval was one of the major objectives of that programme. Women were required to postpone their childbearing, but not to stop births permanently. Therefore, it was still possible to achieve the desired family size but in a longer span. Nevertheless, the average number of children ever borne for women who reached their late thirties and over in the 1970s was smaller than their older counterparts. This confirms that the occurrence of births of very high orders has been eliminated over time. The effects of successful birth control during the 1970s on cohort fertililty will be seen more fully in the next several decades.

Cohort–Period Comparison

From China's 1982 Fertility Survey data, age-specific fertility rates can be calculated for every single year of age and time span. These

TABLE 4.12. *Comparison of cohort and period fertility rate*

	P/F ratios in periods									
	1952–4	1955–7	1958–60	1961–3	1964–6	1967–9	1970–2	1973–5	1976–8	1979–81
National										
15–19	1.001	1.079	1.203	0.912	1.058	1.051	1.090	1.121	1.118	1.011
20–4	0.914	0.996	1.372	0.963	0.936	1.104	1.113	1.255	1.338	1.070
25–9	—	0.940	1.275	1.012	0.954	0.986	1.085	1.293	1.454	1.261
30–4	—	—	—	0.984	0.944	1.003	1.059	1.292	1.590	1.551
35–9	—	—	—	—	0.906	0.987	1.054	1.357	1.741	1.802
40–4	—	—	—	—	—	—	1.046	1.398	1.888	2.054
45–9	—	—	—	—	—	—	—	—	1.941	2.222
Rural										
15–19	0.985	1.070	1.217	0.909	1.051	1.047	1.087	1.118	1.107	1.025
20–4	0.901	0.987	1.394	0.948	0.912	1.091	1.100	1.242	1.317	1.057
25–9	—	0.938	1.292	0.997	0.915	0.967	1.070	1.263	1.434	1.238
30–4	—	—	—	0.966	0.896	0.968	1.035	1.266	1.558	1.497
35–9	—	—	—	—	0.854	0.936	1.009	1.315	1.708	1.746
40–4	—	—	—	—	—	—	0.984	1.321	1.827	1.994
45–9	—	—	—	—	—	—	—	—	1.835	2.113
Urban										
15–19	1.079	1.135	1.164	0.963	1.166	1.094	1.132	1.105	1.216	0.926
20–4	0.964	1.024	1.297	1.072	1.201	1.265	1.190	1.420	1.426	1.138
25–9	—	0.935	1.206	1.094	1.266	1.207	1.278	1.553	1.527	1.333
30–4	—	—	—	1.071	1.298	1.305	1.346	1.699	1.870	1.864
35–9	—	—	—	—	1.297	1.401	1.455	1.930	2.250	2.416
40–4	—	—	—	—	—	—	1.593	2.210	2.587	2.877
45–9	—	—	—	—	—	—	—	—	2.955	3.331

completed birth histories enable us to estimate the cumulated period fertility as well as cohort fertility rate for each province. The conventional P/F ratio method then can be used to assist in the interpretation of fertility changes,[35] although the general trend of China's fertility transition has already been clearly shown. P here refers to cohort fertility rate, while F refers to period fertility rate. Since the sampling errors of fertility rates from the fertility survey are often unacceptably high when based on a single-year's experience,[36] the P/F ratios presented here are on a three-year basis.

The picture is similar to that shown earlier. The P/F values in 1958–60 and 1961–3 are affected by massive fertility fluctuations. Moreover, the steady declines in P/F ratios by age in the late 1960s, especially for the rural population, reflect the impact of this disturbance. Fertility in urban areas started falling in the early 1960s. The steep decline took place during the mid-1960s, and speeded up in the early 1970s. For the rural population, the sustained fertility decline emerged in the early 1970s, and became sizeable only in the mid-1970s. By the early 1980s the total period fertility rate in urban areas was only about one-third of the cohort fertility rate. In rural areas, the current period fertility in 1979–81 was less than half of the cohort one.

IV. Effects of Nuptiality and Marital Fertility on Overall Fertility

Because of the peculiar features of Chinese marriage already mentioned in earlier sections, illegitimate births can be neglected in examining China's fertility transition. Overall fertility levels, therefore, are determined by women's marital status and fertility within marriage. In this section, the relative importance of changes in these two fertility components on China's fertility transition are examined. We begin with an analysis of changes in marital fertility.

Changes in Period Marital Fertility Rates

Marital fertility can be estimated from age-specific fertility rate and women's marital status. Here, all are period measures. The time series of proportions of women currently married for each age in different time periods are not available. However, the proportion of women ever married can be estimated by summing age-specific first-marriage rates through the cohort diagram. Because of the stability of Chinese

TABLE 4.13. *Total marital fertility rates, China 1954–1981*

Year	TMFR			Year	TMFR		
	Nation	Urban	Rural		Nation	Urban	Rural
1954	6.98	7.02	7.09	1968	7.55	5.27	8.03
1955	6.96	6.87	7.09	1969	6.82	5.40	7.26
1956	6.45	6.23	6.47	1970	6.81	4.97	7.28
1957	7.20	7.14	7.20	1971	6.74	4.78	7.11
1958	6.28	6.25	6.37	1972	6.28	4.44	6.60
1959	4.90	4.97	4.82	1973	5.94	4.99	6.31
1960	4.52	4.96	4.50	1974	5.77	4.28	6.04
1961	3.69	4.58	3.75	1975	5.17	3.98	5.35
1962	6.62	5.99	6.80	1976	4.84	3.71	5.08
1963	8.30	7.61	8.48	1977	4.34	3.27	4.42
1964	7.08	6.10	7.27	1978	4.42	4.35	4.57
1965	6.98	5.75	7.40	1979	4.55	3.17	4.65
1966	7.36	5.30	7.86	1980	3.72	2.70	3.86
1967	6.31	4.31	6.65	1981	4.21	3.27	4.39

marriage and the rapid decline in adult mortality in the past, this alternative approach is reasonable. On this basis, we have calculated the age-specific and total marital fertility rate for China over the past four decades, separating the rural from the urban. Almost all Chinese women aged 40 and over marry. Hence, the age-specific marital fertility rates for women in their 40s are virtually the same as age-specific fertility rates. Total marital fertility rate (TMFR) between 1954 and 1981 is presented in Table 4.13. The TMFR before 1964 is calculated from recorded and estimated age-specific fertility rates.

Table 4.13 shows that the national TMFR declined by 43 per cent from around 6.9 in the mid-1950s to 3.97 in the early 1980s. During this period, the urban TMFR declined by 56 per cent, compared with 41 per cent in the rural areas. The general trends of fertility within marriage were similar to those of total fertility. There were minor rural–urban differences in the TMFR in the late 1950s. During the period of demographic disturbance, the fluctuation of the rural population was more severe. Urban marital fertility started to decline in the mid-1960s and suffered a setback in the early phase of the Cultural Revolution. Since the early 1970s sustained fertility decline has occurred in both rural and urban areas. On the whole, the magnitudes of fertility reduction within marriage were smaller than those of the total female populations.

Changes in Marital Fertility by Duration

We have shown that accompanying the rise of marriage age, the first-birth interval became compressed over time. In this section, changes in duration-specific marital fertility rates are examined. Cumulated duration-specific rates are recorded in Table 4.14.

It is interesting to discover that except for the abnormal fluctuations around 1960, fertility at duration 0–4 rose steadily through the 1950s and reached its highest level in the mid-1960s. There has been virtually no change since then. This is certainly associated with the changes in nuptiality patterns. In the early 1950s the mean age at first marriage for China as a whole was about 18.7 years, rising to 19.7 in 1965, and further jumping to 23 in 1980. Biological studies have proven that the fecundability of women who married in their teens is relatively lower than for slightly older women. As the occurrence of very early marriage diminishes over time, the fertility of women at their early marriage life rises. Therefore, although China's family-planning programme effectively pushed women to get married later, it did not affect childbearing immediately after marriage. This suggests that the impact of postponing marriage on the overall fertility may be small without other effective controls over the family size.

This early rise in duration fertility can be found at duration 5–9 as well. But fertility at this duration began decline around the mid-1970s and fell sharply afterwards.

For those higher durations, duration fertility reached a peak in the period 1964–5. A steep decline started in the late 1960s and speeded up during the 1970s. By the early 1980s there were almost no births which occurred to women who had married 20 years earlier. Births were highly concentrated during the first several years of marriage.

Urban China also experienced the early rise in duration fertility rate at duration 0–9 in the 1950s. However, while fertility at duration 0–4 remained constant throughout the 1970s, sustained decline occurred in the urban areas. Trends at longer durations were similar. By the early 1980s there were very few children who were born to mothers at the duration 10–14 (and higher) in the urban areas, whereas rural women at this duration were still very active in terms of childbearing.

Generally speaking, the movement of marital fertility has been similar to that of total fertility. Decline in marital fertility was earlier and steeper for the urban population, which indicates that the family-planning campaigns were carried out more successfully in the urban areas.

TABLE 4.14. *Cumulated duration fertility rate up to the end of duration*

Marital duration	1949–51	1952–4	1955–7	1958–60	1961–3	1964–6	1967–9	1970–2	1973–5	1976–8	1979–81
National											
0–4	1.34	1.56	1.59	1.19	1.45	1.71	1.74	1.78	1.77	1.74	1.72
5–9	2.74	3.05	3.11	2.41	2.94	3.30	3.34	3.28	3.07	2.74	2.56
10–14	—	4.37	4.44	3.44	4.23	4.67	4.63	4.47	3.94	3.29	2.92
15–19	—	—	5.52	4.29	5.24	5.75	5.65	5.36	4.51	3.61	3.10
20–4	—	—	—	—	5.83	6.43	6.25	5.91	4.84	3.77	3.19
25–9	—	—	—	—	—	6.67	6.44	6.06	4.95	3.83	3.22
30+	—	—	—	—	—	6.71	6.47	6.08	4.96	3.84	3.23
Rural											
0–4	1.30	1.54	1.55	1.12	1.40	1.72	1.74	1.79	1.79	1.76	1.80
5–9	2.71	3.03	3.08	2.31	2.93	3.42	3.43	3.38	3.18	2.84	2.71
10–14	—	4.37	4.42	3.36	4.25	4.93	4.88	4.73	4.15	3.45	3.12
15–19	—	—	5.51	4.23	5.31	6.12	6.03	5.77	4.83	3.84	3.33
20–4	—	—	—	4.37	5.94	6.88	6.72	6.40	5.24	4.03	3.44
25–9	—	—	—	—	—	7.14	6.93	6.58	5.36	4.09	3.48
30+	—	—	—	—	—	7.19	6.96	6.59	5.37	4.11	3.48
Urban											
0–4	1.51	1.65	1.74	1.52	1.65	1.64	1.76	1.74	1.63	1.60	1.33
5–9	2.87	3.12	3.27	2.83	3.04	2.80	2.89	2.68	2.33	2.09	1.62
10–14	—	4.36	4.54	3.82	4.14	3.56	3.53	3.19	2.65	2.24	1.68
15–19	—	—	5.47	4.56	4.89	4.08	3.90	3.44	2.78	2.30	1.69
20–4	—	—	—	—	5.30	4.36	4.09	3.57	2.82	2.31	1.70
25–9	—	—	—	—	—	4.46	4.15	3.60	2.83	2.32	1.70
30+	—	—	—	—	—	4.47	4.16	3.60	2.84	2.32	1.70

Source: Computed from A. Coale and Chen Shengli 1986.

Marriage versus marital fertility

It is instructive to ask what are the net effects of changing nuptiality and marital fertility on China's fertility transition. To answer this question, a decomposition procedure has been adopted. The age-specific marital fertility rate and the proportion of women ever married up to certain age in 1964 are taken as references, along with the TFR. The equation used here for the decomposition is:

$$TFR^i - TFR^r = \Sigma\ [1/2(M_a^{\,i} + M_a^{\,r})(G_a^{\,i} - G_a^{\,r}) + 1/2(G_a^{\,i} + G^{ar})(M_a^{\,i} - M_a^{\,r})]$$

Where:

$M_a^{\,i}$ is the proportion of women ever married up to age *a* in year *i*

$G_a^{\,i}$ is the age-specific marital fertility rate for age *a* in year *i*

r refers to reference

The first part of the right-hand side of the equation indicates the effect of changes in marital fertility and the second part refers to the impact of nuptiality changes. The advantage of using this equation is that it can simplify the work and eliminates the interactive effects. Results of the decomposition are presented in Table 4.15.

Table 4.15 shows that both changes in nuptiality and fertility within marriage contributed to the decline in total fertility rate. During the period between the mid-1960s and the early 1980s, China's total fertility declined by about 60 per cent. While change in nuptiality accounted for about 20 per cent of this decline, reduction of marital fertility alone was responsible for the remaining 80 per cent. In other words, changes in marital fertility rates played the most important role in TFR changes.

China's fertility fluctuated during the second half of the 1960s, probably because of the Cultural Revolution. The 1967 trough was certainly caused by the massive marriage deficit and fewer conceptions during the previous year 1966 when the country was caught up in the mass movement. On the other hand, the 1968 peak reflected the anarchic situation in 1967. On the whole, fertility remained more or less constant for China as a whole and in the rural areas as well during this period. However, an average 23 per cent fertility reduction was recorded in the urban areas; 78 per cent of this decline was due to fertility changes within marriage. Compared with the first half of the 1970s, the importance of marriage change on TFR was smaller in the late 1960s. This may reflect the effects of the Cultural Revolution. After a sharp increase in the mid-1960s, the age at marriage fell slightly in the following few years, although it was still higher than that of the

TABLE 4.15. *Changes in TFR and the effects of components changes* (%)

Year	National			Urban			Rural		
	TFR	Marital Fertility	Marriage	TFR	Marital Fertility	Marriage	TFR	Marital Fertility	Marriage
1965	−1.6	26.0	74.0	−15.7	81.7	18.3	+0.5	—	—
1966	+1.3	—	—	−31.7	82.4	17.6	+5.9	—	—
1967	−14.0	78.3	21.7	−36.6	82.6	17.4	−10.9	74.8	25.2
1968	+4.6	—	—	−12.8	50.3	49.7	+7.0	—	—
1969	−7.3	58.0	42.0	−26.7	75.8	24.2	−4.6	38.7	61.3
1970	−5.9	34.2	65.8	−27.7	68.8	31.2	−0.27	-24.7	124.7
1971	−11.9	55.6	44.4	−37.1	69.1	30.9	−0.84	45.2	54.8
1972	−19.4	65.6	34.4	−43.2	71.1	28.9	−16.1	64.4	35.6
1973	−26.8	68.2	31.8	−49.3	64.3	35.7	−23.7	69.0	31.0
1974	−32.7	68.2	31.8	−59.4	69.6	30.4	−29.2	69.1	30.9
1975	−42.6	72.3	27.7	−64.0	67.4	32.6	−39.6	74.2	25.8
1976	−48.0	73.2	26.8	−68.5	71.9	28.1	−45.3	75.2	24.8
1977	−54.4	75.0	25.0	−69.2	67.8	32.2	−52.4	77.4	22.6
1978	−56.5	74.0	26.0	−69.9	60.4	39.6	−54.7	76.6	23.4
1979	−56.0	72.4	27.6	−74.1	68.5	31.5	−53.5	74.9	25.1
1980	−64.3	78.7	21.3	−79.8	78.4	21.6	−62.1	80.9	19.1
1981	−57.8	77.2	22.8	−73.9	75.1	24.9	−55.4	79.3	20.7

Note: The average of 1964 and 1965 has been taken as the reference.

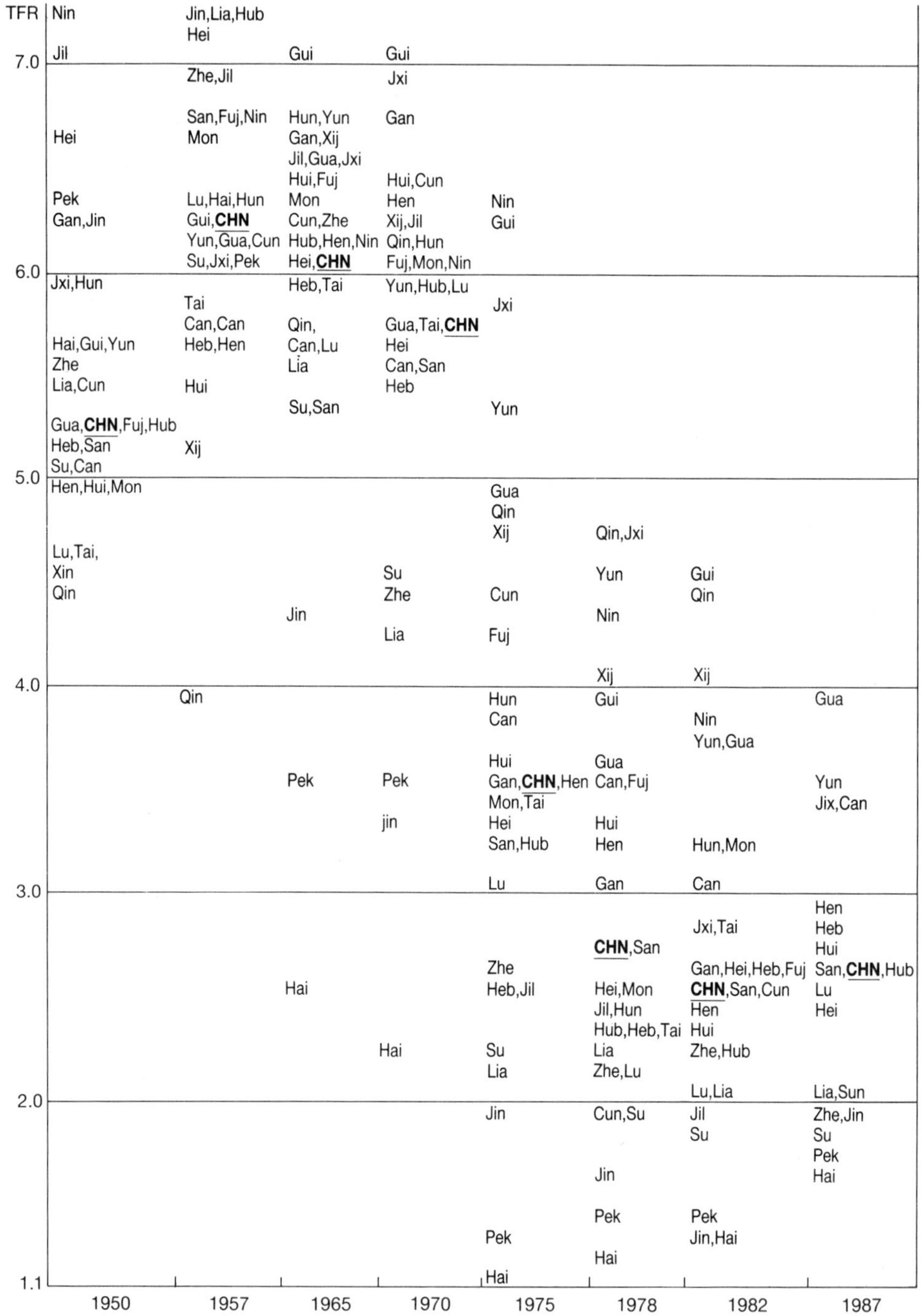

Fig. 4.7 China's fertility trends by province (1950–1987)

INDEX	PROVINCE	INDEX	PROVINCE
CHN	China	Lu	Shandong
Pek	Beijing	Hen	Henan
Jin	Tianjin	Hub	Hubei
Heb	Hebei	Hun	Hunan
Tai	Shanxi	Can	Guangdong
Mon	Nei monggol (MAR)	Gua	Guangxi (MAR)
Hei	Heilongjiang	Yun	Yunnan
Jil	Jilin	Gui	Guizhou
Lia	Liaoning	Cun	Sichuan
Hai	Shanghai	San	Shaanxi
Su	Jiangsu	Gan	Gansu
Zhe	Zhejiang	Nin	Ningxia (MAR)
Hui	Anhui	Qin	Qinghai
Fuj	Fujian	Xij	Xinjiang (MAR)
Jxi	Jiangxi		

Note: MAR refers to Minority Autonomous Region

Sources: Data for 1987 from Jiang Zhenghua 1988.
Others from A. J. Coale and Chen Sheng Li 1987.

early 1960s. Consequently, the continuous decline in urban fertility rate then was mainly brought about by massive fertility decline within marriage.

Astonishing fertility reduction occurred during the 1970s. The net effect of changes in marriage patterns on TFR reduction was great—the result of the rapid increase of age at marriage in the first half of the 1970s. However, its importance declined as time passed. At the beginning of that decade, more than 40 per cent of fertility decline can be attributed to changes in marriage pattern, compared with only slightly above 20 per cent in the early 1980s. The trends in the urban and rural were similar.

It is not surprising that the effect of marriage pattern on overall fertility reduction was relatively small. As was discussed above, despite the great postponement of marriage, Chinese women did eventually get married. Hence, changes in marriage pattern only affects fertility at young ages. Moreover, although marriage patterns were quite different between the early 1980s and the mid-1960s, marital fertility, particularly those older ages and higher marital durations, changed more significantly due to the effective implementation of family-planning programmes. As a result, the reduction of marital fertility was four times more important than changes in marriage patterns.

V. Summary

From the above discussion, some conclusions can be reached. Over the past several decades, dramatic fertility changes have occurred in China.

In the 1950s and 1960s, the fertility level for China as a whole and for the rural population remained more or less constant except during the famine period. During that period, however, fertility at young ages fell steadily as a result of delayed marriage, though this was offset by increased fertility of women in their twenties. Since 1970 China has experienced a sustained and steep fertility decline. Childbearing is more and more concentrated in a compressed age interval and the proportion of higher order births has fallen over time. Compared with the impact of the delayed marriage, the reduction of fertility within marriage, especially at longer durations, played a much more important role in reducing the total fertility level. The fertility transition occurred much earlier, say about one decade, in urban areas. It seems that the urban population is more willing, in some cases may be under pressure, to accept the family-planning programme. Nevertheless, changes in fertility and nuptiality in both the urban and rural populations have been accelerated by the government's determined efforts on population control.

In addition to considerable rural–urban differentials, there are great regional diversities in fertility and nuptiality changes. This will be discussed in later chapters. But the general picture may be presented at this point.

In Figure 4.7, provinces are ranked according to their levels of the total fertility rates in the selected years. Generally speaking, China's regional fertility transition is a process of diffusion. Sustained fertility decline started in a few large municipalities and some eastern provinces. Thereafter the transition gradually spread to the interior. By the later 1970s fertility in eastern China had been reduced to around replacement level. In contrast, the area covering the northwest and southwest of China entered the transition much later and relatively high fertility has persisted to the present.

NOTES

1. See e.g. A. J. Coale, *Rapid Population Change in China 1952–1982* (Washington DC: National Academy Press, 1984).
2. See e.g. J. Hobcraft *et al.*, 'Advances in the P/F Ratio Method for the Analysis of Birth Histories', *Population Studies*, 36 (2), 291–316 (1982).
3. Technical discussion of that method can be found in a special issue of the *Renkou yu jingji (Population and Economy)* (Beijing, 1983), 35.
4. A. J. Coale and Chen Shengli, *Basic Data on Fertility in the Provinces of China, 1940–82* (Honolulu: East–West Population Institute, 1987).
5. For instance, the directly calculated incomplete fertility rate up to age 39 for China as a whole between 1954 and 1956 was 5.51, Coale and Chen's estimate of TFR for

the same period was 5.86. This means that the 40–49 age group contributed less than 6% of the TFR. This figure is certainly too low bearing in mind that there was apparently no birth control effort at that time.

6. G. Barclay *et al.*, 'A Reassessment of the Demography of Traditional Rural China', *Population Index*, 42 (4), 606–35 (1976).
7. State Statistical Bureau of PRC, *Statistical Yearbook of China, 1986*.
8. Ma Yinchu, 'Xin renkou lun (New Population Theory)', *People's Daily*, 5 July 1957.
9. See Tian Xueyuan, 'A Survey of Population Growth since 1949', in Liu Zheng *et al.*, *China's Population: Problems & Prospects* (Beijing: New World Press, 1981), 52.
10. See *People's Daily*, 25 May 1958.
11. A detailed analysis of the fertility consequence of the Great Leap Forward can be found in Xizhe Peng, 'The Demographic Consequences of the Great Leap Forward in China's Provinces', *Population and Development Review*, 13 (4), 639–70 (1987).
12. Quoted from Jiang Zhenghua, 'Reasons for Fertility Decline in China', paper presented at the Seminar on Fertility Transition in Asia: Diversity and Change, Bangkok, 28–31 Mar. 1988.
13. See *Liao Wang (Outlook Weekly)*, No. 28 (July 1987).
14. 'Constitution of the People's Republic of China', see Editorial Committee, *1983 Zhonghua renmin gongheguo nianjian (1983 People's Republic of China Yearbook)* (Beijing: Xinhua, 1984), 419–36.
15. P. C. Smith, 'The Impact of Age at Marriage and Proportions Marrying on Fertility', in R. A. Buiatao and R. D. Lee (eds.), *Determinants of Fertility in Developing Countries* (New York: Academic Press, 1983), ii. 473.
16. E. J. Croll, *The Politics of Marriage in Contemporary China* (Cambridge: Cambridge University Press, 1981).
17. C. K. Yang, *The Chinese Family in the Communist Revolution* (Cambridge, Mass.: MIT Press, 1965).
18. Croll, *Politics of Marriage*.
19. There is a considerable literature in Chinese sources on the subject. See e.g. 'Booming Marriage Introduction Services', *Beijing Review*, 18 (4 May 1981), 27–8.
20. Yang, *Chinese Family*.
21. See e.g. W. L. Parish and M. K. Whyte, *Village and Family in Contemporary China* (London: University of Chicago Press, 1978).
22. Li Ning, 'How does China deal with Divorce?', *Beijing Review*, 5 (4 Feb. 1985), 18–21.
23. Zeng Yi, 'Marriage and Marriage Dissolution in China: A Marital Status Life Table Analysis', paper presented at the 20th general conference of IUSSP, Florence, Italy, 5–12 June 1985.
24. *Zhongguo Funu (Women of China)*, No. 9 (1987).
25. J. Hobcraft, 'Family-Building Patterns', in J. Cleland and J. Hobcraft (eds.), *Reproductive Change in Developing Countries* (Oxford: Oxford University Press, 1985), 64–86.
26. Barclay *et al.*, 'Reassessment of the Demography', cited in n. 6 above.
27. Zhao Weigang and Yu Huilin, 'Changes of Women's Age at First Marriage since the Liberation', in the special issue of *Population and Economy* (Beijing, 1983).
28. Croll, *Politics of Marriage*.
29. E. Snow, *China's Long Revolution* (London: Penguin Books, 1972).
30. Zhao Weigang and Yu Huilin, 'Changes of Women's Age'.
31. Coale, *Rapid Population Change in China*.
32. Coale and Chen Shengli, *Basic Data on Fertility*.

33. See e.g. M. Kendall, 'The World Fertility Survey: Current Status and Findings', *Population Report*, Series M, No. 3 (1979).
34. W. R. Lavely, 'The Rural Chinese Fertility Transition: A Report from Shifan Xian, Sichuan', *Population Studies*, 38 (3), 365–84 (1986).
35. Hobcraft *et al.*, 'Advances in the P/F Ratio Method'.
36. See e.g. R. Little, 'Sampling Errors of Fertility Rates from the World Fertility Survey', WFS Tech. 1589 (1981).

5

Fertility Transition in Urban China

I. Introduction

Compared with many other developing countries, the level of urbanization in China is low: only 20.5 per cent of its total population lived in urban areas in 1982. China is generally considered to be a rural country; however, it is also a country of great cities. There are more than 200 million urban dwellers, a figure larger than the total population of either Japan or Indonesia.

Having analysed China's national trends in nuptiality and fertility, our focus now turns to the provincial patterns of the fertility transition. In the previous chapter we saw that the fertility trends in the urban and rural areas were similar during the 1950s, but that urban fertility was always slightly lower. Both the rural and urban populations experienced a massive fertility fluctuation during the period 1958–63. Urban fertility started its decline immediately following the peak in 1963, which was the result of fertility compensation, while rural fertility remained more or less constant until the early 1970s. There is roughly a one-decade time-lag between the urban and rural areas. Although the general trends are similar, the urban–rural differences in fertility changes are substantial.

Besides other socio-economic factors, the earlier implementation of the family-planning programme in the urban areas is one of the most important factors responsible for this urban–rural difference. The first two of China's birth-control campaigns were urban-orientated and left the vast rural areas almost untouched in the 1950s and 1960s. In addition, overall fertility in individual provinces is inevitably affected by the level of urbanization which varies greatly between provinces.

Historically, China's economy and population were highly concentrated in the eastern provinces. This led to a relatively high level of urbanization along China's eastern seaboard. Since 1949 great efforts have been made to develop the inland areas. Immigration to large cities along the coastal areas was strictly controlled, while the movement to the inland urban areas was relatively encouraged.[1] Consequently, the inland provinces in general experienced a relatively faster process of urbanization, while changes in the eastern provinces were small. Affected by government policies, the degree of urbanization is not closely connected with the provincial economic situation nor the population density.

Apart from the three major municipalities, Beijing, Tianjin, and Shanghai, the proportion of the urban population in 1982 varied from a high of 42 per cent for Liaoning province to a low of 11.8 per cent for Guangxi autonomous region. The northeast is the most urbanized area.

Such factors dictate that the provincial patterns of fertility transaction are considered separately for rural and urban population. In this chapter, the urban fertility transition at the provincial level is discussed, including the impact of marriage and other relevant factors.

In China's 1982 Fertility Survey, women were classified according to their current place of residence, as were their maternity histories. The implication of this procedure is that there was no migration between the rural and the urban areas throughout the last four decades. Because of the very slow process of urbanization in China, especially during the 1960s and 1970s, this assumption is probably close to reality. However, the fertility level for the urban population in the 1950s may be exaggerated because of the rapid urban expansion at that time.[2] Therefore, the urban fertility in the 1950s should be treated with some caution.

Qinghai and Ningxia provinces are sometimes excluded from the general comparison, because of their abnormal fertility fluctuations, which are believed to be caused mainly by reporting and sampling errors.[3] The population in these two provinces is only 0.8 per cent of the national total in 1982. Thus the general picture will not be distorted by their exclusion.

The fertility level is sometimes measured by the Partial Total Fertility Rate (PTFR) which is defined as accumulated period fertility rate up to age 39. As noted earlier, the upper-age limit of China's Fertility Survey is 67. The complete sets of fertility rates are only available from 1964 onwards. Many indirect techniques can be used to replenish the fertility rate prior to 1964. But because the massive fertility fluctuation happened in the late 1950s and the early 1960s, the risk of distortion is more likely to occur when an effort is made to reconstruct the complete sets of TFRs by employing extrapolation methods.

My preference here is for accuracy rather than completeness. Therefore, only original data are used at the cost of omitting the fertility for the 40–9 age group. This may slightly underestimate the magnitude of the overall fertility decline.

II. General Patterns

China's provincial fertility trend for the urban population is presented in Figure 5.1. Provinces, except for Qinghai and Ningxia, are ranked in accordance with their PTFRs for the selected years.

One can see from the figure that all provinces experienced great fertility decline over the last three decades or so. However, such a transition was by no means homogeneous. There were substantial regional differences in the original level of fertility, the timing, and the path of the decline.

Provincial Fertility Trend

In the mid-1950s (which here refers to 1954–7), high urban fertility was a national phenomenon. The provincial PTFRs were around 5.2 and the regional differences in the PTFR were relatively small compared with those in later years. There was no clear-cut geographical pattern, but the PTFRs in three northeastern provinces were among the highest 25 per cent of provinces.

The massive fertility crisis in the later 1950s also hit China's urban areas. Generally speaking, the crisis was less severe in urban than in rural areas. Compared with the pre-crisis level, urban China lost or postponed one normal year's total births over the crisis period. However, there existed great regional diversities. For instance, the urban population in Guizhou province was hit most severely by the crisis: its massive fertility deficit started in 1959 and continued until 1962. During this four-year period, lost or postponed births in Guizhou's urban area amounted to 1.7 times its annual total births under the normal conditions at that time. On the other hand, the crisis in Jiangsu was moderate: it lasted 2 years and the total fertility loss was equivalent to half a year's normal births. Most provinces recovered from the crisis in 1962 and their fertility returned to the pre-crisis level in 1963.

The sustained urban fertility decline began immediately after the massive fertility fluctuations. In late 1962 the Chinese government launched its second, or the first effective, birth-control programme. Partly as a result of the swift response to the programme, two-thirds of all 26 provinces had experienced a more than 20 per cent fertility decline from their pre-transition level by 1964. Five of them, including Shanghai, Tianjin, Beijing, Zhejiang, and Fujian, had achieved a more than 30 per cent fertility reduction. By contrast, the partial total

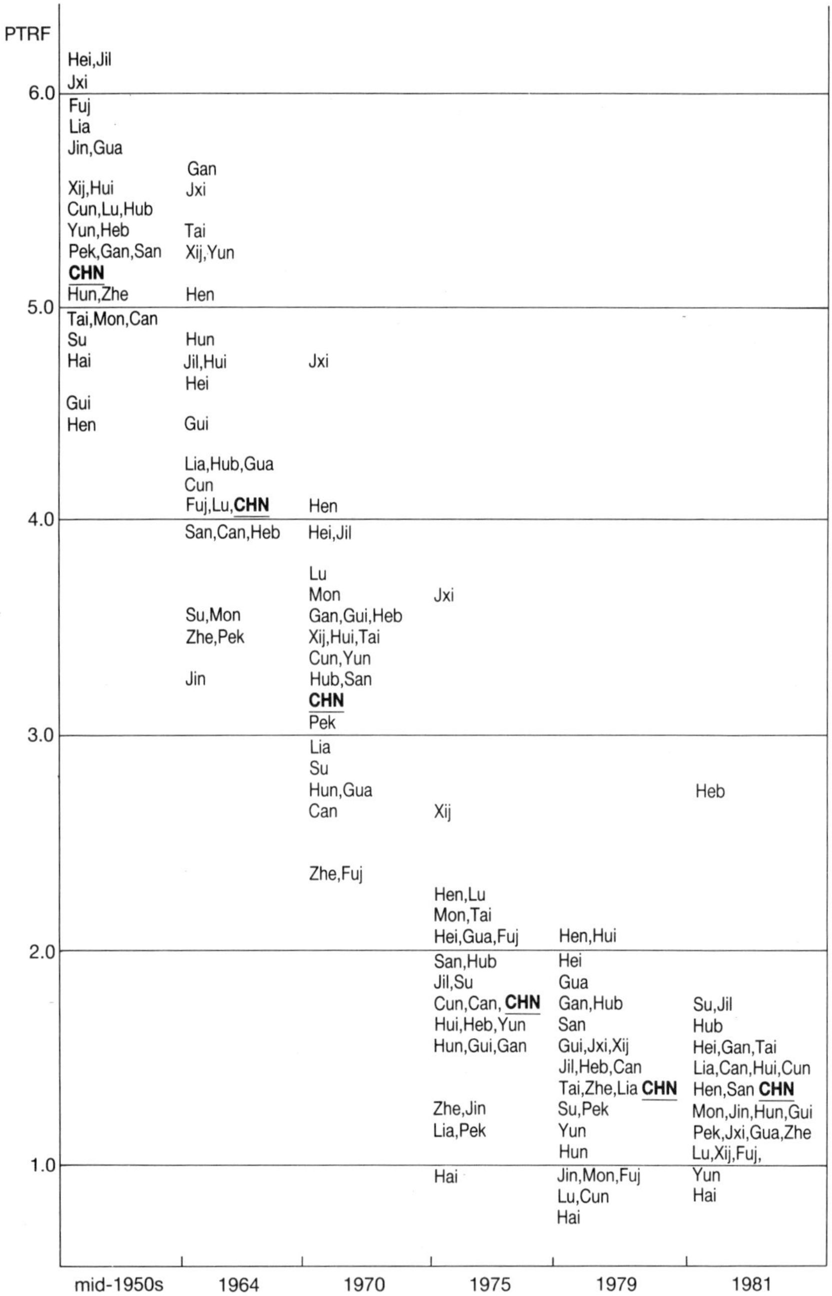

Fig. 5.1 China's urban fertility trends (mid-1950s–1981)

1). Keys for the figures 5.1 and 6.1 illustrating China's urban and rural fertility trends are the same as for the figure of the national fertility trends.

CHN : China national,	Hui : Anhui	San : Shaanxi
Can : Guangdong	Hub : Hubei	Su : Jiangsu
Cun : Sichuan	Hun : Hunan	Tai : Shanxi
Fuj : Fujian	Jil : Jilin	Xij : Xinjiang
Gui : Guizhou	Jin : Tianjin	Yun : Yunnan
Hai : Shanghai	Jxi : Jiangxi	Zhe : Zhejiang
Gan : Gansu	Lia : Liaoning	Qin : Qinghai
Gua : Guangxi	Lu : Shandong	Nin : Ningxia
Heb : Hebei	Mon : Neimonggu	
Hei : Heilongjiang	Pek : Beijing	
Hen : Henan		

fertility rate in Henan, Gansu, and Shanxi increased above the mid-1950s' level. A 12.3 per cent fertility increase was recorded in Henan province, which was clearly the combined outcome of the province's very low PTFR in the mid-1950s and prolonged fertility compensation after the crisis. The fertility levels of the remaining provinces were more or less unchanged.

It is interesting to note that fertility transition in Shanghai started much earlier than in other areas. Shanghai's fertility began to fall markedly in 1958 and the decline has continued ever since. While all other provinces experienced some kind of fertility compensation in 1962 and 1963, Shanghai's fertility remained at a very low level, and its PTFR was already below 2 in 1964. Thus it is likely that the fertility crisis in Shanghai was moderate. Hence we can say without being misleading that Shanghai's fertility transition started as early as the late 1950s.

During the period 1964–70 provincial fertility showed another major fluctuation, although not as large as the previous one. This phenomenon was clearly related to the process of the Cultural Revolution. In most provinces, the fertility reached a trough in 1966–7. This may reflect the continuation of the downward trend that had started several years before. On the other hand, it may also result from the chaotic events of the Cultural Revolution, which was launched in the summer of 1966. Following that, a small period fertility peak in 1968 was observed in almost all provinces. This peak is undoubtedly associated with social disturbances and destruction of government functions in 1967. We will discuss this later.

The difference between the highest and the lowest TFR was 2.7 fold in 1970. Nevertheless, we can see from the figure that, except for Jiangxi, the total fertility rate was everywhere lower than the lowest value 15 years earlier. All nine provinces with a TFR lower than 3 in

TABLE 5.1. *China's urban fertility trends by provinces*[a]

Province	1950s[b]	1964			1970		1975		1980	
	PTFR	PTFR	% Change	TFR	TFR	% Change	TFR	% Change	TFR	%Change
CHINA	5.18	4.08	–21.2	4.40	3.27	–25.7	1.78	–45.6	1.15	–35.4
Heilongjiang	6.07	4.64	–23.6	5.15	4.14	–19.6	2.09	–49.5	1.51	–27.8
Jilin	6.02	4.78	–20.5	5.42	4.02	–25.8	1.86	–53.7	1.05	–43.5
Jiangxi	6.00	5.58	–7.0	6.01	5.24	–12.8	3.65	–30.3	1.22	–66.6
Fujian	5.98	4.04	–32.4	4.32	2.35	–45.6	2.02	–14.0	1.05	–48.0
Liaoning	5.88	4.29	–27.0	5.55	2.94	–47.0	1.16	–60.5	1.20	3.4
Tianjin	5.78	3.27	–43.4	3.54	1.83	–48.3	1.26	–31.1	1.17	–7.1
Guangxi	5.73	4.22	–26.4	5.20	2.95	–43.3	2.11	–28.5	0.96	–54.5
Xinjiang	5.42	5.26	–3.0	5.26	3.69	–29.8	2.67	–27.6	0.94	–64.8
Anhui	5.41	4.71	–12.9	5.36	3.57	–33.4	1.85	–48.2	1.59	–14.1
Sichuan	5.39	4.13	–23.4	4.51	3.59	–20.4	1.82	–49.3	0.83	–54.4
Shandong	5.39	4.04	–25.0	4.29	3.93	–8.4	2.27	–42.2	1.08	–52.4
Hubei	5.35	4.28	–20.0	4.50	3.50	–22.2	1.94	–44.6	1.32	–32.0
Hebei	5.27	3.93	–25.4	4.29	3.78	–11.9	1.69	–55.3	1.38	–18.3
Yunnan	5.27	5.22	–1.0	5.68	3.37	–40.7	1.71	–49.3	1.00	–41.5
Beijing	5.26	3.46	–34.3	3.58	3.05	–14.8	1.13	–63.0	1.29	14.2
Gansu	5.24	5.63	+7.5	5.85	3.78	–35.4	1.53	–59.5	1.03	–32.7
Shaanxi	5.22	3.97	–24.0	4.33	3.40	–21.5	1.99	–41.5	1.46	–26.6
Hunan	5.06	4.86	–4.0	5.11	2.72	–46.8	1.57	–42.3	1.32	–15.9
Zhejiang	5.04	3.46	–31.4	3.59	2.36	–34.3	1.27	–46.2	0.65	–48.8

Nei Monggol	4.98	3.56	–28.5	3.85	3.74	–2.9	2.22	–40.6	1.49	–32.9
Shanxi	4.98	5.36	+7.6	5.90	3.85	–34.7	2.13	–44.7	1.78	–16.4
Guangdong	4.93	3.97	–19.5	4.18	2.63	–37.1	1.78	–32.3	1.62	–9.0
Jiangsu	4.82	3.58	–25.7	3.79	2.95	–22.2	1.81	–38.6	0.84	–53.6
Shanghai	4.75	1.62	–65.9	1.65	1.75	6.1	0.95	–45.7	0.61	–35.8
Guizhou	4.53	4.43	–2.3	4.84	3.76	–22.3	1.68	–55.3	0.89	–47.0
Henan	4.48	5.03	+12.3	5.34	4.32	–19.1	2.40	–44.4	1.20	–50.0
MEAN	5.32	4.28	–19.2	4.66	3.35	–26.7	1.87	–43.8	1.17	–33.7
MEDIAN	5.27	4.250	–23.50	4.675	3.535	–24.07	1.835	–44.62	1.185	–34.34
ST.D.	0.45	0.870	18.65	0.981	0.786	14.47	0.549	11.46	0.299	20.98
MIN.	4.48	1.620	–65.90	1.650	1.750	–48.31	0.950	–62.95	0.610	–66.57
MAX.	6.07	5.630	12.30	6.010	5.240	6.06	3.650	–14.04	1.780	14.16
Q1	4.98	3.842	–27.38	4.097	2.885	–37.98	1.560	–50.57	0.955	–50.61
Q3	5.74	4.903	2.47	5.375	3.797	–18.03	2.115	–37.06	1.400	–16.31

[a] Changes are compared with the fertility in the previous period.
[b] Refers to the average of 1954–7.

1970 were located along China's coastal areas, from Liaoning in the north to Guangxi in the south.

The total fertility rate for Shanghai in 1970 was 1.75 which was about 6 per cent higher than that in 1964. Nevertheless, 1.75 was still the national lowest record at that time. About one-third of all provinces witnessed a more than 40 per cent fertility reduction during the period 1964–70. Only in Shandong and Nei Monggol were the reductions less than 10 per cent.

During the first half of the 1970s with the implementation of China's third family-planning programme, known as 'Later, Longer, and Fewer', fertility decline accelerated. Nineteen out of 26 provinces experienced more than 40 per cent fertility reduction in this five-year period. The fertility level halved in six provinces, including Beijing, Liaoning, Gansu, Guizhou, Hebei, and Jilin. The fertility decline in these latter four provinces had been moderate in the 1960s, but now they caught up. The smallest decline, 14 per cent, was recorded in Fujian province. This was partly owing to the fact that its TFR had already decreased by 46 per cent in the previous period 1964–70, one of the sharpest falls nationally at that time.

In 1980 urban fertility in all provinces was below the replacement level. The TFR in seven provinces was lower than one. The lowest was again in Shanghai, its TFR being as low as 0.61. By contrast, the TFRs in Anhui, Shanxi, and Guangdong provinces were above 1.5. The highest TFR of 1.78 in Shanxi was 2.9 times the lowest in Shanghai.

The sharpest decline, about 65 per cent, in this period was found in Jiangxi and Xinjiang. Fertility levels in these two provinces were consistently among the highest nationally in the 1960s and the 1970s. In 1980, however, Xinjiang became one of the seven provinces with a TFR below unity.

One can see that in general fertility transition continued through the late 1970s. Provinces where the sustained decline started later speeded up their transition and matched the national pattern.

In the first two years of the 1980s China's urban fertility generally remained at the 1979 level. The decline continued in provinces with a relatively higher fertility rate. However, fertility rates in more than half of all provinces increased slightly, despite success in implementation of the 'one-child policy'. This was mainly caused by the marriage boom following the promulgation of the new marriage law. It seems to suggest that the potential fertility decline for China's urban population is very small. Indeed, merely to consolidate this achievement will be a hard job.

Fertility Variation between Provinces

China's urban fertility differs enormously between provinces. Table 5.2 shows the urban fertility and ratios of provincial fertility rate to the national one for different periods. The provincial diversities are further illustrated in Figure 5.2. Figures for the mid-1950s (1954–7) reflect the situation in the pre-transition period. The fertility variation during the period 1958–63 is not included because of its unusual features. Data are three-year averages in order to smooth the trend and eliminate fluctuations caused by sampling errors.

Differences in regional fertility were not simply caused by the different patterns of fertility transition. The fertility level varied greatly among provinces even in the pre-transition period, perhaps a reflection of differences in natural fertility. In the mid-1950s the provincial PTFR ranged from a high of 6.07 in Heilongjiang to a low of 4.48 in Henan province. The fertility level for Henan and Guizhou province in the mid-1950s was suspiciously low. However, we have not found any plausible explanations for this.

There were seven provinces where fertility was more than 10 per cent higher than the national level, including three northeast provinces: Liaoning, Jilin, and Heilongjiang. Tianjin was among the highest quarter with a PTFR of 5.78. The fertility rate in 15 out of 26 provinces was around the national level with the difference less than 5 per cent. It can be seen that fertility in urban Shanghai and Jiangsu was already very low compared with other provinces.

The period of 1964–6 witnessed a steep urban fertility decline. The regional diversity seems to have widened in this period, which is clearly associated with the difference in the timing of the transition in different provinces. Whereas the ratios for Jiangxi and Gansu exceeded 140, the ratio for Shanghai was as low as 40. Apart from Shanghai, there were another 5 provinces, Beijing, Tianjin, Jiangsu, Zhejiang, and Guangdong, where the total fertility rate was at least 10 per cent below the national level. The total fertility rate for Jiangxi province was the highest—some 2.6 times higher than that for Shanghai in the period 1964–6.

The downward trend continued through the late 1960s. There were 11 provinces with the total fertility rate lower than the national level. Almost all of them were coastal provinces. On the other hand, the total fertility rate in Jiangxi, Henan, and Shanxi remained very high in contrast to the sharp decline elsewhere.

The transition process speeded up through the 1970s. Although the fertility rate dropped in every province, the pace was quite varied.

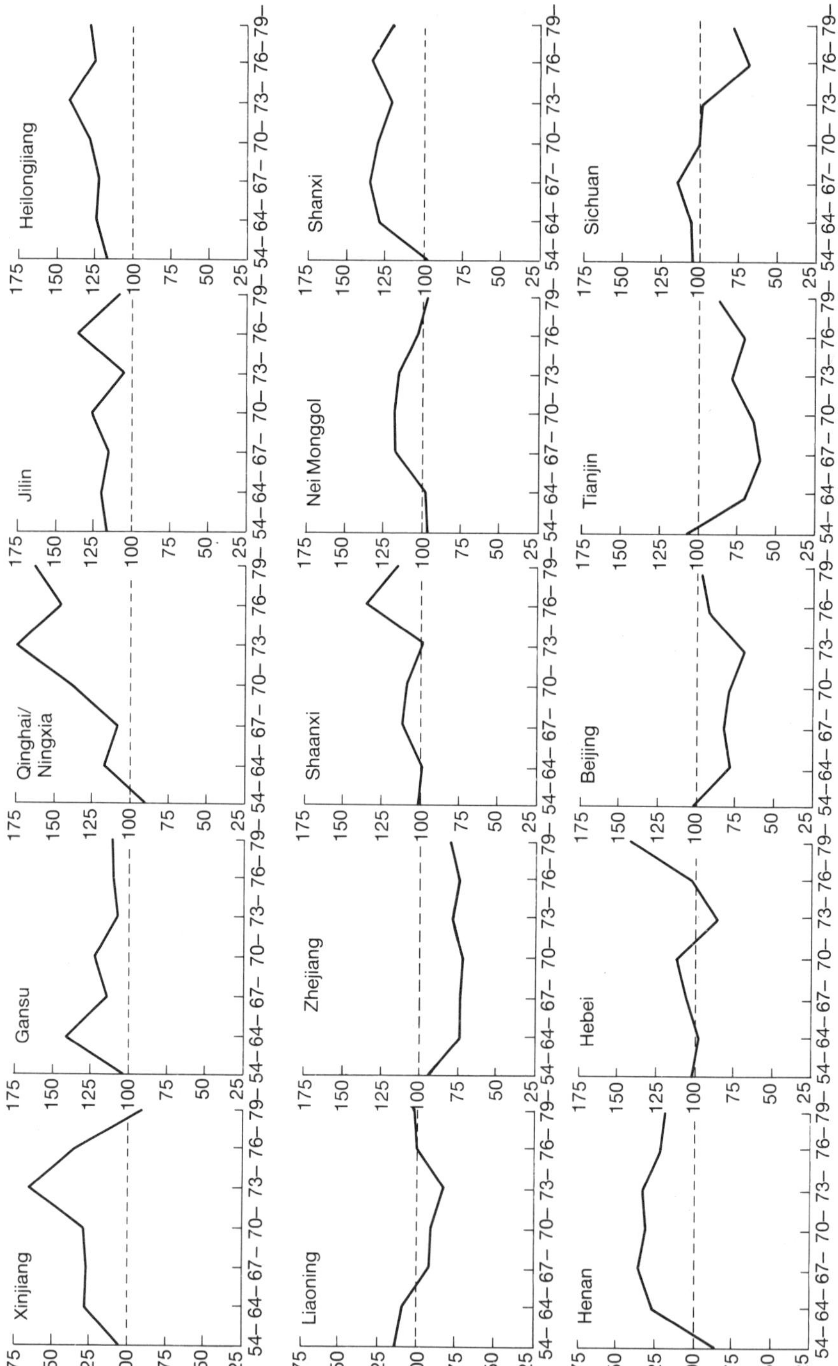
Xinjiang
Gansu
Qinghai/ Ningxia
Jilin
Heilongjiang
Liaoning
Zhejiang
Shaanxi
Nei Monggol
Shanxi
Henan
Hebei
Beijing
Tianjin
Sichuan
175
150
125
100
75
50
25
54– 64– 67– 70– 73– 76– 79–

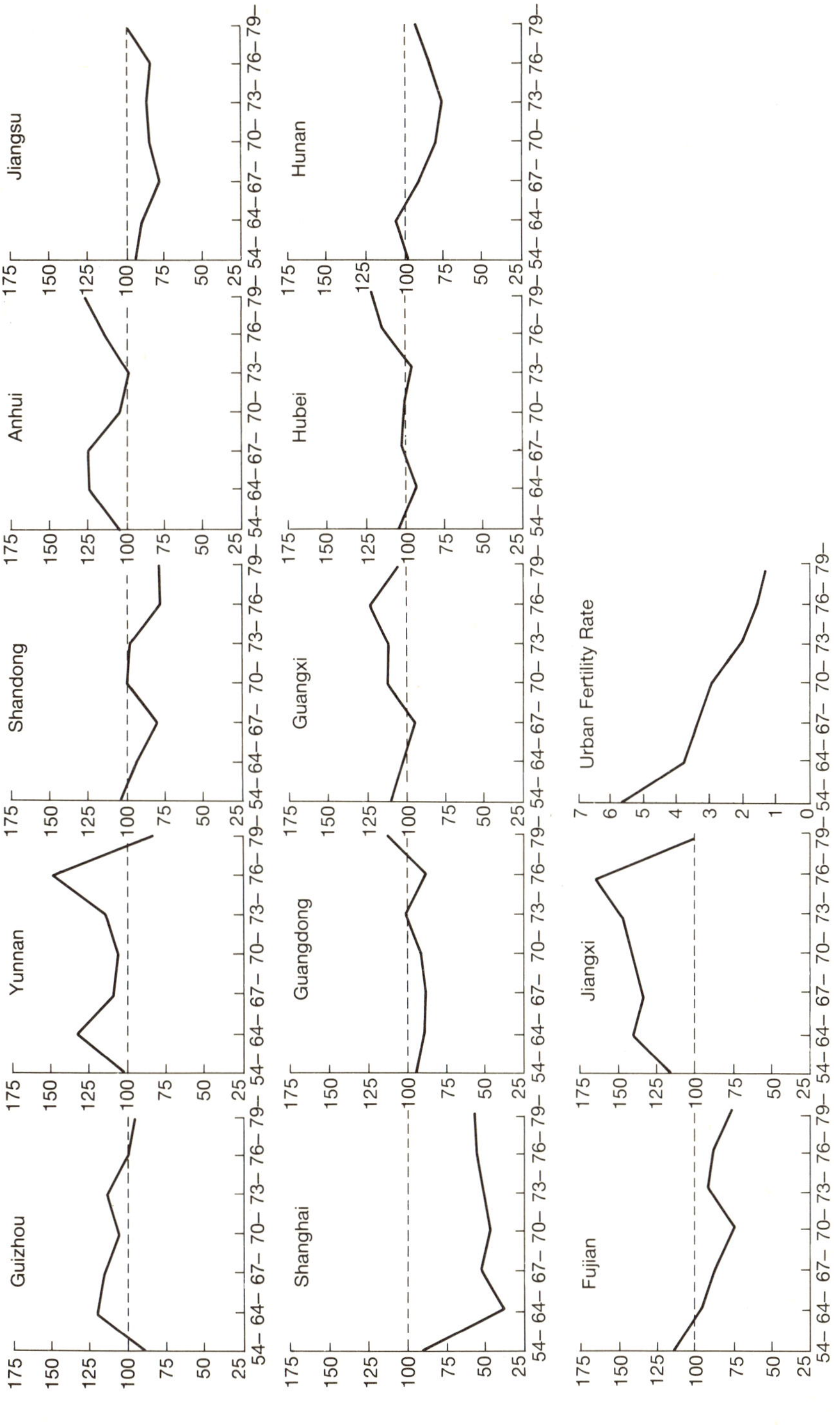

Fig. 5.2 Ratios of provincial fertility rates to national ones, urban 1950–1981

TABLE 5.2. *Urban fertility rates and ratios of provincial fertility to the national rate*[a]

Province	1954–7		1964–6		1967–9		1970–2		1973–5		1976–8		1979–81	
	PTFR[b]	Ratio	TFR	Ratio	TFR	Ratio	TFR	Ratio	TFR	Ratio	TFR	Ratio	TFR	Ratio
CHINA	5.18	100	3.75	100	3.36	100	2.93	100	2.05	100	1.58	100	1.30	100
Heilongjiang	6.07	117	4.66	124	4.08	122	3.76	128	2.92	142	1.98	125	1.68	129
Jilin	6.02	116	4.49	120	3.86	115	3.70	126	2.15	105	2.14	135	1.41	108
Jiangxi	6.00	116	5.31	142	4.52	135	4.15	142	3.04	148	2.63	166	1.31	101
Fujian	5.98	115	3.62	97	2.94	88	2.23	76	1.90	93	1.40	89	1.00	77
Liaoning	5.88	113	4.10	109	3.09	92	2.66	91	1.70	83	1.60	101	1.34	103
Tianjin	5.78	112	2.64	70	2.01	60	1.91	65	1.60	78	1.10	70	1.14	87
Guangxi	5.73	111	3.86	103	3.19	95	3.30	113	2.30	112	1.97	124	1.37	105
Xinjiang	5.42	105	4.80	128	4.28	127	3.79	129	3.37	165	2.13	135	1.17	90
Anhui	5.41	104	4.66	124	4.20	125	3.04	104	2.01	98	1.80	114	1.67	128
Shandong	5.39	104	3.52	94	2.70	80	2.92	100	2.00	98	1.23	78	1.02	79
Sichuan	5.39	104	3.94	105	3.83	114	2.92	100	2.01	98	1.07	68	1.02	78
Hubei	5.35	103	3.48	93	3.44	102	2.94	100	1.95	95	1.82	115	1.58	122
Hebei	5.27	102	3.67	98	3.56	106	3.29	112	1.75	85	1.60	101	1.85	142
Yunnan	5.27	102	5.00	133	3.65	109	3.11	106	2.34	114	2.36	149	1.08	83
Beijing	5.26	102	2.93	78	2.76	82	2.34	79	1.41	69	1.46	92	1.26	97
Gansu	5.24	101	5.28	141	3.82	114	3.58	122	2.20	107	1.74	110	1.44	111
Shaanxi	5.22	101	3.73	99	3.72	111	3.17	108	2.00	98	2.13	135	1.48	114
Hunan	5.06	98	3.98	106	3.06	91	2.33	80	1.56	76	1.33	84	1.20	93
Zhejiang	5.04	97	2.83	75	2.51	75	2.14	73	1.63	80	1.20	76	1.06	82
Nei Monggol	4.98	96	3.69	98	3.93	117	3.47	118	2.35	115	1.63	103	1.25	96
Shanxi	4.98	96	4.83	129	4.52	135	3.80	130	2.49	121	2.11	134	1.55	119
Guangdong	4.93	95	3.39	90	3.00	89	2.71	92	2.08	102	1.39	88	1.48	114
Jiangsu	4.82	93	3.33	89	2.62	78	2.49	85	1.78	87	1.33	84	1.31	101
Shanghai	4.75	92	1.48	40	1.85	55	1.45	49	1.10	54	0.92	58	0.77	59
Guizhou	4.53	88	4.56	121	3.88	116	3.12	106	2.33	114	1.59	100	1.23	95
Henan	4.48	86	4.81	128	4.59	137	3.85	132	2.74	134	1.93	122	1.55	119
MEAN	5.32		3.946		3.447		3.007		2.103		1.676		1.316	
ST.D.	0.45		0.898		0.756		0.677		0.517		0.430		0.251	

[a] All figures are averages of the period.
[b] PTFR: Partial total fertility rate.

Consequently, there was no sign of diminishing the regional variability. For most of the 1970s the highest provincial urban fertility was recorded in Jiangxi province. During this decade, Jiangxi, like other provinces, experienced a sharp fertility decline. In the 1976–8 period its total fertility rate was 2.63, which was roughly 40 per cent lower than its record 10 years earlier. Nevertheless, compared with the national trend the fertility transition in Jiangxi was well behind the other provinces. Its total fertility rate was more than 40 per cent above the national level in the first half of the 1970s and 66 per cent higher in the 1976–8 period.

Shanghai's fertility level has been the lowest in the country since the mid-1960s. Its total fertility rate never exceeded 60 per cent of the national figure over this entire period.

Even ignoring these two extremes, the provincial variation was still substantial. Provinces can be classified into several groups according to the movement of their ratios.

The first consists of Heilongjiang, Jilin, Jiangxi, Anhui, Xinjiang, Gansu, Shanxi, Yunnan, and Guangxi. Fertility rates in these provinces were above the national level throughout the entire period considered here. Guizhou and Henan can also be classified into this group, except for their very low fertility in the mid-1950s. These provinces are scattered in the northeast, the northwest, the southwest, and the central parts of China.

Urban fertility in Shanghai, Jiangsu, and Zhejiang provinces was consistently below the national level. Except for the high fertility in the mid-1950s, Tianjin, Beijing, Fujian, and Shandong in many ways were similar to these three provinces. All seven are neighbouring provinces in the eastern coastal areas. Ratios in other provinces varied from time to time, but they were more or less close to unity, implying similarity to the national pattern of fertility transition.

In summary, one can see that there was always marked regional diversity in terms of China's urban fertility. The original picture of the regional variation changed a lot with the progress of the transition. Nevertheless, some historical patterns remained: fertility in the eastern coastal provinces was lower than the national level, while fertility in the northeast, the northwest, and the southwest provinces was commonly higher than the rest.

The Onset of Fertility Transition

Studies on European fertility transition show that once an initial decline had begun, fertility then continued to fall.[4] It is, therefore, of particular interest to estimate the approximate date of onset of China's urban fertility transition in each province. To avoid the effect of stochastic variation, these estimates are not the turning-point of the initial fertility decline, but are the dates at which certain decline was achieved. Because of the large variation in original fertility level, two criteria have been employed: the date at which the PTFR was more than 15 per cent below the initial level, and the date when the PTFR was for the first time lower than 4.5. The initial fertility level is set in this study as the PTFR in the period 1954–7. We know that the national figure of the urban PTFR in the mid-1950s was about 5.2. Therefore, a PTFR lower than 4.5 undoubtedly marks the beginning of the transition from the national point of view.

Using the PTFR as the fertility measurement may make the estimate of the date of onset slightly later than it might be, since women in their 40s are probably the age group reducing childbearing earliest. However, due to the small contribution of the ASFR for the 40–9 age groups to the TFR, the general picture should not be significantly affected.

The choice of criteria is of course arbitrary, but it is sufficient to indicate that a substantial fertility decline is on the way. Moreover, such a date should also indicate an irreversible trend of the fertility decline in order to avoid misleading by single-year fluctuation or other unusual circumstances. Hence we further define the first criterion as the date at which the PTFR declined by more than 15 per cent from the reference level and remained so for at least the next two consecutive years. The same restriction is added to the second criterion too.

It is very difficult to identify the exact time at which China's urban fertility transition started. The problem here is how to treat the massive fertility deficit which occurred in the period 1958–62. The fertility decline during that period is obviously abnormal. However, we can not ignore the possibility that the massive fertility fluctuation was related to the real fertility regulation. In other words, the real fertility limitation may be concealed by the fertility crisis in a few places.

Annual deviations of the partial total fertility rate from the average value of the index for 1954–7, which is taken as a reference, for 25 provinces, separating the province total, the rural from the urban population, are illustrated in Figure 5.3. In that figure, the index of TL refers to Total Fertility Loss which is defined as the sum of significant (i.e. in excess of 15 per cent) negative differences during the years of crisis for the province. This index (TL) can be viewed as a measure of severity of the fertility crisis. In most provinces, as can be seen from the figure, the massive fertility deficit lasted for about three years from 1959 to 1961. The severity of the crisis varied greatly, the TL ranging

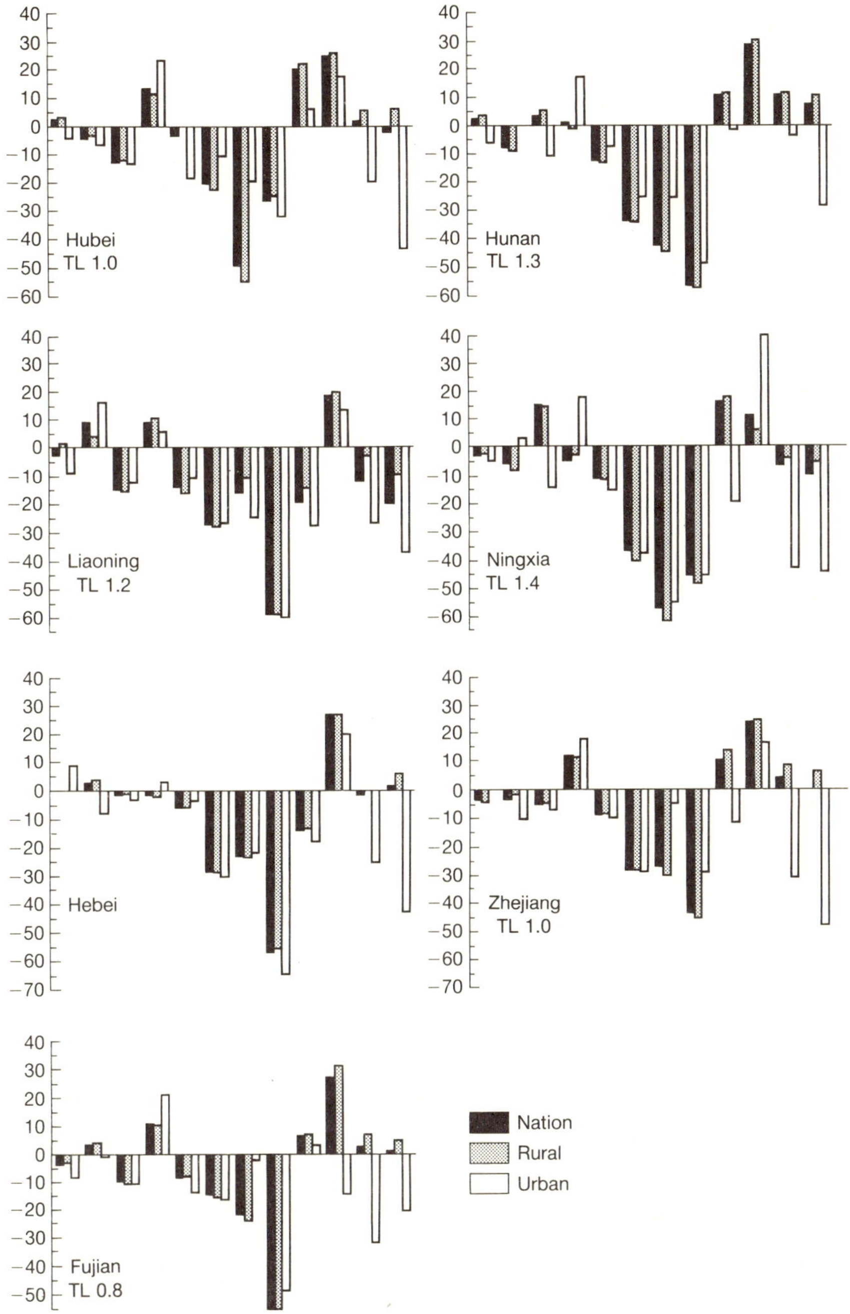
Hubei
TL 1.0
Hunan
TL 1.3
Liaoning
TL 1.2
Ningxia
TL 1.4
Hebei
Zhejiang
TL 1.0
Fujian
TL 0.8
Nation
Rural
Urban

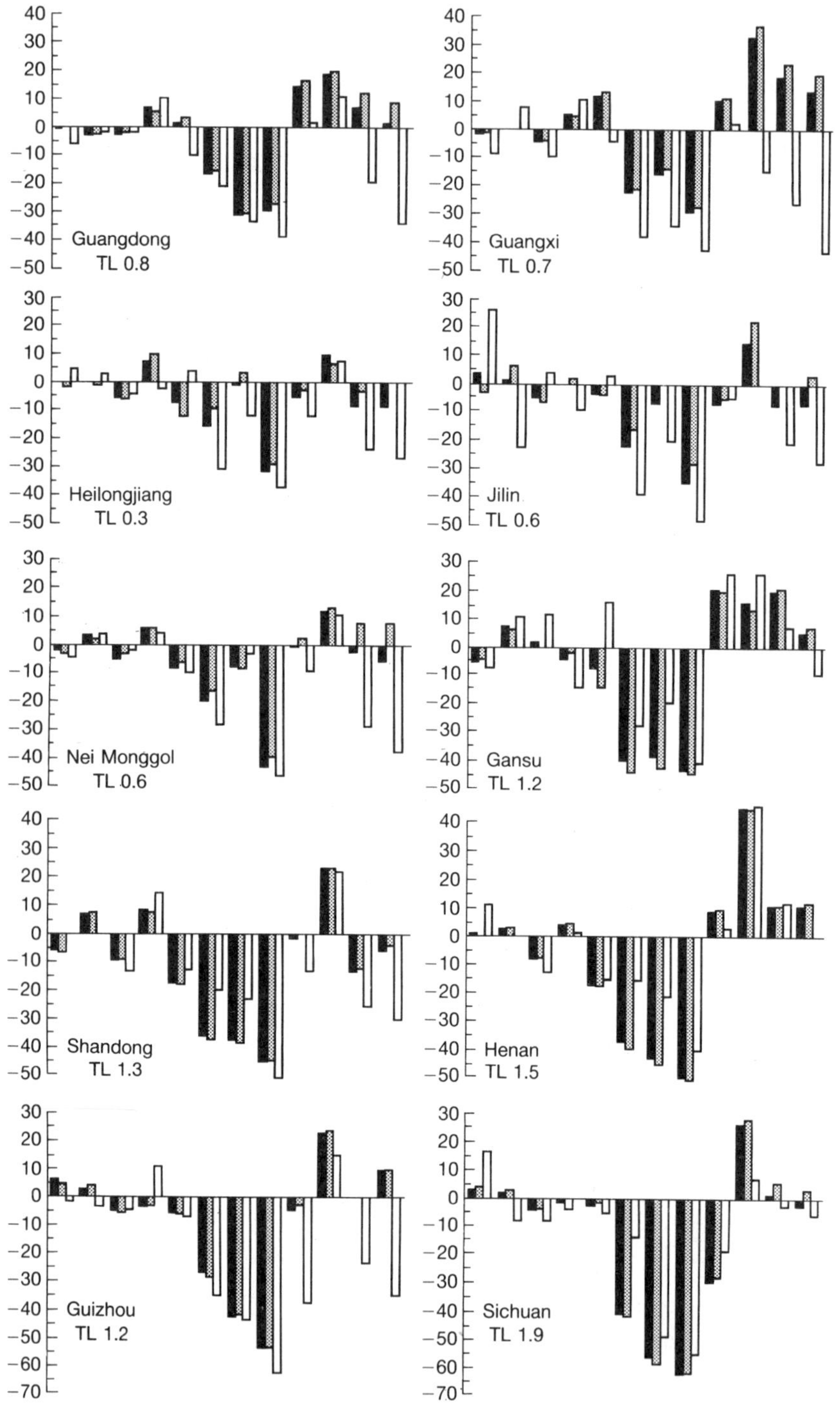
Guangdong
TL 0.8
Guangxi
TL 0.7
Heilongjiang
TL 0.3
Jilin
TL 0.6
Nei Monggol
TL 0.6
Gansu
TL 1.2
Shandong
TL 1.3
Henan
TL 1.5
Guizhou
TL 1.2
Sichuan
TL 1.9

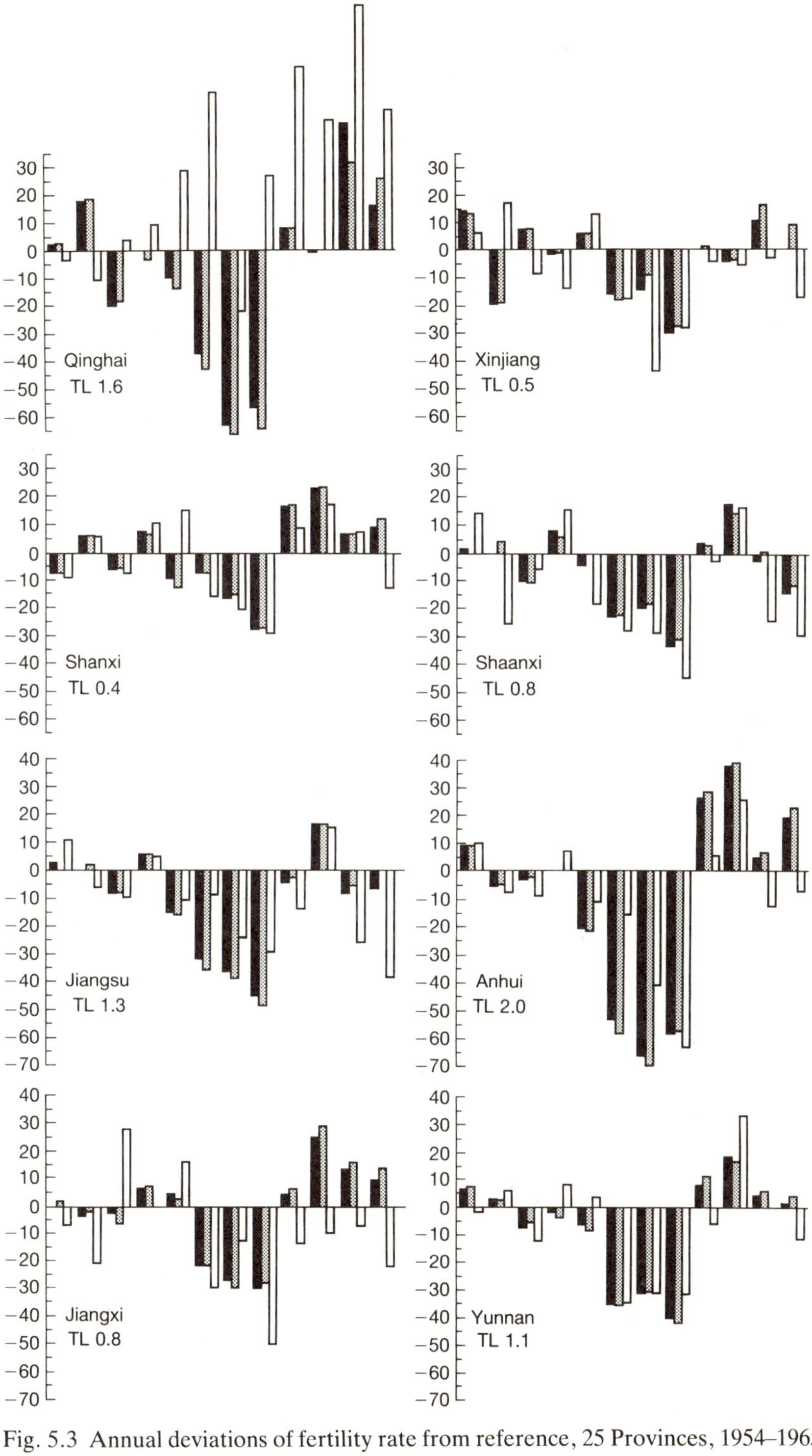

Fig. 5.3 Annual deviations of fertility rate from reference, 25 Provinces, 1954–1965

from a high of 200 per cent in Anhui to a low of 31 per cent in Heilongjiang. This means that in Anhui province the equivalent of two normal years' annual births to women aged 15–39 were lost or postponed during the crisis period. Generally speaking, the broad band of provinces which runs across the central part of China from Sichuan to Jiangsu, but with a gap in the centre, was the area most severely affected by the fertility crisis. In contrast, the far northern and southern parts of China suffered relatively less.

Figure 5.3 also suggests that there was a short time-lag in the fertility crisis between the rural and the urban areas. It seems likely that the urban population did relatively better at the early stage of the crisis. But by 1961, the fertility situation in the majority of towns was as bad as, or even worse than, that of the countryside. The rural population recovered from the crisis more quickly than did urban residents. This picture may reflect the real situation, but may also be slightly distorted by the early start of sustained fertility transition in towns. It is impossible to separate these two different phenomena. Therefore, we have to assume that this abnormal fertility deficit is not the onset of the prolonged fertility transition unless our study proves otherwise.

Estimates of the year when the PTFR declined by more than 15 per cent from the initial level are given for each province in chronological order in Table 5.3, together with the estimates of the second criterion: PTFR < 4.5.

There was no clear linkage between the severity of the fertility crisis and the onset of the sustained fertility transition. The steep fertility decline in most provinces began in 1964, as is indicated by both criteria. While all other provinces witnessed some fertility compensation immediately after the fertility crisis, fertility in urban Shanghai remained at a very low level and was never reversed. It is safe to say that fertility transition in urban Shanghai must have begun in the late 1950s.

The PTFR began to fall below 4.5 one or two years later in Heilongjiang, Jilin, and Fujian provinces. Jiangxi recorded a more than 15 per cent fertility decline first in 1965, but it took about six years for its PTFR to reach the 4.5 level in 1971. Because the original fertility level was very low, Henan's sustained fertility decline started as late as 1971, even though its PTFR first fell below 4.5 much earlier in 1965. The onset date of fertility transition in Gansu province was very late, no matter which criterion is used.

It seems likely that apart from a few exceptions, China's urban fertility transition started around the same time, say the mid-1960s, in each province. But the pace of this transition differed. The total

TABLE 5.3. *Onset date of China's urban fertility transition*

Province	Date at which			
	Drop > 15%	PTFR < 4.5	TFR < 4	TFR < 2
CHINA (urban)	1964	1964	1965	1974
Shanghai	1958	1958	1964	1964
Tianjin	1964	1964	1964	1972
Beijing	1964	1964	1964	1972
Zhejiang	1964	1964	1964	1972
Jiangsu	1964	1964	1964	1972
Hebei	1964	1964	1965	1974
Liaoning	1964	1964	1965	1974
Hubei	1964	1964	1965	1974
Sichuan	1964	1964	1965	1975
Guangdong	1964	1964	1965	1975
Nei Monggol	1964	1964	1964	1979
Guangxi	1964	1964	1965	1978
Shaanxi	1964	1964	1965	1979
Shandong	1964	1964	1966	1976
Guizhou	1964	1964	1970	1975
Fujian	1964	1966	1966	1977
Jilin	1964	1965	1971	1978
Heilongjiang	1964	1965	1971	1978
Hunan	1965	1965	1965	1973
Xinjiang	1965	1965	1972	1978
Jiangxi	1965	1971	1971	1979
Yunnan	1966	1966	1970	1978
Anhui	1966	1966	1966	1975
Shanxi	1966	1965	1970	1978
Gansu	1967	1969	1969	1975
Henan	1971	1965	1967	1976

fertility rate in six provinces, Shanghai, Jiangsu, Zhejiang, Beijing, Tianjin, and Nei Monggol, fell below 4 in 1964. The other seven provinces, Shanxi, Yunnan, Guizhou, Jiangxi, Heilongjiang, Jilin, and Xinjiang, reached this point only in the early 1970s. Furthermore, the total fertility rate in one-third of all provinces first fell below 2 in the early 1970s, the next third reaching this level in 1975–7, and the remaining third in the late 1970s.

Progress of the Urban Fertility Transition

If the date of initial decline was similar in most provinces, the course of China's urban fertility transition was quite different. In this section, we try to document the progress of the provincial fertility transition.

The average of the PTFR in 1979–81 has been treated as the achieved fertility, in order to avoid single-year fluctuations. The total amount of the fertility reduction can be derived by comparing this achieved fertility with the pre-transition level which is set as the average of the PTFRs in 1954–7.

The total fertility reduction during this entire period is calculated for each province and measured in percentage terms. The national figure for the total reduction was 74 per cent. The provincial figures varied from the highest of 84 per cent in Shanghai to the lowest of 66 per cent in Henan province. Although these figures are affected by the variation of the original fertility level, they do provide a measure of the magnitude of the fertility transition at the province level.

Among the lowest quarter are Henan, Shanxi, Anhui, Guangdong, Hubei, and Shaanxi. The fertility decline in these provinces is less than 72 per cent. Shanghai, Sichuan, Fujian, Shandong, Tianjin, and Yunnan compose the highest quarter with a decline of 82 per cent on average.

Taking the total fertility reduction between the mid-1950s and the average of 1979–81 as unity, the progress of the provincial fertility transition can be approximately estimated. By assuming the transition is a continuous process, the amount of fertility reduction up to certain years from the initial level is treated as a percentage of the total fertility reduction throughout the entire period. This is a measure similar to the cumulated fertility rate up to certain ages by assuming the TFR equals 1. The indices of progression are presented in Table 5.4.

At the national (average) level, the fertility reduction between the mid-1950s and the mid-1960s accounted for 43 per cent of the total fertility reduction over the entire period. By the period 1964–6, more than 40 per cent of their total fertility reductions had already taken place in 17 provinces. The top ten of those provinces were all located in eastern China. In Shanghai, the index was as high as 82 per cent, which means that more than four-fifths of Shanghai's fertility transition had already been completed by then. Indeed, if some fluctuations were discounted, the downward tendency of the PTFR was already visible in the late 1950s, at least in those provinces. On the other hand, the fertility decline in Henan, Gansu, Guizhou, Shanxi, Yunnan, and Xinjiang was very insignificant, as indicated by a ratio smaller than 20 per cent.

By the end of the 1960s the fertility transition had passed the half-way mark in 15 provinces, indicated by a ratio higher than 50 per cent. All these provinces were located in the eastern and the southern parts of China, while most of the remaining provinces were situated in the

TABLE 5.4. *Progress of urban fertility transition by province*

Province	PTFR		Total	Progress of the transition[a] (%)				
	Mid-50s[b]	1980[c]	reduction (%)	1964–6	1967–9	1970–2	1973–5	1976–9[d]
CHINA (urban)	5.18	1.29	73.6	43	51	60	82	93
Shanghai	4.75	0.75	84.2	82	73	83	92	96
Fujian	5.98	1.00	83.3	50	65	76	82	92
Sichuan	5.39	1.02	81.1	41	41	60	79	99
Shandong	5.39	1.02	81.0	48	62	58	78	95
Yunnan	5.27	1.03	80.4	16	42	53	70	69
Tianjin	5.78	1.14	80.3	72	82	84	90	101
Zhejiang	5.04	1.06	79.0	57	65	73	86	97
Xinjiang	5.42	1.17	78.4	19	31	41	50	77
Jiangxi	6.00	1.31	78.2	21	38	43	64	72
Liaoning	5.88	1.34	77.2	51	65	72	93	95
Guangxi	5.73	1.32	76.9	53	59	58	80	86
Jilin	6.02	1.40	76.7	43	53	53	84	85
Hunan	5.06	1.20	76.2	34	54	72	91	97
Beijing	5.26	1.26	76.1	62	63	75	96	95
Nei Monggol	4.98	1.25	75.0	42	33	43	71	90
Hebei	5.27	1.40	73.4	50	50	56	91	95
Jiangsu	4.82	1.30	73.0	49	64	68	87	99
Guizhou	4.53	1.23	72.8	10	27	47	72	90
Heilongjiang	6.07	1.67	72.5	42	53	57	73	94
Gansu	5.24	1.44	72.4	7	44	46	83	95
Shaanxi	5.22	1.48	71.6	47	48	59	88	83
Hubei	5.35	1.57	70.7	55	56	67	92	93
Guangdong	4.93	1.48	70.0	48	59	66	83	103
Anhui	5.41	1.67	69.1	28	37	66	92	98
Shanxi	4.98	1.55	68.8	12	17	43	75	84
Henan	4.48	1.53	65.8	3	13	31	62	90
MEAN	5.32	1.31	75.2	40	50	60	81	92
ST.D.	0.45	0.25	0.05	20	17	14	12	9

[a] All figures are three-year averages, in percentages. [b] Refers to the average of 1954–7.

[c] Refers to the average of 1979–81. Due to abnormally high PTFR in 1981, the average of 1979–80 is used for Hebei province.

[d] Figures higher than 100 indicate the PTFR in 1977–9 was lower than that in 1979–81.

north and the southwest. This finding, together with findings revealed from the earlier discussion, suggests that the fertility transition started earlier in the eastern and southern provinces.

The course of the fertility transition, on the whole, had reached the 81-per-cent point by 1973–5. There were eight provinces for which the ratio was higher than 90 per cent. This means that no massive fertility reduction took place afterwards. The lowest quarter consists of Henan, Guizhou, Yunnan, Jiangxi, Nei Monggol, and Xinjiang. Ratios for them were below 73 per cent at that time. Xinjiang's ratio in that period, say 50 per cent, was the lowest in the country, indicating that half of Xinjiang's total fertility decline occurred after the mid-1970s.

The fertility decline in the first half of the 1970s in Henan, Anhui, Guizhou, and Shanxi was dramatic, accounting for more than 40 per cent of their total fertility falls for the entire 25 years. In Shanxi province, about 58 per cent of the total fertility decline took place in this period. This seems to suggest that the fertility transition in the western and northern parts of China was moderate prior to 1970 and accelerated during the first several years of the 1970s.

Since 1976 the urban fertility transition by and large has been drawing to a close. Only in Yunnan, Jiangxi, and Xinjiang, was more than 30 per cent of their total fertility reduction attributable to declines in the late 1970s.

To conclude, China's urban fertility transition shows some kind of diffusive feature: it started from the coastal provinces with Shanghai as the leading place, then gradually spread to the interior. Although China's urban fertility transition did accelerate in the first half of the 1970s, the reductions in the period prior to 1970 played a very important role. The dramatic fertility decline was virtually over by the later 1970s.

III. Nuptiality Changes

Over the last three decades, China experienced a remarkable change in its marriage pattern, especially for the urban population. Late marriage became one of the major objectives not only of family-planning programmes but also of other social reform initiatives.[5] Marriage has been significantly postponed, but it is still virtually universal. Early marriage was one of the strong features of China's traditional marriage pattern. The resistance to late marriage mainly arose from this tradition, though socio-economic factors should not be ignored. On the other hand, marriage events were frequently affected by China's socio-political changes, which resulted in great fluctuations in marriage over the period.

The Mean Age at First Marriage

Since China's first marriage law was put into effect in 1950, the postponement of marriage has been very impressive in the urban areas. The mean age at first marriage for China's urban female population has risen from 19.46 in the early 1950s to 24.87 in the early 1980s, an increase of 5.41 years during this thirty-year period. The increase was moderate in the 1950s and sharp in the 1970s.

On the whole, the provincial patterns were similar to the national one. Late marriage was achieved in all localities. In Table 5.5, changes in mean age at first marriage are presented by provinces. Several points emerge from the table.

The upward trend of marriage age started from different base levels. The legal minimum age of marriage set by China's 1950 marriage law was 18 for women and 20 for men. Although there was no province in which the average age at first marriage in the early 1950s was below this, the MAFM in a few provinces was only marginally above it. In Shanxi, Henan, Gansu, and Xinjiang, urban women got married on average before they reached the age of 18.5. This means that a certain proportion of women married below the legally required age. In addition, the lowest quarter also includes Jiangxi, Hubei, Fujian, Shaanxi, and Heilongjiang. The average MAFM for these nine provinces in the early 1950s was 18.50. On the other hand, women married relatively later in Guizhou, Jiangsu, Shandong, Shanghai, Guangdong, and Tianjin. The MAFM in all these provinces was above 20 at that time.

The average age at marriage then rose steadily during the 1950s at an average annual increase of 0.17 per year. The sharpest rise was recorded in Shanghai, Zhejiang, and Nei Monggol. By the end of that decade, marriage in these three provinces had taken place at least two years later than before.

This upswing continued through the period 1959–61. The rise was slightly greater than that in the 1950s. This may reflect the population's response to the famine. Regional diversity was at its greatest, as indicated by the large standard deviation.

The steep increase in marriage age occurred in almost all provinces during the mid-1960s. This can partly be attributed to the success of the second family-planning programme which started in the early 1960s. Although there was no unified requirement, the proposed age for

TABLE 5.5. *Mean age at first marriage, urban China 1950–1981*

Province	Mean age at first marriage in period[a]											Total
	1950–2	1953–5	1956–8	1959–61	1962–4	1965–7	1968–70	1971–3	1974–6	1977–9	1980–1	rise
CHINA (urban)	19.46	19.98	20.50	21.01	21.57	22.62	22.41	23.02	24.10	25.12	24.87	5.41
Guangdong	20.45	21.41	21.90	21.83	22.13	22.79	23.05	23.10	24.86	25.55	25.23	4.78
Guangxi	19.48	19.77	20.31	21.43	22.08	23.03	22.33	22.29	24.37	24.91	25.32	5.84
Hubei	18.61	19.32	19.92	20.39	21.26	22.47	22.63	23.63	24.76	25.26	24.90	6.28
Hunan	19.69	20.16	20.21	20.37	21.73	22.16	21.76	22.39	24.18	25.19	24.66	4.97
Jiangxi	18.51	18.70	19.39	19.19	19.79	21.07	20.82	22.11	22.51	24.08	24.29	5.78
Fujian	18.55	18.59	19.92	19.33	20.20	20.47	20.69	21.75	23.10	24.80	24.90	6.35
Zhejiang	18.93	20.13	21.06	21.49	21.10	22.94	21.87	23.72	23.93	25.48	25.25	6.32
Shanghai	20.42	21.25	22.67	23.58	23.95	24.75	23.91	25.03	25.91	26.83	26.95	6.53
Jiangsu	20.57	20.48	21.04	21.56	22.18	23.02	22.44	23.72	23.68	25.22	24.93	4.35
Anhui	19.15	20.02	19.89	20.25	21.41	22.49	21.54	21.87	22.97	24.35	24.39	5.24
Shandong	20.48	20.51	21.31	21.82	22.59	23.52	23.09	23.58	24.61	25.75	24.94	4.46
Sichuan	20.01	20.39	20.94	21.83	21.45	22.66	21.64	22.09	24.07	25.47	24.67	4.66
Guizhou	20.72	21.15	22.07	22.03	22.81	22.05	21.22	22.73	23.84	25.17	25.10	4.38
Yunnan	18.78	19.42	20.45	19.69	21.78	20.98	21.02	21.88	22.10	23.99	23.13	4.34
Shaanxi	18.67	19.09	19.83	20.31	21.69	22.60	21.95	22.86	23.61	24.93	24.58	5.91
Nei Monggol	19.16	20.06	21.51	21.97	22.29	24.08	23.16	23.32	24.50	25.11	24.92	5.76
Shanxi	18.18	19.22	19.33	19.89	19.99	20.95	21.07	20.80	22.56	24.08	24.02	5.84
Henan	18.38	18.89	19.55	20.14	20.85	22.27	22.24	23.43	23.64	24.58	24.81	6.43
Hebei	19.22	20.42	20.62	21.28	22.03	23.06	23.62	23.45	24.52	25.26	24.36	5.14
Beijing	18.87	19.17	20.26	21.92	22.16	22.41	22.79	24.22	24.93	25.62	25.31	6.43
Tianjin	20.07	19.99	20.86	21.61	22.31	23.67	24.30	24.96	25.73	26.31	25.80	5.73
Liaoning	19.58	20.18	20.31	21.10	22.11	23.30	23.03	23.85	25.00	25.29	24.86	5.27
Heilongjiang	18.72	19.38	19.51	20.34	20.67	22.06	21.98	21.94	23.05	23.97	23.63	4.91
Jilin	19.20	19.23	19.89	19.96	20.91	22.68	22.45	23.21	24.65	25.12	24.57	5.37
Gansu	18.41	18.00	18.76	19.07	19.39	20.56	21.88	22.61	24.12	24.43	24.43	6.02
Ningxia/Qinghai	19.40	20.51	20.45	20.34	21.71	22.45	22.23	22.32	22.74	24.08	24.08	4.68
Xinjiang	18.48	19.19	19.30	20.39	20.51	21.78	22.41	22.64	23.53	24.96	24.94	6.46
MEAN	19.29	19.80	20.42	20.86	21.52	22.45	22.26	22.94	23.98	25.03	24.78	5.49
MEDIAN	19.16	19.99	20.31	20.39	21.71	22.49	22.24	22.86	24.07	25.12	24.86	5.73
ST.D.	0.77	0.843	0.932	1.071	1.013	1.028	0.923	0.996	0.965	0.699	0.704	0.74

[a] Figures are three-year averages.

marriage was put forward in various provinces.[6] The rises in provinces with lower MAFM originally was very remarkable. In Jilin province, the mean age at first marriage rose by about 2.7 years over the first half of the 1960s.

There was a backlash in the late 1960s. The estimated marriage age fell in 17 out of 27 provinces compared with the previous period. Only Gansu province witnessed a marked increase: by 1.31 years. This setback was no doubt associated with the Cultural Revolution, since the pressures and incentives for delaying marriage were removed. In addition, the youngsters were closely involved in 'revolutionary activities', which gave them more opportunities to choose their own mates. This in turn brought about a temporary increase in fertility level for the corresponding period.

The sharp increase in urban marriage ages took place throughout the 1970s and reached a peak at the end of the decade. The increase in almost all provinces exceeded 2 years, and the MAFM rose by 2.7 years during this decade for urban areas as a whole. Urban women in Guizhou, Sichuan, Hubei, Jiangxi, and Fujian who got married at the end of the 1970s were at least three years older than they would have been ten years earlier.

This was certainly the result of the vigorous implementation of the later marriage campaign. The minimum age at marriage was put forward by local authorities and often reached an unrealistic level. There was no nation-wide standard for the marriage age, but it was usually around 25 for urban females. To get married so late created a lot of problems, not least because of China's moral tradition.[7]

In addition, during this period about 17 million urban youngsters were sent to the countryside, usually when they graduated from the middle school.[8] Since this migration was regarded as a temporary arrangement, and these youngsters would eventually return to the urban areas from which they came, marriages were voluntarily postponed until they got back.[9]

In the early 1980s as China entered a new era of reconstruction of the legal system, a new marriage law was passed and went into effect in January 1981. The minimum legal age at marriage was set at 20 for females and 22 for males, both substantially lower than the age targets for marriage enforced through the 1970s. Although late marriage was still encouraged, getting married at an older age was no longer a legal requirement. Consequently, a marriage boom occurred across the country.[10] A large number of young women got married, who would not have been eligible in the 1970s. The mean age at first marriage declined slightly in 20 provinces, but it was still a very high level.

Provincial Variation

Table 5.5 also shows that although all provinces experienced a considerable rise in the average age at first marriage, the overall magnitude of this increase varied. In 8 provinces, Shanghai, Fujian, Zhejiang, Hubei, Henan, Beijing, Gansu, and Xinjiang, the mean age at first marriage rose by more than 6 years over the previous three decades. Urban women in Shanghai in the early 1980s got married on the average 6.5 years later than women who had married thirty years before. By contrast, the increase in another third of the provinces, Yunnan, Guizhou, Sichuan, Jiangsu, Shandong, Guandong, Hunan, Heilongjiang, Ningxia, and Qinghai, was less than 5 years. The smallest increase was in Yunnan where women in the early 1980s married 4.34 years later than those marrying in the early 1950s. This differing achievement is certainly related to the original level of the marriage age, but also resulted from changes over the previous thirty years.

The regional difference in the mean age at first marriage changed over time (Table 5.6). The difference widened through the 1950s and reached the highest in the famine period 1959–61. In the period 1950–2 the age gap in terms of marriage age between the highest and the lowest province was 2.5 years, but rose to 4.5 in 1959–61 and 1962–4. Afterwards, the gap gradually narrowed and returned to the early 1950s' level in 1977–9. But this provincial gap may have widened again in the early 1980s.

TABLE 5.6. *Statistics of mean age at first marriage, urban*[a]

Period	Mean	Median	St.d.	Min.	Max.	Diff.[b]	Q1	Q3
1950–2	19.285	19.16	0.774	18.18	20.72	2.54	18.61	20.01
1953–5	19.801	19.99	0.843	18.00	21.41	3.41	19.19	20.42
1956–8	20.417	20.31	0.932	18.76	22.67	3.91	19.83	21.04
1959–61	20.856	20.39	1.071	19.07	23.58	4.51	20.14	21.82
1962–4	21.521	21.71	1.013	19.39	23.95	4.56	20.85	22.16
1965–7	22.454	22.49	1.028	20.47	24.75	4.28	22.05	23.03
1968–70	22.264	22.24	0.923	20.69	24.30	3.61	21.64	23.03
1971–3	22.944	22.86	0.996	20.80	25.03	4.23	22.11	23.63
1974–6	23.980	24.07	0.965	22.10	25.91	3.81	23.10	24.65
1977–9	25.029	25.12	0.699	23.97	26.83	2.86	24.43	25.47
1980–1	24.777	24.86	0.704	23.13	26.95	3.82	24.39	25.10

[a] For 27 provinces (Qinghai and Ningxia are combined).
[b] Difference between the highest and the lowest.

The uneven progress of the marital transition among provinces must have been responsible for this change. Although the provincial trends in general were similar, the timing of the change was different. For instance, the marked increase in the MAFM had already taken place in Shanghai by the late 1950s, and by the mid-1960s in Tianjin, Hubei, and Liaoning. But it occurred only in the early 1970s in Fujian, Jiangxi, Guizhou, and many other provinces.

In the late-marriage campaigns, especially during the 1970s, the age target for marriage was set by local authorities and varied between provinces. The difference in these target ages was small, but it did account to some extent for the provincial variation of the mean age at marriage. In addition, this phenomenon not only reflected the timing factor of the local performance of the late-marriage campaign, but was also related to local marriage customs. The change to late marriage seems to have been much more difficult to introduce in places where early marriage prevailed in the past.

This is supported by an examination of the ratios of the provincial MAFM to the national figure over the period under study. The results are illustrated graphically in Figure 5.4.

These ratios show some consistency over time. Generally speaking, women in provinces for which the MAFM was lower than the national average in the 1950s got married relatively earlier in the late 1970s. For example, the marriage of the urban women took place earlier in Fujian, Jiangxi, Heilongjiang, and Jilin than their counterparts in other provinces throughout the last several decades. On the other hand, the marriage age in Shanghai, Guangdong, Shandong, and Jiangsu was consistently higher than the national average. This suggests that the local background condition, or tradition, is very important in understanding provincial differences in the marital transition.

The provincial difference in terms of marriage age seems to be closely associated with geographical locations. In the early 1950s provinces with low MAFM were adjacent and located in the north and southeast part of China, while the high MAFM concentrated along China's eastern coast. This geographic pattern persisted until the 1980s.

Universal Marriage

Marriages have been considerably delayed in urban China, but women universally still got married. The proportion of women ever married at the age of 32 is estimated for each province through the last thirty years.

Table 5.7 shows that almost all women were married by the time they

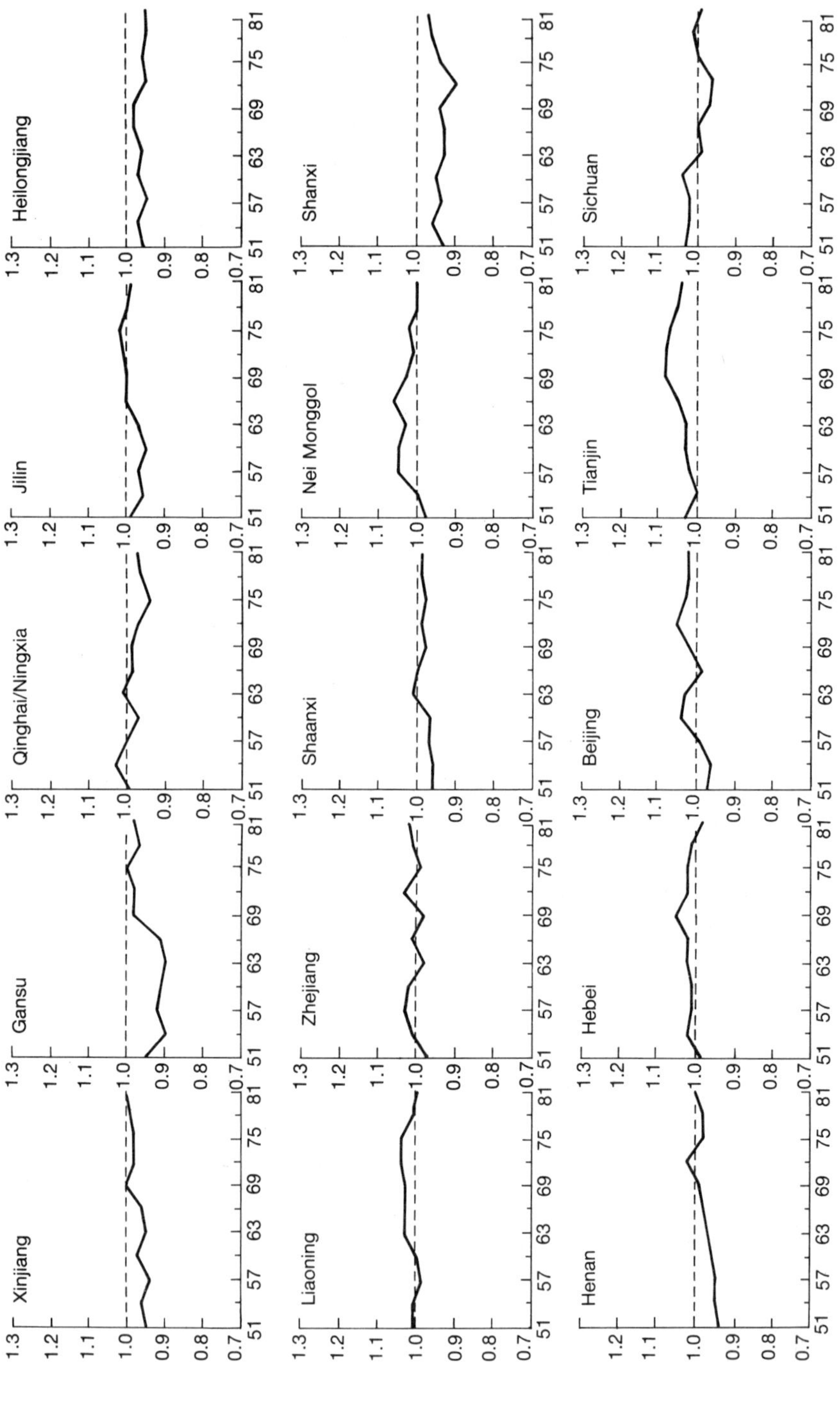
Xinjiang
Gansu
Qinghai/Ningxia
Jilin
Heilongjiang
Liaoning
Zhejiang
Shaanxi
Nei Monggol
Shanxi
Henan
Hebei
Beijing
Tianjin
Sichuan
51 57 63 69 75 81
0.7 0.8 0.9 1.0 1.1 1.2 1.3

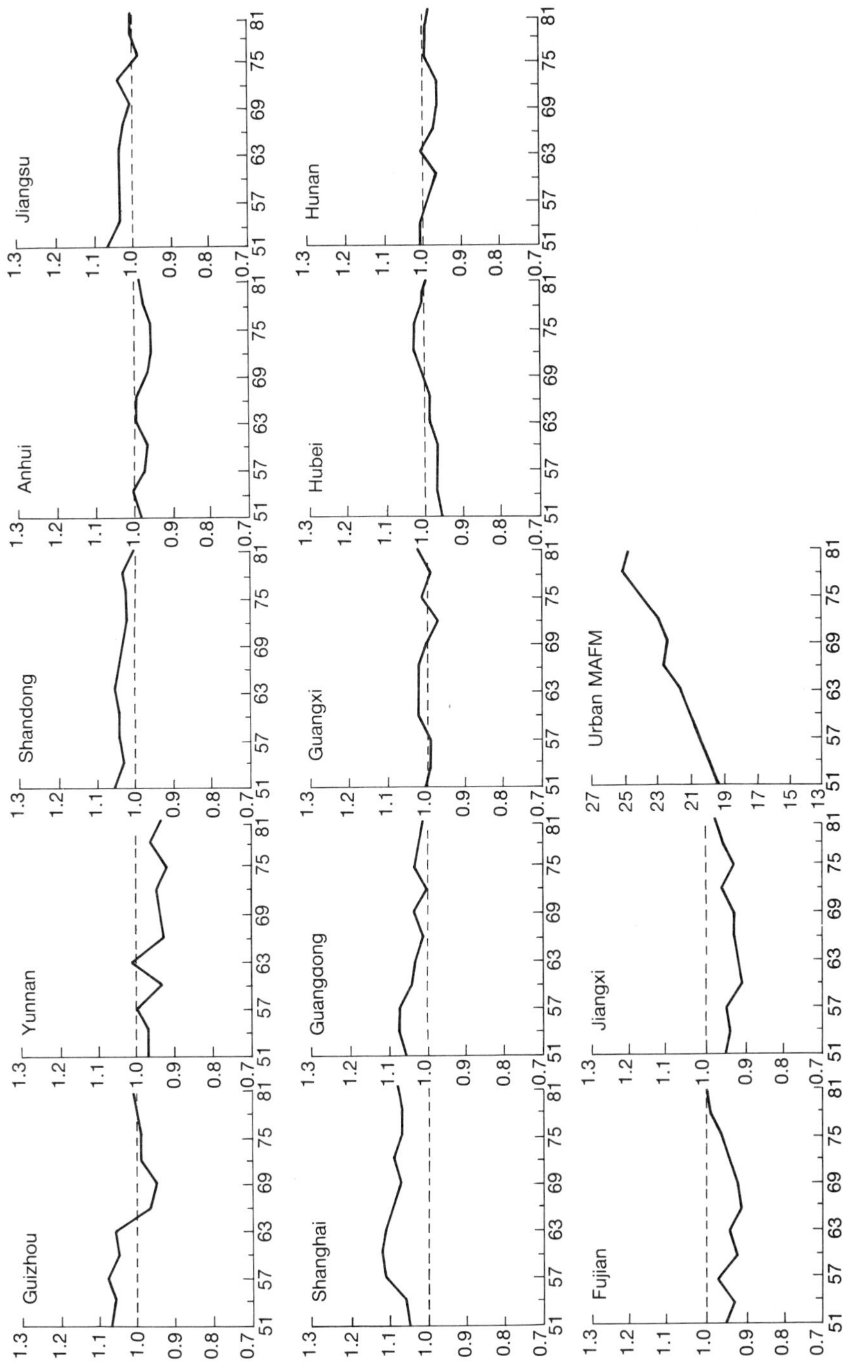

Fig. 5.4 Ratios of provincial MAFM to national onces, urban China 1950–1981

TABLE 5.7. *Proportion of women ever married, urban 1949–1981*

Province	1949–51	1952–4	1955–7	1958–60	1961–3	1964–6	1967–9	1970–2	1973–5	1976–8	1979–81
CHINA (urban)	99.0	99.5	99.4	99.6	99.9	99.8	99.9	99.9	99.7	99.4	98.1
Guangdong	92.3	97.5	96.4	97.3	97.7	99.4	100.0	98.4	100.0	99.0	97.9
Guangxi	100.0	100.0	100.0	100.0	100.0	100.0	97.6	97.8	96.4	100.0	100.0
Hubei	100.0	100.0	100.0	100.0	100.0	100.0	100.0	100.0	100.0	100.0	99.4
Hunan	96.9	98.0	100.0	100.0	100.0	99.1	100.0	100.0	98.8	97.0	96.1
Fujian	100.0	100.0	100.0	100.0	100.0	100.0	100.0	100.0	100.0	97.4	95.8
Jiangxi	100.0	100.0	100.0	100.0	100.0	100.0	100.0	100.0	100.0	100.0	100.0
Zhejiang	100.0	100.0	97.8	98.7	100.0	100.0	100.0	100.0	100.0	100.0	97.1
Shanghai	100.0	100.0	97.7	98.3	100.0	98.9	100.0	99.0	99.1	98.3	90.7
Jiangsu	98.9	100.0	99.1	100.0	100.0	100.0	100.0	100.0	100.0	100.0	97.8
Anhui	100.0	97.6	100.0	100.0	100.0	99.1	100.0	100.0	100.0	100.0	100.0
Shandong	100.0	100.0	100.0	100.0	100.0	100.0	100.0	100.0	100.0	100.0	100.0
Yunnan	97.2	100.0	100.0	100.0	100.0	100.0	100.0	100.0	100.0	96.2	97.4
Guizhou	100.0	100.0	98.3	100.0	100.0	100.0	100.0	100.0	98.0	100.0	95.6
Sichuan	100.0	99.1	99.5	99.6	99.5	100.0	100.0	100.0	100.0	100.0	99.7
Shaanxi	100.0	97.8	100.0	100.0	100.0	100.0	100.0	100.0	100.0	100.0	100.0
Nei Monggol	100.0	100.0	100.0	100.0	100.0	100.0	100.0	100.0	100.0	100.0	100.0
Shanxi	100.0	100.0	100.0	100.0	100.0	100.0	100.0	100.0	100.0	92.1	97.4
Henan	100.0	100.0	100.0	100.0	100.0	100.0	100.0	100.0	100.0	100.0	100.0
Hebei	100.0	100.0	100.0	100.0	100.0	100.0	100.0	100.0	100.0	100.0	100.0
Beijing	100.0	100.0	100.0	100.0	100.0	100.0	100.0	100.0	100.0	99.0	99.0
Tianjin	100.0	100.0	100.0	100.0	100.0	100.0	100.0	100.0	100.0	98.9	97.1
Xinjiang	100.0	100.0	100.0	100.0	100.0	100.0	100.0	100.0	100.0	100.0	100.0
Gansu	100.0	100.0	100.0	100.0	100.0	100.0	100.0	100.0	100.0	98.6	97.0
Jilin	100.0	100.0	100.0	100.0	100.0	100.0	100.0	100.0	100.0	100.0	99.4
Heilongjiang	100.0	100.0	100.0	100.0	100.0	100.0	100.0	100.0	100.0	100.0	99.4
Liaoning	100.0	100.0	100.0	100.0	100.0	99.1	99.2	100.0	98.9	99.5	97.6

Note: All figures are three-year averages.

reached their early thirties. Until the mid-1970s 100 per cent entry into marriage was virtually uniform across the country, except for Guangdong in which the proportion of women still unmarried at age 32 was consistently high. Some other studies have suggested that female celibacy was part of the peculiar social subculture in Guangdong province.[11] Even so, an overwhelming majority of urban women in Guangdong got married before reaching the age of 32.

In the early 1980s women who remained unmarried at the age of 32 exceeded 2 per cent of all women in this age group in 12 provinces. In Shanghai, the proportion was as high as 10 per cent. Whether this indicates a new tendency to remain single permanently, or simply reflected very late marriage is not clear. But it is likely that in the case of China, if women were still single in their early thirties the chances for them to get married were limited. Urban women in their early thirties at the time of China's 1982 Survey belonged to the generation who were commonly sent to rural areas during the late 1960s and the early 1970s when they were about 20 years old. Their education, career, and family formation were all affected by this movement. They differed in many ways from other generations.[12] Therefore, the high proportion of women remaining unmarried may be a phenomenon of this generation only. In my opinion, although the proportion of women never married may rise, the virtual universality will continue to be one of the prominent features of Chinese marriage in the near future.

IV. Age Patterns of the Fertility Transition

Closely linked with the changes in nuptiality are the changes in the age patterns of childbearing. In this section, the age pattern of urban fertility transition is examined. Changes in fertility rates by age group are considered first, followed by analyses of the age group and the parity contributions to the overall fertility.

Changes in Fertility Rates by Age Group

In Table 5.8, changes in fertility rates by age group are recorded. To simplify the work, women in their reproductive ages are classified into four age groups: 15–19, 20–9, 30–9, and 40–9.

The age-specific fertility rate of the 15–19 age group declined well before that of any other age group. While the fertility of other ages

TABLE 5.8. *Changes in urban fertility rates by age group (%)*

Province	Mid-50s–64[a]				1964–70[a]					1970–80[a]			
	PTFR	15–19	20s	30s	TFR	15–19	20s	30s	40s	TFR	15–19	20s	30s
CHINA (urban)	−26	−53	−18	−34	−25	−60	−13	−33	−65	−61	−91	−55	−70
Beijing	−43	−79	−37	−47	−42	−64	+19	−44	−53	−57	−100	−54	−60
Tianjin	−50	−80	−42	−54	−42	−100	−25	−50	−90	−41	—	−39	−39
Hebei	−34	−40	−29	−40	−22	−67	−9	−32	−50	−63	—	−56	−69
Nei Monggol	−33	−20	−21	−47	+1	−71	+5	+20	−77	−67	−100	−66	−62
Shanxi	−3	+73	−3	−21	−33	−74	−18	−24	−56	−59	−85	−45	−65
Heilongjiang	−25	−52	−10	−38	−26	−30	−13	−35	−59	−58	−86	−48	−73
Jilin	−24	−51	−17	−28	−27	−47	−15	−23	−89	−69	−100	−63	−78
Liaoning	−32	−59	−23	−41	−48	−87	−21	−42	−85	−56	−68	−54	−57
Shanghai	−68	−84	−59	−79	+9	−36	+11	+10	−54	−59	−100	−70	−35
Shandong	−27	−62	−18	−37	−20	−70	0	−40	−72	−75	−100	−71	−79
Jiangsu	−32	−27	−24	−44	−30	−66	−12	−45	−81	−63	−100	−60	−64
Zhejiang	−40	−54	−35	−45	−33	+22	−27	−46	−43	−56	−95	−44	−67
Anhui	−10	−29	−3	−16	−27	−59	−25	−5	−80	−49	−33	−30	−73
Fujian	−26	−51	−12	−42	−38	+8	−33	−41	−75	−57	−92	−51	−56
Jiangxi	−14	−63	−16	+3	−21	−5	−8	−45	+11	−73	−43	−63	−87
Guangdong	−26	−40	−22	−32	−35	−54	−23	−45	−82	−42	−92	−32	−57
Guangxi	−34	−50	−21	−49	−42	−65	−19	−50	−81	−50	−100	−40	−61
Hubei	−32	−78	−28	−29	−20	−72	−14	−31	−30	−56	−100	−47	−64
Hunan	−16	−78	+2	−33	−43	−39	−40	−43	−69	−55	−100	−47	−72
Henan	+6	−57	+17	+3	−17	+1	14	−27	+12	−61	−100	−56	−65
Sichuan	−28	−77	−22	−29	−14	−2	+7	−31	−61	−77	−100	−70	−87
Guizhou	−4	−39	+6	−11	−15	−12	−15	−15	−31	−67	−85	−44	−89
Yunnan	−6	−14	−5	−7	−34	−55	−4	−54	−70	−66	−100	−61	−83
Shaanxi	−26	−68	−18	−33	−18	−100	−5	−23	−39	−54	—	−41	−66
Gansu	−1	−51	−1	+13	−42	−62	−31	−59	+2	−63	−100	−46	−85
Xinjiang	−10	−55	+4	−18	−20	−69	−1	−43	−12	−66	−100	−53	−90
MEAN	−24	−49	−17	−32	−27	−49	−13	−33	−54	−60	−90	−52	−69
ST.D	16	31	17	18	14	33	14	19	30	9	18	11	14

[a] The averages of the ASFR in 1964 and 1965, 1969 and 1970, 1979 and 1980 are taken as the numerators respectively.

remained more or less constant, or even increased, births to women in their teens were already sharply reduced. By 1964 the age-specific fertility rate of the 15–19 age group had already declined by more than 50 per cent from the mid-1950s' level in more than two-thirds of the provinces. The three major cities, Shanghai, Beijing, and Tianjin, together with Hubei, Hunan, and Sichuan, took the lead with a drop of more than 75 per cent. Only in Shanxi was the fertility rate for the 15–19 group in the mid-1960s higher than a decade earlier. This is probably the result of sampling fluctuation. The trend in general is certainly attributable to the move towards later marriage.

The ASFR of the 15–19 age group declined further during the late 1960s. The elimination of the teenage birth was finally achieved by the end of the 1970s. At present, almost no births occur to urban women in their teens. This is undoubtedly attributable mainly to the success of the policy of postponed marriage. However, since the share of the 15–19 to the TFR is very small, especially after 1964, the fertility decline of this group contributed only a small part of the total reduction.

The situation for the 40–9 age group prior to 1964 is not very clear. Available data indicate that the trend of this age group was in general similar to that of the 15–19 age groups, though the decline occurred a little later. The fertility rates for women in their forties dropped by more than 75 per cent during the second half of the 1960s in 9 provinces. Most of these provinces were located along China's coastal areas. By the late 1970s the age-specific fertility rate for this age group was already negligible in all provinces.

Changes in fertility rates for women in their twenties, particularly the later twenties, were relatively moderate before 1970, in contrast to the steep declines that were taking place for the 15–19 and 40–9 age groups. By the mid-1960s, only half of all provinces, and mostly coastal ones, had experienced a decline of more than 20 per cent. For the remaining provinces, the ASFR for the 20–9 group was more or less unchanged. A similar situation continued until the early 1970s. The 1970s, however, witnessed a breakthrough. By the early 1980s, the ASFR of the 20–9 group in 14 out of 26 provinces was half of the level prevailing in 1970. The smallest reduction was in Anhui province, but even there the decline was about 30 per cent. Because of the fact that women in their twenties are most fecund, a 50 per cent decline is really a great achievement in terms of the fertility transition. So far as the 30–9 age group is concerned, the extent of their fertility decline was between the extremes of the groups mentioned above.

Changes in Percentage Contribution to the Total Fertility

The age pattern of fertility can also be examined by looking at changes in the percentage contributions to the total fertility rate of the various age groups. These contributions are three-year averages and estimated from 1965 onwards.

It can be seen from Figure 5.5 that the general trends were similar among most provinces. Childbearing in urban China was more and more concentrated in the 20–9 age group. On the other hand, births to women aged 15–19 and 40–9 fell sharply, so that their shares to the TFR are negligible at present. The share of the 30–9 age group declined as time passed. This trend is common to all provinces.

In the period 1965–7 teenage births had accounted for less than 3 per cent of the total fertility in the overwhelmingly majority of provinces. The exceptions were Yunnan (11 per cent) and Shanxi (8 per cent). This is not surprising since the MAFM in these two provinces for the corresponding period, as was shown in the earlier section, was among the lowest nationally (below 21 years of age). However, the MAFM in Gansu and Fujian for the same period was even lower than that of Yunnan and Shanxi, but the contributions of the 15–19 age group to the total fertility in the former two provinces were 4 and 3 per cent respectively. This is probably due to the difference in birth interval between marriage and first birth between these provinces.[13] By the early 1980s teenage births in no province exceeded 1 per cent of the total fertility.

In the mid-1960s the ASFR for women aged 20–9 accounted for about half of the total fertility rate. The percentage in the early 1980s increased to more than 85 per cent in Yunnan, Gansu, Xinjiang, Sichuan, Shandong, Jiangsu, Hebei, and three northeast provinces Liaoning, Jilin, and Heilongjiang. In Yunnan, all births in the urban areas in 1980–1 were to women in their twenties. However, the contribution of the 20–9 group in Shanghai and Tianjin was exceptionally low and was accompanied by a relatively big share for the 30–9 group. The extremely late marriage and subsequently late birth by Chinese standards in these two great cities must be responsible for this phenomenon.

As early as 1965–7, the contribution of the 40–9 age group to total fertility was already below 10 per cent in more than half of provinces. In Shanghai, Zhejiang, Hubei, Beijing, and Gansu, less than 5 per cent of the total fertility rate was attributable to the 40–9 group. By contrast,

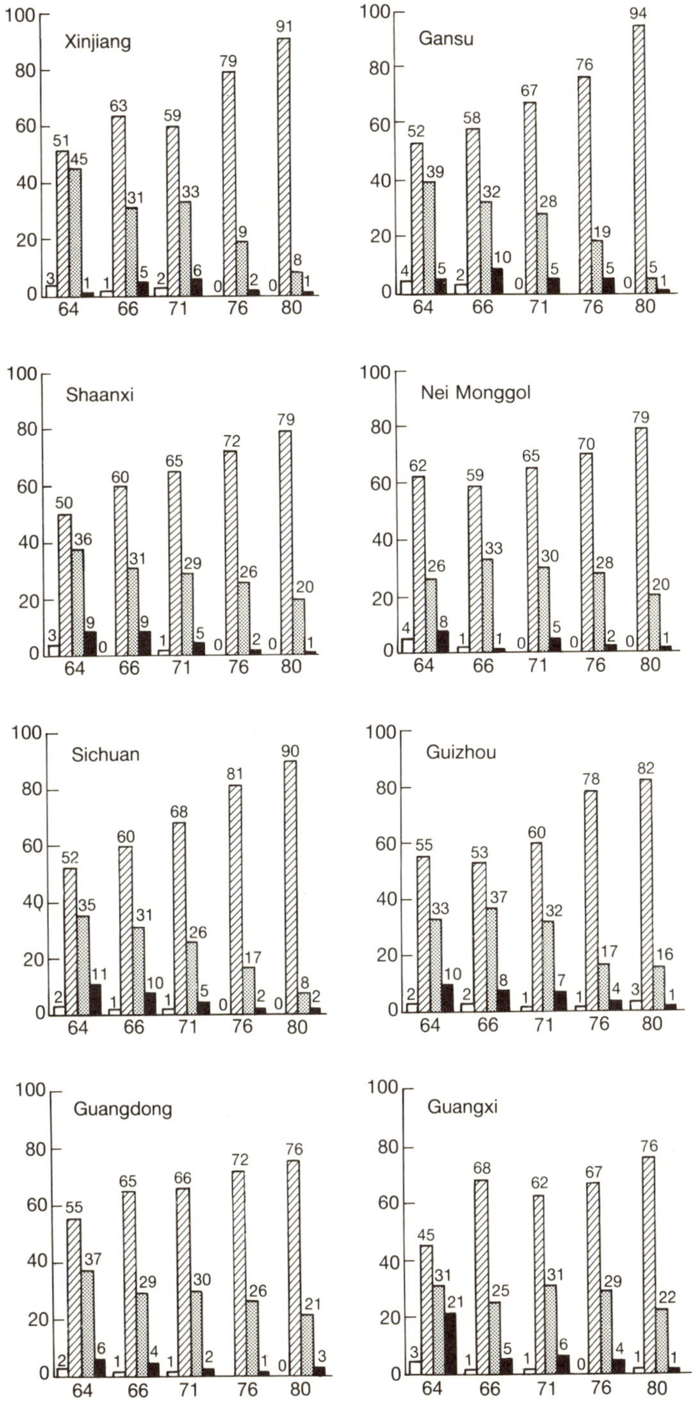
Xinjiang
3 51 45 1 / 1 63 31 5 / 2 59 33 6 / 0 79 9 2 / 0 91 8 1
Gansu
4 52 39 5 / 2 58 32 10 / 0 67 28 5 / 76 19 5 / 0 94 5 1
Shaanxi
3 50 36 9 / 0 60 31 9 / 1 65 29 5 / 0 72 26 2 / 0 79 20 1
Nei Monggol
4 62 26 8 / 1 59 33 1 / 0 65 30 5 / 0 70 28 2 / 0 79 20 1
Sichuan
2 52 35 11 / 1 60 31 10 / 1 68 26 5 / 0 81 17 2 / 0 90 8 2
Guizhou
2 55 33 10 / 2 53 37 8 / 1 60 32 7 / 1 78 17 4 / 3 82 16 1
Guangdong
2 55 37 6 / 1 65 29 4 / 1 66 30 2 / 72 26 1 / 0 76 21 3
Guangxi
3 45 31 21 / 1 68 25 5 / 1 62 31 6 / 0 67 29 4 / 1 76 22 1
0 20 40 60 80 100
64 66 71 76 80

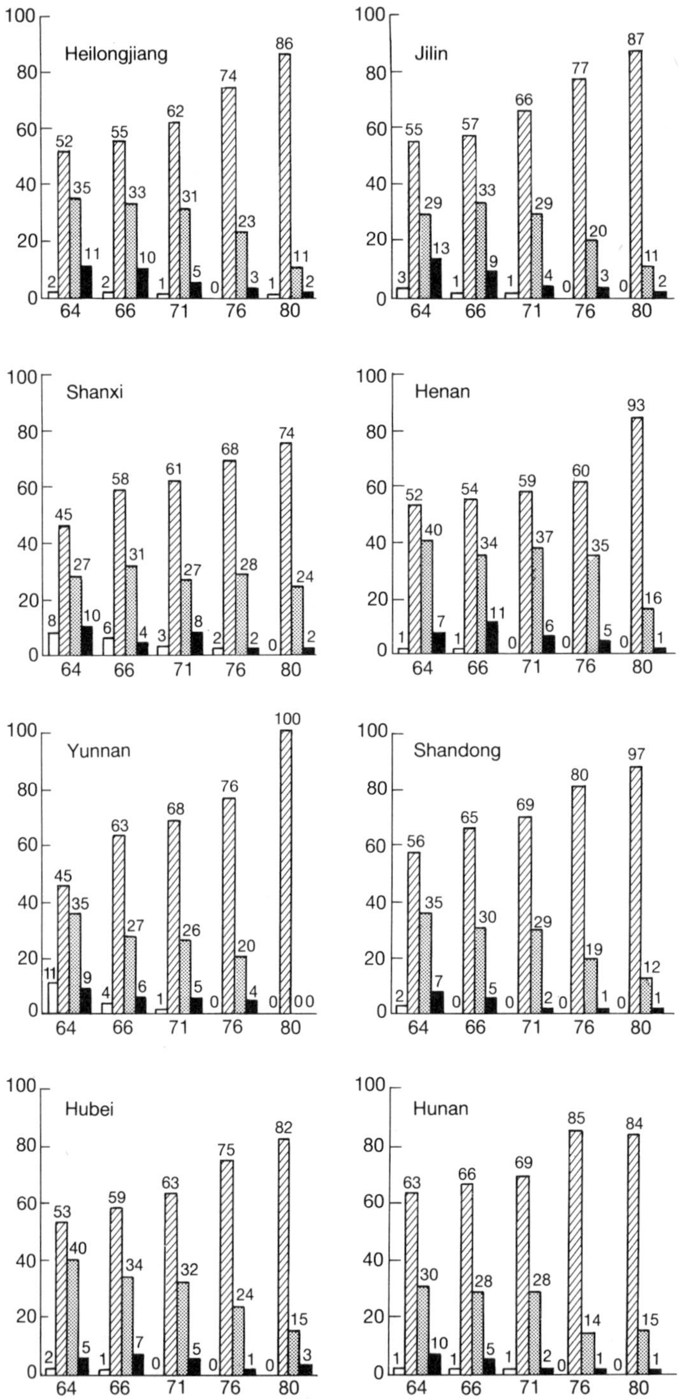
Heilongjiang
Jilin
Shanxi
Henan
Yunnan
Shandong
Hubei
Hunan
64
66
71
76
80

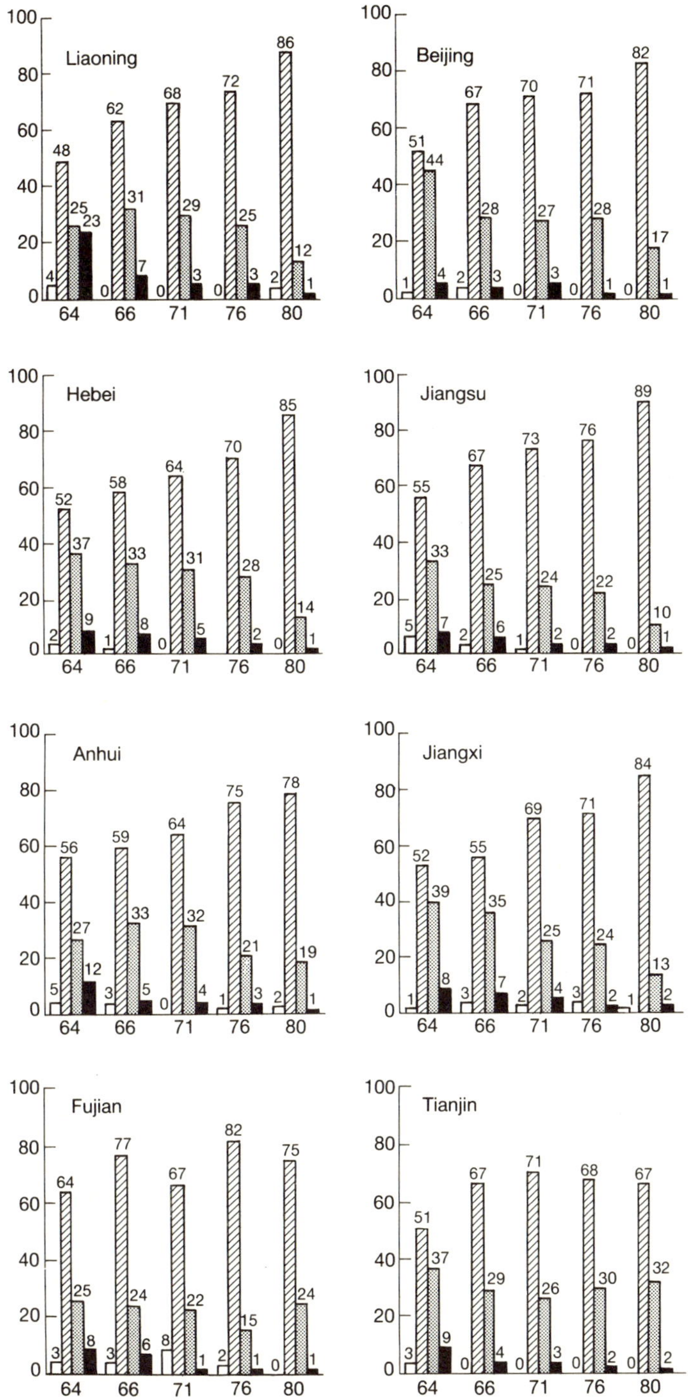
Liaoning
Beijing
Hebei
Jiangsu
Anhui
Jiangxi
Fujian
Tianjin
64
66
71
76
80

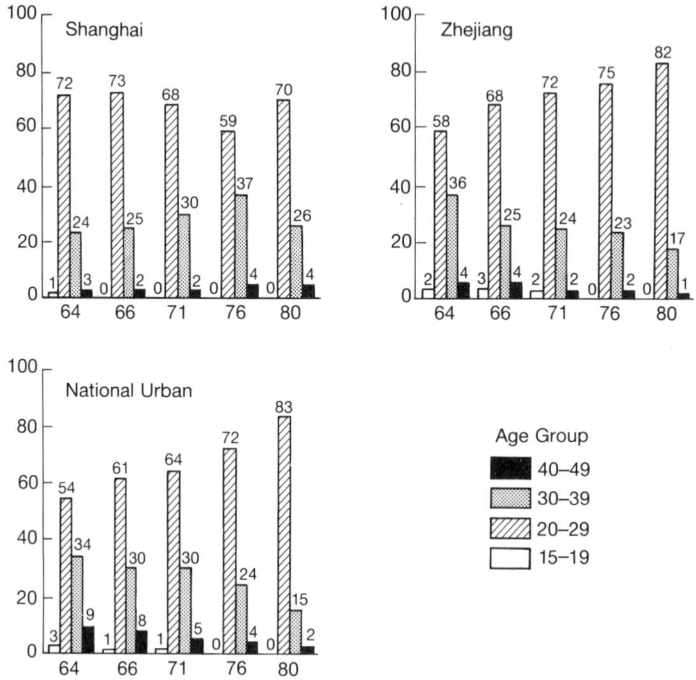

Fig. 5.5 Contribution to the TFR by age group, urban

childbearing to women in their forties in some northeast and the southwest provinces still contributed a significant proportion of the total fertility in 1964. Shares of the 40–9 group fell as time passed. By the early 1980s, only a very tiny proportion of the TFR was produced by this group.

Cumulated Period Fertility

The 80-per-cent interval (A_{80}), which has been defined in the previous chapter, has been estimated for each province. The calculated indices of A_{10} and A_{90}, which indicate the ages at which the cumulated period total fertility rate reaches 10 and 90 per cent respectively, are presented in Figure 5.6.

Figure 5.6 shows that, although there were small fluctuations, the index of A_{10} increased over time, especially in the 1970s. The increment was commonly about 3 years over the entire period. However, the index declined in most provinces in the early 1980s, no doubt because of the decline in age at marriage for the corresponding period.

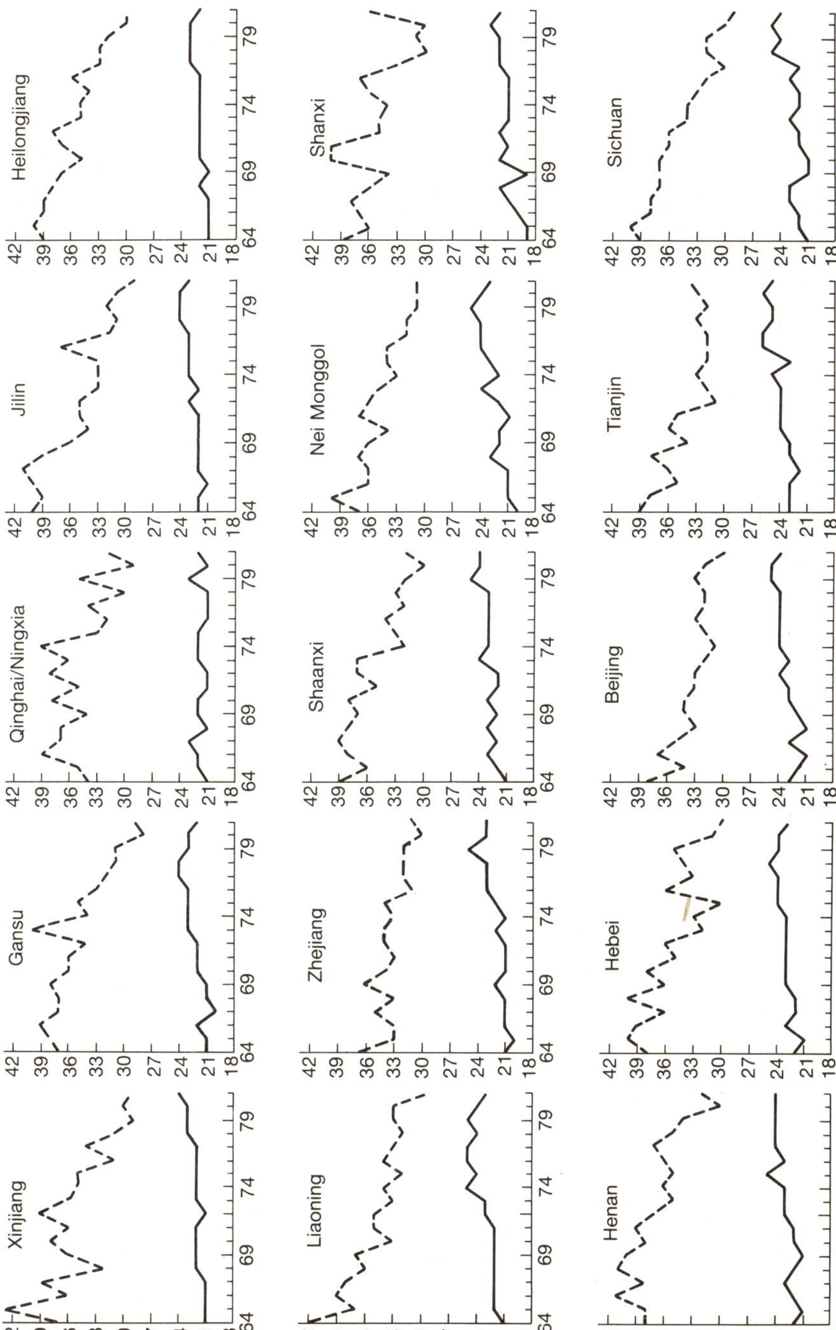
Xinjiang
Gansu
Qinghai/Ningxia
Jilin
Heilongjiang
Liaoning
Zhejiang
Shaanxi
Nei Monggol
Shanxi
Henan
Hebei
Beijing
Tianjin
Sichuan
42
39
36
33
30
27
24
21
18
64
69
74
79

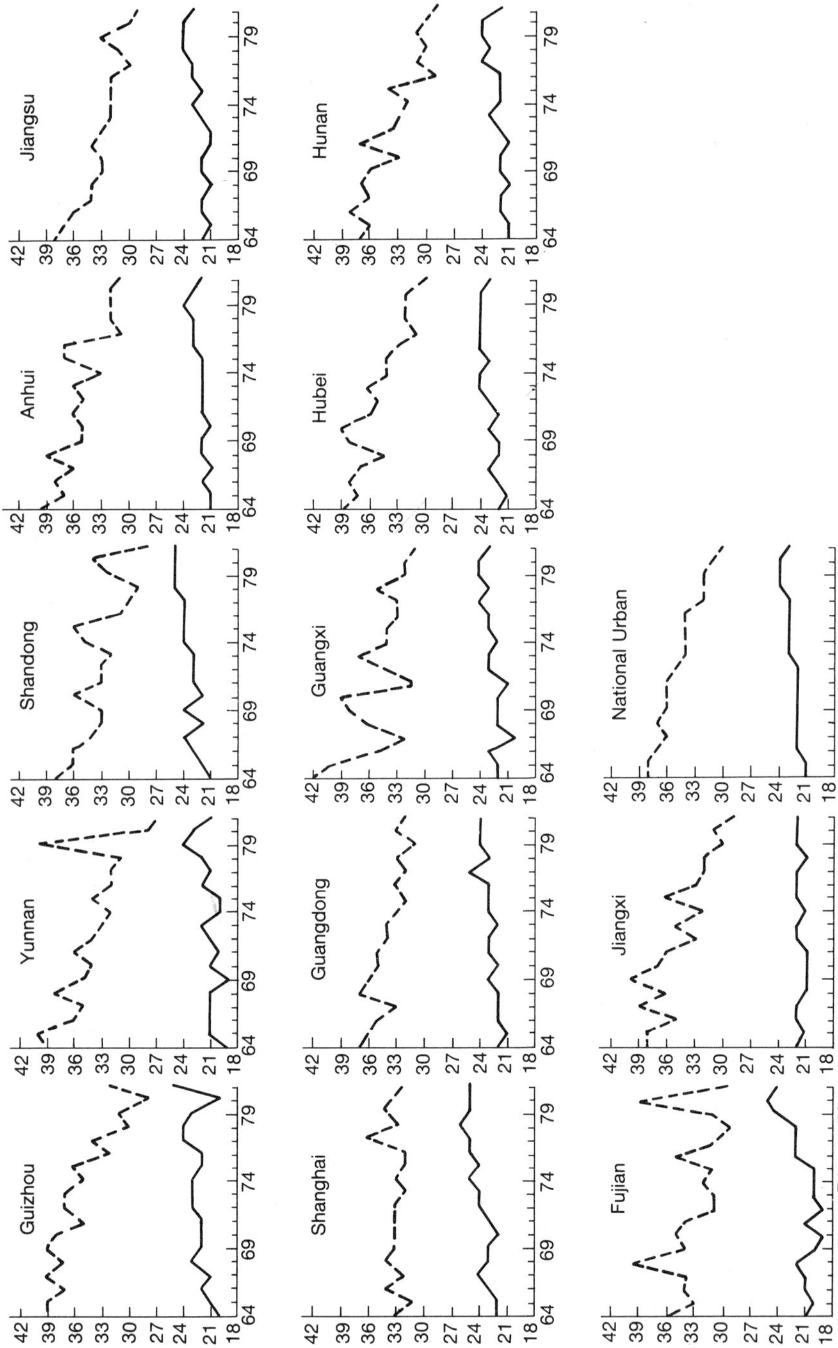

Fig. 5.6 Provincial indices of A_{10} and A_{90} urban 1964–1981

The decline in the index of A_{90} was more impressive and varied widely between provinces. In general, the A_{90} was around the age of 40 in the mid-1960s and fell to 30 in the early 1980s. The timing of these changes also differed. The index of A_{90} in Shanghai was already as low as 33 in 1964, and there has been no change since then. This seems to suggest that the fertility transition in Shanghai was virtually completed by the mid-1960s. The major decline in A_{90} occurred during the late 1960s in Tianjin, Liaoning, Jilin, and Jiangsu province. In contrast, the steep drop took place only in the second half of the 1970s in Gansu and Guizhou, and probably in Henan and Shanxi as well. This regional variation is clear evidence of the timing difference in the fertility transition.

These graphs firmly support the point made earlier that reproductive activities in urban China gradually became concentrated in a very narrow age span. The 80-per-cent interval (A_{80}) was usually about 15–20 years in the mid-1960s, and shortened to less than 10 years in the early 1980s in a majority of provinces. This interval was only 3 years between 25 and 28 in Shandong, one of the model provinces in implementation of the family-planning programme.

Data from China's 1982 Fertility Survey show that the interval between marriage and first birth also narrowed over time. The proportion of births within the first three years of marriage for China's urban females rose from 38 per cent in 1957, to 52 per cent in 1970, and 67 per cent in 1980. This clearly indicates that at present, Chinese urban females get married in their 20s and bear their children soon after marriage. When they reach their early 30s, they have already completed their family formation.

The change in the index A_{10} is closely associated with the trend towards delayed marriage. However, the reduction of the childbearing for women in their older ages seems more significant, as indicated by the greater changes in the index of A_{90}. Since the mean age at first marriage for Chinese urban women is around 24 at present, births to women in their late thirties are obviously high orders. The reduced share of this age group to the TFR and the shortened 80-per-cent interval suggest that births of higher order have been avoided.

Changes in Parities

To support this conclusion, percentage contributions to total yearly births by birth order are estimated for 1970, 1977, 1981, and 1984. Data for the former three years come from China's 1982 Fertility Survey, while information for 1984 is obtained from family-planning statistics.

The choice of these four years is made simply on grounds of data availability. But they are representative. The parity contributions in 1970 reflect the situation before the strict implementation of the nation-wide family-planning programme. Nineteen seventy-seven is the year before the launching of the 'one-child policy'. The 1981 data indicate the early achievement of the policy. Finally, information for 1984 shows more recent progress. The results of these calculations are shown in Figure 5.7.

The picture that emerges is very remarkable. It shows that the contributions of the first birth to total births increased from about 30 per cent in 1970 to 90 per cent in 1981. There were marked regional differences. In 1981, while the percentage of the first birth to total births in 11 out of 26 provinces exceeded 90, it was lower than 70 in Jiangxi and Shanxi.

On the other hand, the occurrence of births of higher orders (defined as birth of the third and higher orders) declined sharply. In 1970 more than half of the total births in 10 provinces were of higher orders. This contribution fell to below 5 per cent in all but Henan province in 1981. The higher order births in Henan accounted for 10 per cent of total births in 1981. Once again, the performance in the coastal provinces was relatively better than in other places.

On the whole, these graphs indicate clearly the success of the one-child policy in China's urban areas. It seems certain that females living in urban areas desire a small family and are more likely to accept the one-child limitation. The very high proportion of first births for urban areas in Shanghai and a few other provinces in 1970 and 1977 does confirm that the acceptance of a one-child family pre-dates the policy itself, as some other surveys have noted.[14]

There was a setback in 1984 when the percentage of the higher order births rose in most provinces. In Xinjiang, Guizhou, and Guangxi, more than 20 per cent of the total births were higher orders. We have already shown that the one-child policy was modified in 1984. Nevertheless, this setback reflects the difficulty in sustaining the policy, especially in remote provinces.

In conclusion, it can be said that China's urban fertility transition started with the youngest age group, which was largely the consequence of postponement of marriage. It is conspicuously clear that higher order births have been eliminated, which has in turn concentrated the reproductive activities for the urban female population in a very narrow age span. Once again, changes in age patterns took place earlier in the urban areas of eastern provinces.

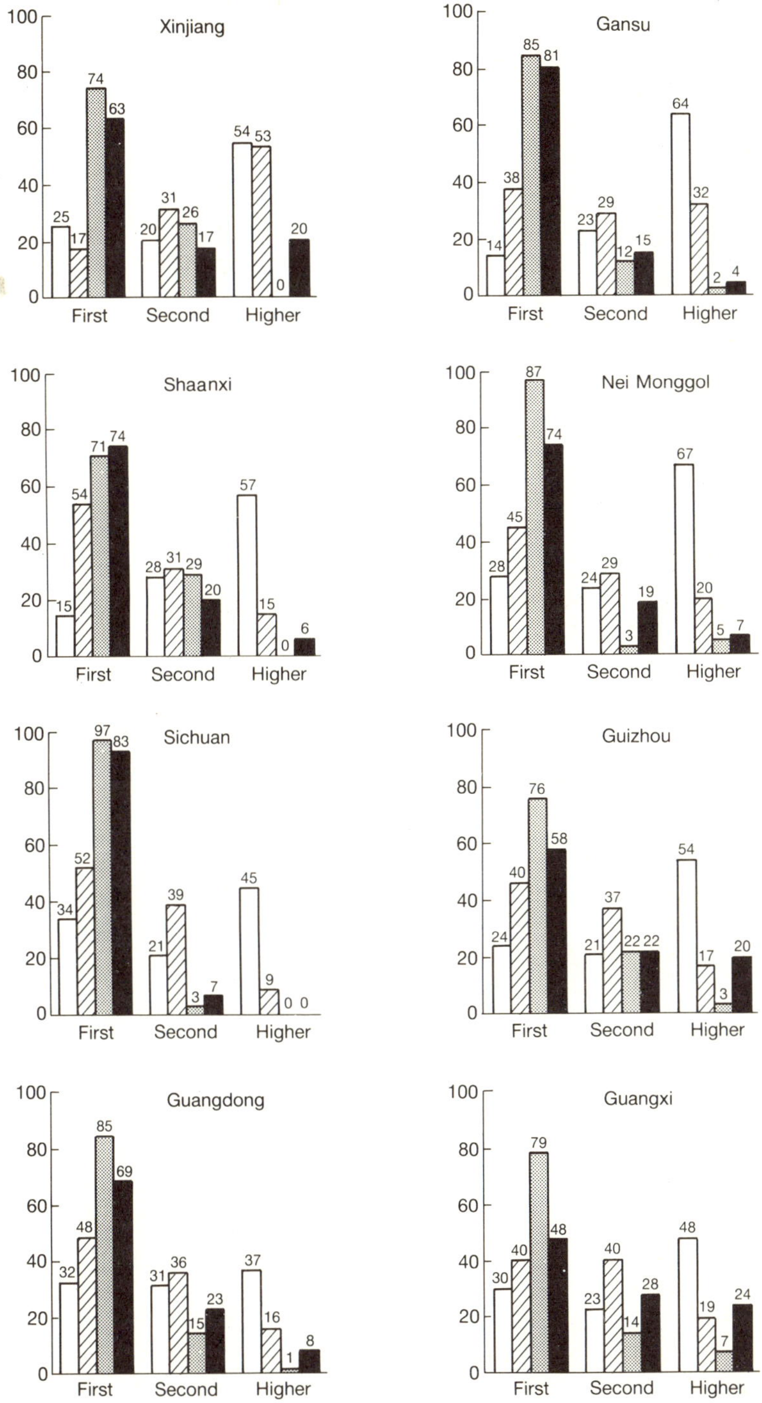
Xinjiang
0 20 40 60 80 100
25 17 74 63
20 31 26 17
54 53 0 20
First Second Higher
Gansu
0 20 40 60 80 100
14 38 85 81
23 29 12 15
64 32 2 4
First Second Higher
Shaanxi
0 20 40 60 80 100
15 54 71 74
28 31 29 20
57 15 0 6
First Second Higher
Nei Monggol
0 20 40 60 80 100
28 45 87 74
24 29 3 19
67 20 5 7
First Second Higher
Sichuan
0 20 40 60 80 100
34 52 97 83
21 39 3 7
45 9 0 0
First Second Higher
Guizhou
0 20 40 60 80 100
24 40 76 58
21 37 22 22
54 17 3 20
First Second Higher
Guangdong
0 20 40 60 80 100
32 48 85 69
31 36 15 23
37 16 1 8
First Second Higher
Guangxi
0 20 40 60 80 100
30 40 79 48
23 40 14 28
48 19 7 24
First Second Higher

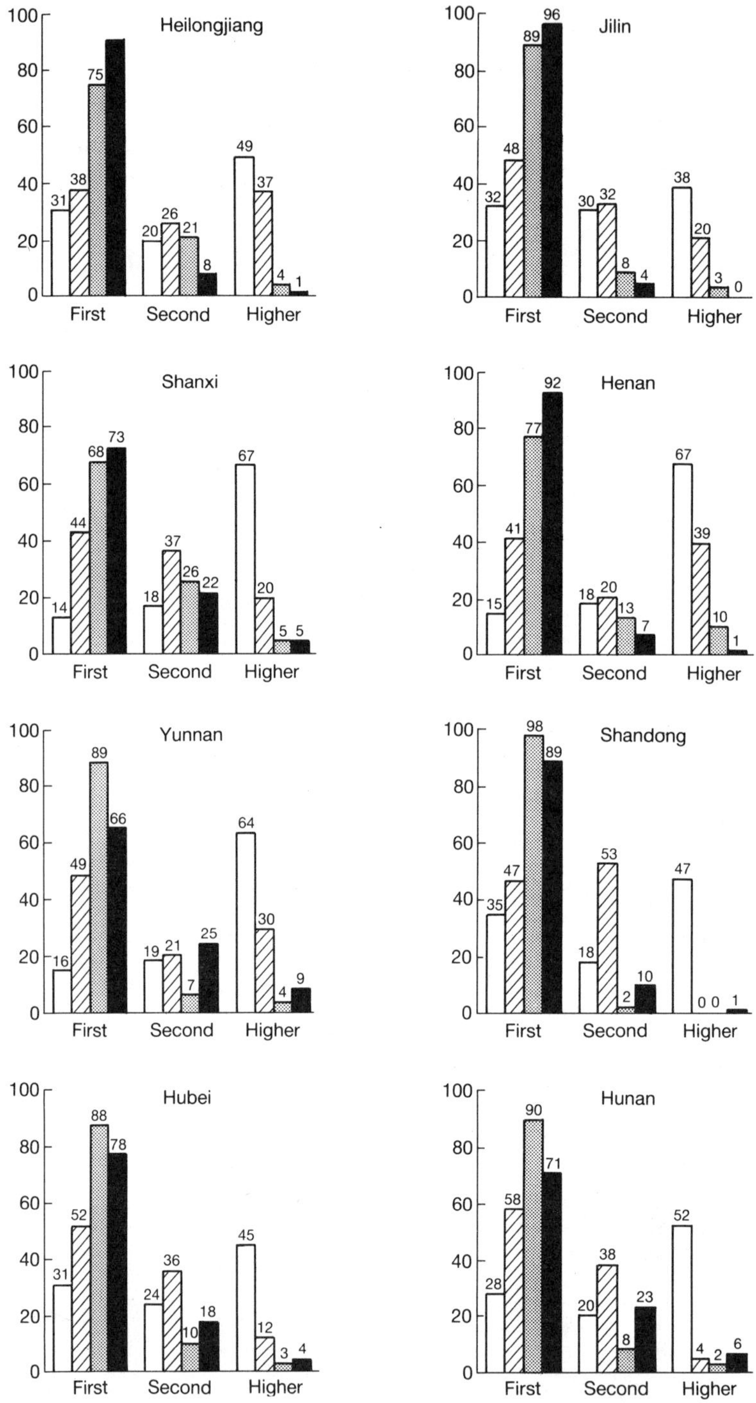
Heilongjiang
100
80
60
40
20
0
31 38 75
20 26 21 8
49 37 4 1
First Second Higher
Jilin
100
80
60
40
20
0
32 48 89 96
30 32 8 4
38 20 3 0
First Second Higher
Shanxi
100
80
60
40
20
0
14 44 68 73
18 37 26 22
67 20 5 5
First Second Higher
Henan
100
80
60
40
20
0
15 41 77 92
18 20 13 7
67 39 10 1
First Second Higher
Yunnan
100
80
60
40
20
0
16 49 89 66
19 21 7 25
64 30 4 9
First Second Higher
Shandong
100
80
60
40
20
0
35 47 98 89
18 53 2 10
47 0 0 1
First Second Higher
Hubei
100
80
60
40
20
0
31 52 88 78
24 36 10 18
45 12 3 4
First Second Higher
Hunan
100
80
60
40
20
0
28 58 90 71
20 38 8 23
52 4 2 6
First Second Higher

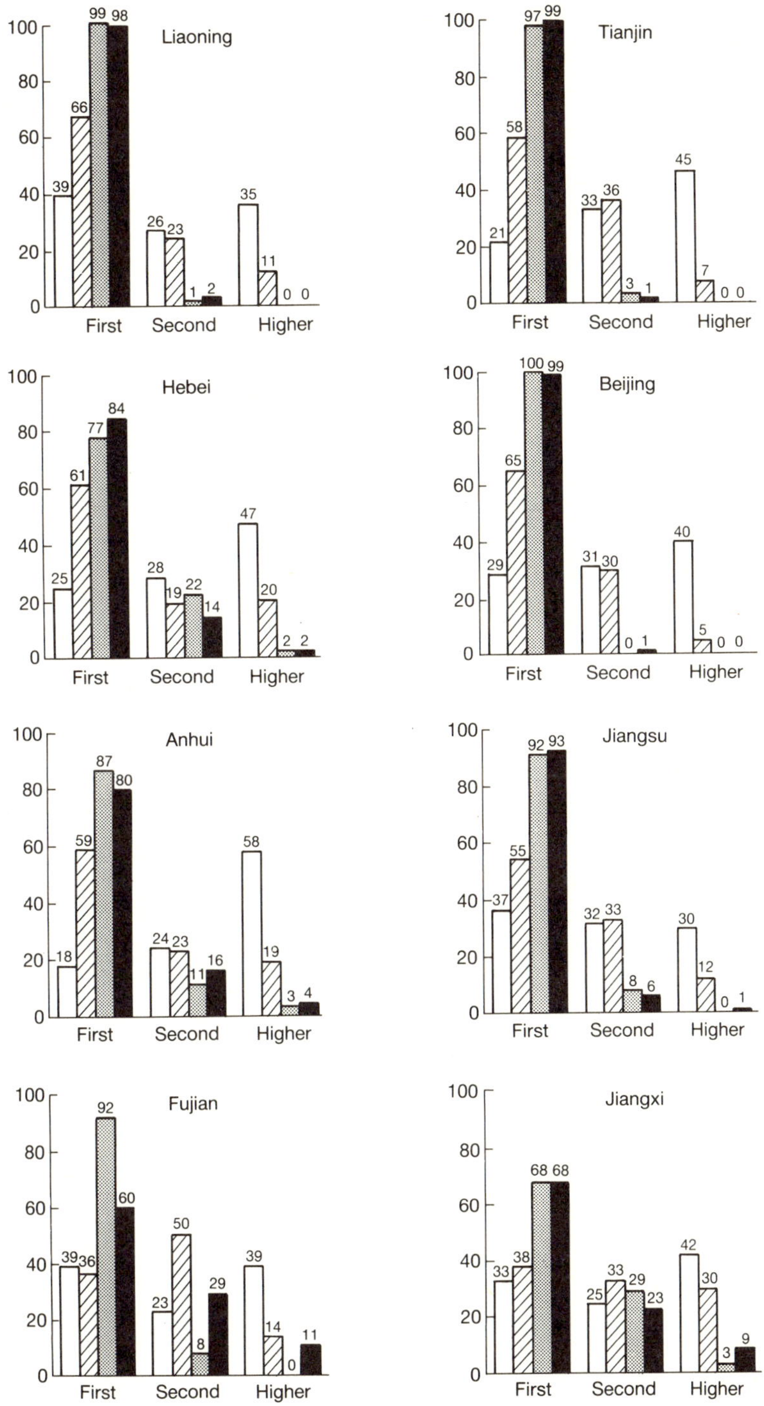
Liaoning
39 66 99 98
26 23 1 2
35 11 0 0
First Second Higher
Tianjin
21 58 97 99
33 36 3 1
45 7 0 0
First Second Higher
Hebei
25 61 77 84
28 19 22 14
47 20 2 2
First Second Higher
Beijing
29 65 100 99
31 30 0 1
40 5 0 0
First Second Higher
Anhui
18 59 87 80
24 23 11 16
58 19 3 4
First Second Higher
Jiangsu
37 55 92 93
32 33 8 6
30 12 0 1
First Second Higher
Fujian
39 36 92 60
23 50 8 29
39 14 0 11
First Second Higher
Jiangxi
33 38 68 68
25 33 29 23
42 30 3 9
First Second Higher
0 20 40 60 80 100

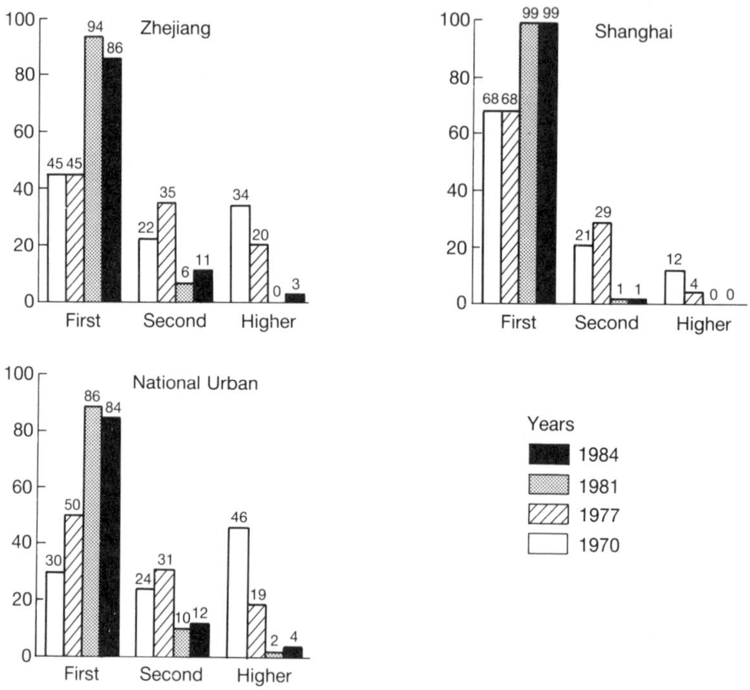

Fig. 5.7 Contribution to total births by birth order, urban

V. Nuptiality versus Marital Fertility

We have analysed changes in the overall fertility and marital patterns over the last thirty years. The logical question is what is the importance of the nuptiality change on the fertility transition. In a country like China, childbearing outside marriage forms no part of the cultural tradition and illegitimate births can safely be excluded from the current analysis. The overall fertility level is, therefore, determined mainly by the proportion of women married and by fertility within marriage. We begin with the examination of the changes in marital fertility through the period concerned.

Marital Fertility Rates

We have calculated the age-specific fertility rate and the age-specific first marriage rate for each province during the last three decades. The marital fertility rate can also be estimated for ever married women based on the above two sets of data. The calculated marital fertility rates correspond to the years of births of the children rather than to the marriage cohorts. Because of this method of calculation, the single-year variation of these marital fertility rates is even greater than that of the total fertility rates. Therefore, three-year averages are used to smooth the fluctuation. The trends in marital fertility (here the total marital fertility rate in 1964 has been taken as the reference) for each province are estimated and shown in Table 5.9.

Variation in trends in marital fertility among the provinces is evident. The substantial fall in marital fertility started considerably earlier in Shanghai than in other provinces. In 1964 the total marital fertility rate in Shanghai was only about half of that in the mid-1950s. Apart from Shanghai, the marital fertility rates in Beijing, Shandong, and Zhejiang had, by 1964, already declined by about 40 per cent. In contrast to these reductions, marital fertility actually increased in Henan, Gansu, Yunnan, Shanxi, and Hubei. Although a decline in overall fertility did take place, the level of marital fertility remained practically constant until 1964 in many other provinces.

Marital fertility in the early 1970s was lower than in 1964, but the decline was moderate in most provinces, compared with the sharp reduction in total fertility rate. In Xinjiang, Fujian, Shandong, and Shanxi, the decline in marital fertility was less than 10 per cent during the late 1960s. The sharpest fall, more than 40 per cent from the 1964 levels, occurred in Tianjin and Liaoning.

The downward tendency has continued and speeded up since the mid-1970s. By the early 1980s the marital fertility rate had, on average, declined by more than 50 per cent. The decline in Yunnan, Sichuan, and Shandong was dramatic: their marital fertility rates in the early 1980s were less than 30 per cent of the values for 1964.

The regional variation in marital fertility was larger than for total fertility. There was no province with a total fertility rate above 2 in the early 1980s, but about one-third of all provinces had a total marital fertility rate above 3. The geographical pattern with respect to the marital fertility was less conspicuous.

Table 5.9 also shows that in 1982, the average number of children ever born to Chinese women at the age of 35 in the urban areas was 2.2. In other words, despite the strong commitment of the 'one-child policy' by the Chinese government which started in 1979, urban women still managed to bear enough children to replace themselves by their mid-thirties. Only 6 out of 28 provinces reported a number lower than 2, including Shanghai, Tianjin, Fujian, Zhejiang, Hunan, and Shandong. As we have documented, all these provinces are situated in the eastern coastal area and the onset of the fertility transition there was earlier

TABLE 5.9. *Trends in marital fertility rate[a], urban China*

Province	1964	Mid-50s		1964–6		1967–9		1970–2		1973–5		1976–8		1979–81		No. of children at age 35[d]
	TMFR	PMFR[b]	Ratio[c]	TMFR	Ratio	TMFR	Ratio	TMFR	Ratio	TMFR	Ratio	TMFR	Ratio	TMFR	Ratio	
CHINA (urban)	6.07	6.24	115	5.70	94	4.98	82	4.79	79	4.40	73	3.81	63	2.99	49	2.22
Shanghai	3.20	6.23	196	3.04	95	3.02	94	2.92	91	2.84	89	2.49	78	1.92	60	1.34
Beijing	4.18	5.99	147	4.84	116	4.10	98	3.73	89	2.52	60	2.42	58	1.79	43	2.12
Zhejiang	4.64	6.32	140	4.72	102	3.63	78	3.78	81	2.53	55	2.40	52	3.15	68	1.84
Shaanxi	4.77	5.71	130	4.08	85	4.24	89	4.45	93	2.94	62	3.34	70	1.79	37	2.33
Shandong	4.98	6.57	139	4.67	94	3.61	72	4.64	93	3.09	62	1.81	36	1.32	26	1.88
Tianjin	5.47	6.64	128	4.32	79	3.35	61	2.88	53	3.14	57	1.65	30	2.00	36	1.86
Jiangsu	5.53	5.98	112	5.27	95	3.76	68	4.07	74	3.25	59	2.74	49	1.97	36	2.13
Jiangxi	5.57	6.87	109	4.87	87	4.13	74	3.80	68	4.05	73	3.37	61	1.81	32	2.89
Guangdong	5.66	6.24	115	4.80	85	5.01	89	4.49	79	4.45	79	3.37	60	2.49	44	2.19
Hebei	5.71	6.15	115	5.06	89	5.11	89	4.38	77	3.04	53	2.76	48	2.42	42	2.34
Qinghai/ Ningxia	5.73	4.11	72	5.08	88	4.53	79	4.88	85	5.19	91	3.80	66	3.01	53	2.22
Nei Monggol	5.77	6.15	112	5.14	89	4.95	86	4.84	84	3.37	58	4.02	70	1.88	33	2.55
Henan	5.82	5.05	92	5.77	99	5.63	97	4.76	82	4.08	70	3.14	54	3.03	52	2.40
Sichuan	5.88	6.63	120	5.28	90	4.83	82	4.47	76	3.49	59	2.66	45	1.71	29	2.17
Heilongjiang	5.94	6.70	123	5.89	99	5.35	90	4.98	84	4.63	78	4.12	69	3.09	52	2.61
Xinjiang	5.96	6.14	103	5.51	92	5.13	86	5.59	94	4.50	76	3.35	56	2.41	40	3.16
Hunan	6.03	6.15	106	5.17	86	4.08	68	3.98	66	3.04	50	3.35	56	2.05	34	1.86
Guizhou	6.23	6.05	104	5.85	94	5.12	82	5.12	82	3.75	60	2.63	42	3.07	49	2.15
Gansu	6.39	5.56	90	6.03	94	4.84	76	4.94	77	2.81	44	2.74	43	1.98	31	2.40
Anhui	6.44	6.51	112	6.03	94	5.31	82	4.25	66	3.67	57	4.00	62	3.18	49	2.73
Hubei	6.61	6.08	95	5.38	81	4.59	69	4.97	75	3.47	52	4.44	67	3.54	54	2.38
Fujian	6.75	6.77	130	6.68	99	5.50	82	6.26	93	5.18	77	4.19	62	2.63	39	1.83
Jilin	6.76	6.94	114	5.84	86	5.65	84	5.26	78	3.83	57	4.13	61	2.02	30	2.20
Yunnan	7.14	6.07	91	6.13	86	4.44	62	4.79	67	3.60	50	3.99	56	1.70	24	3.00
Shanxi	7.29	5.77	85	5.95	82	6.01	82	5.31	73	4.47	61	3.65	50	3.00	41	2.82
Guangxi	7.67	6.62	99	5.31	69	4.81	63	4.82	63	4.54	59	4.17	54	2.53	33	2.64
Liaoning	7.81	6.75	103	5.67	73	4.56	58	4.63	59	4.29	55	2.86	37	2.99	38	2.15
MEAN	5.93	6.26	114	5.29	90	4.65	79	4.56	78	3.69	63	3.26	55	2.41	41	2.30
ST.D.	1.07	0.44	24	0.74	9	0.74	11	0.74	11	0.77	12	0.76	12	0.60	11	0.41

[a] All ratios are estimated by taking the total marital fertility rate in 1964 as 100.
[b] Partial total marital fertility rate (up to age 39).
[c] Compared with the PMFR in 1964.
[d] Refers to number of children ever born to ever married women at the age of 35 in 1982.

than in the others. The average number of children for urban women aged 35 in Shanghai was only 1.34, which was the lowest in the country in 1982. By contrast, the number of children was as high as 3.16 and 3.00 for Xinjiang and Yunnan provinces. Both of these provinces have a relatively large proportion of ethnic minorities. This may be due in part to differences in population policy towards minority populations, as discussed earlier.

Women aged 35 in 1982 were born in 1947, and entered their childbearing period in the mid-1960s. This cohort has been the principal target of the family-planning programme since the early 1970s. In spite of the large falls, the earlier figures suggest that Chinese urban females did not fail to replace themselves on the whole. Women born in the early 1950s are more likely to be the targets of the current single-child programme. Since they have not completed their reproductive circles, it is hard to say with certainty what will be the case for this cohort.

Decomposition

During the last three decades in China's urban areas, marital fertility declined substantially and marriage was widely postponed. It is instructive to ask what had been the net effect of nuptiality changes on China's urban fertility transition? To answer this question, a decomposition procedure has been adopted. The equation used here for the decomposition is the same as that used in the analysis of the national patterns. The age-specific marital fertility rate and the proportion of women ever married up to a certain age in the mid-1950s and 1964 are taken as two reference points. To refresh our memory, the decomposition equation is presented below.

$$\mathrm{TFR}^{i} - \mathrm{TFR}^{i} = \Sigma\,[1/2\,(\mathrm{M}_{a}^{\,i} + \mathrm{M}_{a}^{\,r})\,(\mathrm{G}_{a}^{\,i} - \mathrm{G}_{a}^{\,r}) + 1/2\,(\mathrm{G}_{a}^{\,i} + \mathrm{G}_{a}^{\,r})\,(\mathrm{M}_{a}^{\,i} - \mathrm{M}_{a}^{\,r})]$$

Where:

$\mathrm{M}a_{a}^{\,i}$ is the proportion of women ever married up to age *a* in year *i*.
$\mathrm{G}_{a}^{\,i}$ is the age-specific marital fertility rate for age *a* in year *i*.
R refers to the reference value.

The national figures show that while changes in nuptiality accounted for about 21 per cent of the decline in total fertility rate, the change in marital fertility alone contributed 79 per cent of this reduction during the period between the mid-1950s and 1964. Compared with the PTFR in the mid-1950s, 18 out of the 26 provinces experienced a more than 10 per cent fertility decline by 1964. The relative contributions of the

TABLE 5.10. *Changes in total fertility and the net effects of component changes*[a], *urban China* (%)

Province	1964[b]			1965–9			1970–4			1975–9			1980–1		
	PTFR (1)	F[c] (2)	M[d] (3)	TFR (4)	F[c] (5)	M[d] (6)	TFR (7)	F[c] (8)	M[d] (9)	TFR (10)	F[c] (11)	M[d] (12)	TFR (13)	F[c] (14)	M[d] (15)
CHINA (urban)	–21.2	79	21	–0.23	78	22	–0.40	69	31	–0.64	67	33	–0.71	79	21
Shanghai	–65.5	80	20	+0.02	—	—	–0.19	–11	111	–0.45	34	66	–0.55	60	40
Tianjin	–43.4	61	39	–0.41	103	–3	–0.48	94	6	–0.69	97	3	–0.66	85	15
Beijing	–34.3	79	21	–0.25	74	26	–0.43	68	32	–0.62	76	24	–0.66	83	17
Fujian	–32.4	70	30	–0.29	86	14	–0.52	85	15	–0.67	70	30	–0.76	88	12
Zhejiang	–31.4	71	29	–0.31	79	21	–0.44	77	23	–0.65	69	31	–0.75	62	38
Nei Monggol	–28.5	80	20	–0.01	—	—	–0.21	128	–28	–0.58	85	15	–0.64	92	8
Liaoning	–27.0	51	49	–0.42	93	7	–0.57	79	21	–0.74	85	15	–0.76	82	18
Guangxi	–26.4	30	70	–0.39	100	0	–0.43	81	19	–0.62	86	14	–0.80	91	9
Jiangsu	–25.7	67	33	–0.26	84	16	–0.42	89	11	–0.62	88	12	–0.66	93	6
Hebei	–25.4	62	38	–0.19	92	8	–0.37	89	11	–0.63	86	14	–0.52	94	6
Shandong	–25.0	71	23	–0.33	73	27	–0.42	65	35	–0.68	90	10	–0.75	84	16
Shaanxi	–24.0	82	18	–0.17	71	29	–0.38	62	38	–0.54	76	24	–0.67	86	14
Heilongjiang	–23.6	76	24	–0.18	82	18	–0.30	77	23	–0.61	72	28	–0.70	81	19
Sichuan	–23.4	57	43	–0.17	84	16	–0.43	84	16	–0.74	81	19	–0.75	81	19

Jilin	−20.5	43	57	−0.28	89	11	−0.42	87	13	−0.64	84	16	−0.74	93	7
Hubei	−20.0	14	86	−0.28	83	17	−0.43	81	19	−0.59	81	19	−0.67	87	13
Guangdong	−19.5	64	36	−0.28	91	9	−0.40	70	30	−0.65	77	23	−0.64	78	22
Anhui	−12.9	67	33	−0.20	71	29	−0.49	70	30	−0.65	65	35	−0.72	69	31
Jiangxi	−7.0	—	—	−0.22	82	18	−0.40	70	30	−0.56	77	23	−0.80	86	12
Hunan	−4.0	—	—	−0.37	80	20	−0.61	70	30	−0.74	70	30	−0.75	75	25
Xinjiang	−3.0	81	19	−0.17	99	1	−0.27	69	31	−0.60	80	20	−0.81	93	7
Guizhou	−2.3	77	23	−0.15	78	22	−0.39	67	33	−0.67	73	27	−0.78	72	28
Yunnan	−1.0	—	—	−0.29	92	8	−0.48	80	20	−0.65	89	11	−0.83	87	12
Gansu	+7.5	—	—	−0.27	77	23	−0.46	74	26	−0.71	85	15	−0.78	87	13
Shanxi	+7.6	—	—	−0.25	71	29	−0.43	65	35	−0.67	70	30	−0.72	75	25
Henan	+12.3	—	—	−0.14	58	42	−0.35	69	31	−0.61	70	30	−0.76	79	21
MEAN	−19.2			−0.24	83		−0.41	75		−0.64	78		−0.72	82	
ST.D.	17.2			0.11	11		0.10	22		0.06	12		0.08	9	

[a] All changes are period averages.
[b] Partial fertility rate up to age 39, the mid-1950s as the reference time. For other periods, 1964 has been taken as the reference.
[c] F indicates the net effect of marital fertility change on TFR in percentage.
[d] M indicates the net effect of nuptiality change on TFR in percentage.
— indicates that the contribution of the marital fertility is negative.

decline in marital fertility and the change in nuptiality varied between provinces. The partial total fertility rate for Hubei province in 1964 fell by 20 per cent from the mid-1950s level, 86 per cent of this decline was caused by the marriage factor. In contrast, only 18 per cent of its total fertility decline was brought about by the marriage changes in Shaanxi. On average for these 18 provinces, about 37 per cent of the fertility decline resulted from changes in the marriage pattern, and the remaining 63 per cent was due to the fertility decline within marriage. In the other 8 provinces fertility remained constant, or even increased during this period. The feature common to all of them was that the effects of changes in nuptiality, which could have brought down the fertility, were offset by a rise in the marital fertility rate.

This situation changed little over time. However, the importance of marital fertility change on TFR was greatest during the period 1965–9. If we combine this with the trend in mean age at first marriage, we can see that the MAFM in the later 1960s was constant for most provinces, so that the main source of fertility decline must have been changes in marital fertility rate. In the first half of the 1970s, with the rapid increase of the MAFM, the net effect of changes in marriage patterns on the TFR change also increased. On the other hand, although marriage patterns were quite different in the early 1980s from what they were in 1964, marital fertility changed even more significantly due to the implementation of the one-child policy. As a result, the effect of reductions in marital fertility on the TFR was four times as great as the impact of changes in marriage patterns.

However, there were still 6 provinces, Shanghai, Anhui, Zhejiang, Hunan, Shanxi, and Guizhou, where the changes in nuptiality accounted for more than 25 per cent of total fertility decline. All of these, except Shanxi, are southern provinces.

VI. Summary and Recent Trend

The main features of China's urban fertility transition can be succinctly summarized. The transition started in the great cities, first of all, Shanghai, and then in provinces along the eastern border, gradually diffusing to the interior. Changes in age at marriage took place much earlier than the fertility decline. As a result, the fertility of the 15–19 age group fell ahead of all other age groups. Childbearing in urban China at present is remarkably concentrated in women in their later 20s and births of higher orders have been virtually eliminated. Although marriage has been postponed, the universality of Chinese marriage has persisted. Therefore, the changes in marital fertility have played a more important role in reducing the TFR.

There are no systematic data available for an analysis of the most recent trends in fertility and nuptiality in China's urban areas. However, it is our belief that the general fertility trend, and the regional differentials, persist. In Table 5.11, we present the provincial figures of contribution to total births by birth order for 1984–6. China has expanded its urban population very rapidly since 1984, which is largely because of the re-setting of administrative boundaries and changes in statistical criteria.[15] For the sake of clarity, data in Table 5.11 are for city residents only. The situation in China's towns usually falls between what happens in the cities and countryside.

For China's cities as a whole, the number of first-order births accounts for about 80 per cent of the total births in 1986, although this is actually slightly lower than that in 1984. The three big municipalities are still well ahead of other provinces, and they are followed by the eastern and northeastern provinces. In Shanghai, only less than 1 per cent of its annual births in this period are not first parity. The numbers of second and higher order births in Jiangsu, Liaoning, and Jilin are all below 10 per cent of their total births. On the other hand, provinces with a bad record in fertility transition remain in the group in which the first-order births account for less than 70 per cent of their annual births. These provinces are generally located in the southern and western parts of China, including Guizhou, Yunnan, Guangxi, Jiangxi, Ningxia, Xinjiang, and Guangdong. The largest change during this period happened in Sichuan, Ningxia, Zhejiang, Xinjiang, and Gansu, where the percentage of first births declined by more than 10 percentage points.

Changes in the contribution of the third and higher order births are minor. While the incidence of higher order births continually decreases or remains unchanged in 18 provinces, it rises in the rest, although the magnitude of such a rise is very small. The highest proportion of higher order births can be found in Xinjiang, Guizhou, and Guangxi.

On the whole, the decline in shares of first-order births is offset by the increase in the contribution of second births. This certainly reflects the effect of the modification of the one-child policy in urban areas. It is reasonable to say that China's urban fertility level may have increased slightly, in part because of the rise in second-order births.

It remains difficult to ascertain the effect of changes in age composition of ever married female population on overall fertility. Since the implementation of the 1980 marriage law, the age at marriage has been falling. Available data are not adequate to estimate the

TABLE 5.11. *Contribution to total births by birth order, cities (%)*

Province	First birth			Second birth			Third and Higher		
	1986	Change[a]	Ratio[b]	1986	Change[a]	Ratio[b]	1986	Change[a]	Ratio[b]
CHINA (cities)	79.59	–4.71	100	17.33	5.30	100	3.08	–0.59	100
Beijing	98.35	–0.71	124	1.63	0.70	9	0.02	0.01	1
Tianjin	98.70	–0.65	124	1.29	0.65	7	0.01	0.00	0
Hebei	83.17	–8.30	104	16.05	8.53	93	0.78	–0.23	25
Shanxi	77.79	4.54	98	19.61	–2.07	113	2.60	–2.47	84
Nei Monggol	82.20	3.49	103	16.38	–0.49	95	1.42	–3.00	46
Liaoning	90.56	–7.68	114	9.28	7.55	54	0.16	0.13	5
Jilin	90.03	–7.03	113	9.82	6.93	57	0.15	0.10	5
Heilongjiang	85.88	–7.03	108	12.55	6.26	72	1.57	0.77	51
Shanghai	99.11	–0.38	125	0.87	0.37	5	0.02	0.01	1
Jiangsu	91.26	–2.87	115	8.38	3.24	48	0.36	–0.37	12
Zhejiang	75.77	–10.50	95	22.76	12.03	131	1.47	–1.53	48
Anhui	78.10	–1.51	98	18.29	2.30	106	3.61	–0.79	117
Fujian	70.45	3.71	89	24.78	–1.12	143	4.77	–2.59	155
Jiangxi	64.14	–0.04	81	26.11	0.28	151	9.75	–0.24	317
Shandong	81.63	–8.06	103	17.81	8.67	103	0.56	–0.61	18
Henan	86.55	–7.49	109	12.79	7.62	74	0.66	–0.13	21

Hubei	74.82	–4.93	94	21.50	4.90	124	3.68	0.03	119
Hunan	69.20	–2.60	87	25.70	3.81	148	5.10	–1.21	166
Guangdong	67.71	–1.74	85	25.41	2.82	147	6.88	–1.08	223
Guangxi	63.09	–3.62	79	22.35	3.57	129	14.56	0.05	473
Sichuan	78.45	–14.07	99	20.39	13.41	118	1.16	0.66	38
Guizhou	54.17	–0.01	68	27.65	4.36	160	18.18	–4.35	590
Yunnan	63.58	0.47	80	27.05	0.91	156	9.37	–1.38	304
Shaanxi	74.52	–3.76	94	22.08	3.95	127	3.40	–0.19	110
Gansu	75.14	–10.00	94	22.33	10.15	129	2.53	–0.15	82
Qinghai	80.43	3.63	101	14.86	–1.11	86	4.71	–2.52	153
Ningxia	64.98	–15.56	82	26.71	10.46	154	8.31	5.10	270
Xinjiang	65.51	–10.27	82	17.94	4.81	104	16.55	5.46	537
MEAN	78.05	–4.03		17.58	4.41		4.37	–0.38	
ST.D.	11.80	5.38		7.98	4.24		5.14	2.00	

[a] Change = $\text{Percentage}_{1986} - \text{percentage}_{1984}$

[b] National figure is taken as 100.

Source: Zhongguo renkou ziliao shouche (Handbook of Chinese Population Information), 1985, 1986, and 1987.

TABLE 5.12. *Provincial performance of family-planning programmes, cities*

Province	Late marriage rate (%)				Contraceptive prevalence (%)				One-child certificate rate (%)			
	1986	Change[a]	Ratio 1[b]	Ratio 2[c]	1986	Change[a]	Ratio 1[a]	Ratio 2[c]	1986	Change[a]	Ratio 1[b]	Ratio 2[d]
CHINA (cities)	66.68	–6.40	1.00	1.00	87.60	0.74	1.00	1.00	34.70	0.24	1.00	1.00
Beijing	84.89	–7.70	1.27	1.03	88.31	7.18	1.01	1.03	63.26	10.93	1.82	1.12
Tianjin	77.58	0.20	1.16	1.05	89.16	3.08	1.02	1.02	67.39	7.31	1.94	1.16
Hebei	58.22	–9.51	0.87	1.05	89.26	1.04	1.02	0.99	44.93	2.28	1.29	1.12
Shanxi	70.59	–2.79	1.06	0.96	93.05	3.42	1.06	1.01	29.18	5.41	0.84	0.83
Nei Monggol	75.21	2.53	1.13	1.01	91.03	–0.69	1.04	0.97	25.52	1.43	0.74	0.61
Liaoning	62.34	2.72	0.93	1.04	86.19	–1.20	0.98	1.03	46.26	–1.80	1.33	1.18
Jilin	64.27	–7.68	0.96	0.97	86.61	–0.94	0.99	0.98	38.16	–1.14	1.10	1.01
Heilongjiang	66.66	–14.26	1.00	0.96	89.48	–2.48	1.02	1.01	36.13	0.29	1.04	1.14
Shanghai	90.24	–7.02	1.35	0.90	82.74	–1.82	0.94	1.15	65.70	4.60	1.89	1.03
Jiangsu	72.43	–11.34	1.09	1.04	89.09	–0.23	1.02	0.99	47.15	2.67	1.36	1.09
Zhejiang	66.73	–13.48	1.00	0.94	89.07	–0.43	1.02	0.92	30.64	–1.70	0.88	0.91
Anhui	74.88	–3.40	1.12	1.01	89.75	–0.77	1.02	0.93	28.44	0.81	0.82	0.57
Fujian	57.88	–5.48	0.87	0.95	89.76	–1.49	1.02	1.01	26.55	2.87	0.77	0.72
Jiangxi	54.20	–1.41	0.81	0.98	82.51	0.29	0.94	1.01	16.11	0.60	0.46	0.53
Shandong	69.35	–9.15	1.04	1.06	89.30	–1.20	1.02	1.02	31.84	–4.56	0.92	1.16

Henan	83.74	–5.26	1.26	1.03	86.90	–2.27	0.99	0.99	35.94	0.03	1.04	0.91
Hubei	69.71	–5.29	1.05	0.96	86.38	–0.35	0.99	1.03	24.01	–1.82	0.69	1.04
Hunan	61.64	–5.48	0.92	1.04	89.01	–1.15	1.02	1.01	24.11	–4.73	0.69	1.01
Guangdong	79.06	–1.48	1.19	1.01	89.11	1.62	1.02	0.96	23.17	1.09	0.67	0.74
Guangxi	65.46	–0.84	0.98	—	80.38	2.95	0.92	0.92	32.53	3.58	0.94	0.52
Sichuan	34.60	–11.88	0.52	1.03	87.78	–0.52	1.00	1.02	37.10	–2.01	1.07	1.10
Guizhou	57.78	–8.30	0.87	0.97	78.28	0.16	0.89	0.93	15.44	0.98	0.44	0.35
Yunnan	44.63	–3.57	0.67	0.96	82.89	2.56	0.95	0.87	18.74	2.80	0.54	0.78
Shaanxi	74.06	–6.05	1.11	1.00	85.58	0.16	0.98	1.01	31.52	2.20	0.91	1.15
Gansu	48.61	–13.06	0.73	1.02	90.71	0.11	1.04	0.99	21.48	–7.48	0.62	0.99
Qinghai	63.36	–2.97	0.95	0.88	88.32	6.68	1.01	0.94	27.74	8.44	0.80	0.47
Ningxia	47.15	–2.52	0.71	0.88	90.32	11.23	1.03	0.82	15.62	1.65	0.45	0.23
Xinjiang	75.51	–4.49	1.13	1.01	80.77	35.01	0.92	1.03	23.33	9.83	0.67	0.69
MEAN	66.10	–5.68			87.21	2.14			33.14	1.59		
ST.D.	12.83	4.60			3.61	7.16			14.27	4.25		

[a] Change = $Rate_{1986} - Rate_{1984}$
[b] Ratio 1 refers to ratio of provincial rate to the national one, 1986.
[c] Ratio 2 refers to ratio of provincial rate to the national one, 1979.
[d] Refers to ratio of provincial rate to the national one, 1980.

MAFM. The trend of the late-marriage rate is used here as an alternative and presented in Table 5.12.

Nowadays, Chinese women who get married at an age of 23 or older are classified as late marriage. Table 5.12 shows that more than two-thirds of all urban marriages are taking place in this category. However, it is clear that the number of early marriages is increasing. This is a nation-wide phenomenon to which there were few exceptions. During this three-year period, the incidences of early marriages (women who got married before 23 years old) increased by 6.4 percentage points for cities as a whole, more than 10 points in Heilongjiang, Zhejiang, Gansu, Sichuan, and Jiangsu. Changes in Sichuan province have been dramatic. While about 95 per cent of all first-time brides, no matter whether they lived in cities or the countryside, were more than 23 years old in 1979, only less than 35 per cent of first marriages taking place in Sichuan's cities fulfilled this criterion in 1986. These changes are believed to have been caused mainly by the relaxation of control over the age at marriage, but also reflect the social impact of the recent reform in China.

In Table 5.12, ratios of provincial late-marriage rates to the national rate are calculated for each province for 1979 and 1986. No consistent trend can be found. This may partly result from the fact that there was a standard criterion of late marriage by 1986, which was not so in 1979.

Changes in contraceptive practice in China's cities have been very moderate. About 87.6 per cent of ever married urban women at reproductive ages practised contraception in 1986. The index was 86.7 and 87.2 per cent in 1984 and 1979 respectively. It is interesting to note that most western provinces improved their records of contraceptive prevalence during the period 1984–6. However, the rates in those eastern and northern provinces declined slightly. Compared to 1979, the contraceptive-prevalence rate in China's urban areas remains more or less constant, but the regional difference has diminished. The standard deviation of provincial contraceptive-prevalence rate declined from 5.28 in 1979 to 3.6 in 1986. Birth control in urban China is widely practised. With improvement of quality of birth-control methods, and more acceptance of the norm of 'one child per family' (see Table 5.12), these high rates of contraceptive prevalence will help to keep China's urban fertility at a low level.

NOTES

1. Hu Huanyong & Zhang Shanyu, *Zhongguo renkou dili (Population Geography of China)* (Shanghai: Eastern Normal University Press, 1986).

2. In 1949 the population in the cities and towns was 57.65 million, 10.6% of the total population. This rose to 130.7 million by 1960, to constitute 19.7% of the national total. The increase rate during this period was 7.7% per annum.
3. As was shown in ch. 1, the sample size for the urban areas in Qinghai province is only 283, and 387 in Ningxia autonomous region.
4. A. J. Coale and S. C. Watkins, *The Decline of Fertility in Europe* (Princeton, NJ: Princeton University Press, 1986).
5. E.g. late marriage was viewed as a means of female liberation.
6. See ch. 2.
7. E.g. the number of pre-marital pregnancies and abortions in women before marriage soared during this period. See Five Cities Family Research Project Group, *Family in China's Urban Areas: Collection of Data and Reports on a Family Survey in 5 Cities* (Jinan: Shandong People's Press, 1985).
8. For an analysis of the sent-down youth programme, see e.g. T. P. Bernstein, *Up to the Mountains and Down to the Villages: The Transfer of Youth from Urban to Rural China* (New Haven: Yale University Press, 1977).
9. Five Cities Family Research Project Group, *Family in China's Urban Areas.*
10. In Shanghai, for example, 128,000 couples registered for marriage in 1979, but the figure soared to 282,000 in 1981. See Family Planning Office of Shanghai, 'Causes of Increase in Shanghai's Birth Rate in 1981', internal paper, Apr. 1982.
11. See e.g. L. Moser, *The Chinese Mosaic: The Peoples and Provinces of China* (Boulder: Westview Press, 1985), 210.
12. This generation is regarded as a 'thinking generation' in China.
13. For instance, the median of the first-birth interval for the 1964 marriage cohort was nearly 3 years in Gansu, but only 1.5 years in Yunnan province.
14. See P. Kane, 'The Single-Child Family Policy in the Cities', in E. Croll *et al.* (eds.), *China's One-Child Family Policy* (London: Macmillan, 1985), 83–113.
15. Bai Jianhua, 'Woguo chengxiang renkou de chuangkuang (Rural and Urban Population of China), *Renkou Yanjiu (Population Research)*, No. 2 (1986), 11–14.

6

Provincial Patterns of China's Rural Fertility Transition

In this chapter, rural fertility transition is analysed and compared with the urban transition. The general measures and procedures employed here are the same as those used for the examination of urban patterns.

I. General Patterns

Over the last few decades, the fertility transition has also been taking place in rural China. Decreasing from around 5.64 in the mid-1950s to about 2.61 in the early 1980s, the national figure of the PTFR declined by more than 50 per cent. Most of the reduction occurred in the first half of the 1970s. In spite of the fact that the magnitude of the fertility reduction in rural China is not yet as large as that in the urban sector, such a fertility decline is still a remarkable achievement, especially in a country with 80 per cent of its population living in the countryside.

Levels and Trends

The general patterns of China's rural fertility trends can be seen from Figure 6.1. Provinces are ranked according to their partial total fertility rates (PTFR) in the selected years. Qinghai and Ningxia are left out from the figure once again owing to the large potential sampling errors.

The figure shows that high rural fertility was a common feature across the country in the mid-1950s. The PTFR for rural Tianjin, similar to its urban district, in the period 1954–7 was extremely high at 7.5. We do not know the specific reasons for this situation. Apart from Tainjin, the PTFRs for the all remaining 25 provinces were within the range between 5.1 and 6.9. No clear regional pattern can be identified for this period. But rural fertility in provinces in the northeastern and far northern parts of China was among the highest.

Rural fertility in 1964 was by and large the same as in the mid-1950s, though with a slight increase, which is believed to be the momentum

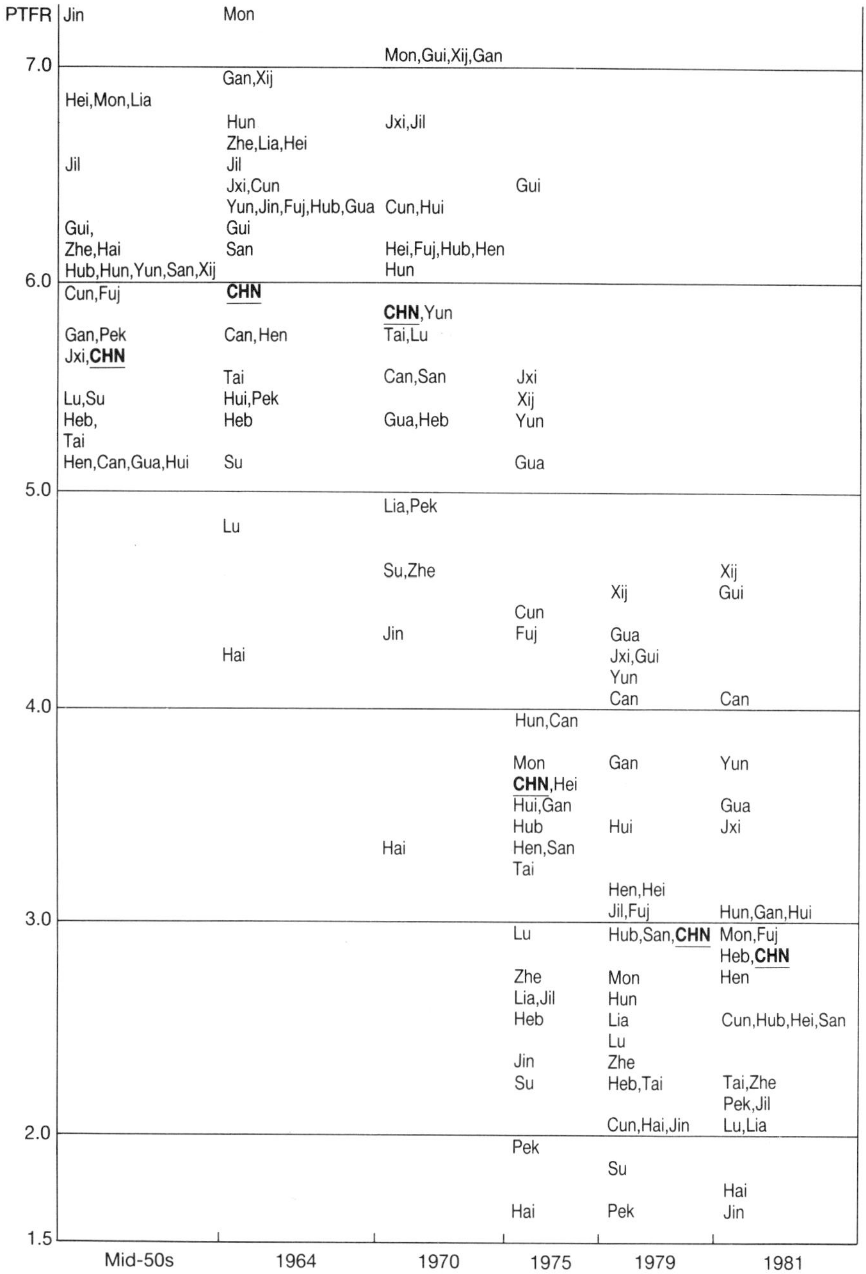

Fig. 6.1 China's rural fertility trends (mid-1950–1981)

effect of the fertility compensation after the massive fertility fluctuation that had occurred in the previous years. Initial fertility transition, nevertheless, had emerged in several places. Early signs of fertility decline can be seen in Tianjin, Jiangsu, and Beijing, and a substantial fertility reduction had already been achieved in Shanghai. The PTFR in rural Shanghai, which was as high as 6.10 in the mid-1950s, had fallen to 4.3 by 1964, a 30-per-cent decline.

The situation during the late 1960s was similar. While the fertility level in a majority of provinces remained high, with some fluctuations, the steep fertility decline accelerated in several provinces. During this period, Shanghai's rural fertility experienced a further reduction, and its PTFR reached 3.4 in 1970. In the 1950s partial total fertility rates were nowhere lower than 5. However, by the end of the 1960s, there were six provinces in which the PTFR was below 5. Among them were three major municipalities, Shanghai, Beijing, and Tianjin, together with Jiangsu, Zhejiang and Liaoning provinces. All these provinces are located along China's eastern coast. This regional variation in the timing of the fertility transition resulted in a widened gap between the highest and the lowest values.

China's third nation-wide family-planning programme ('Wan, Xi, Shao') was launched officially in 1971. This programme, unlike the previous two, penetrated the vast rural areas. During the first half of the 1970s, the national rural PTFR declined by 37 per cent, falling from 5.85 in 1970 to 3.69 in 1975. Although fertility decline occurred in almost all provinces, the speed and extent of the reduction varied greatly. The uneven progress of rural fertility transition was more noticeable than ever. Rural Shanghai was the first to approach a PTFR below 2 as early as 1972: by 1975, it had fallen to 1.45. On the other hand, Guizhou's fertility rate remained almost unchanged until the mid-1970s. Apart from Guizhou, there were another 4 provinces, Jiangxi, Xinjiang, Yunnan, and Guangxi, where the PTFR was still above 5 in 1975. Provinces among the highest third were all located in the southern part of the country except for Xinjiang. In contrast, all of the nine provinces with a PTFR below 3 in 1975 were situated in eastern China. This indicates that during the early stage of the rural transition, the eastern provinces changed distinctly earlier than elsewhere.

The downward trend of rural fertility continued throughout the second half of the 1970s. By 1979 there was no province with a rural PTFR above 5, which was the lowest value two decades earlier. However, the momentum of the decline slowed down in the early 1980s, when only a marginal further reduction occurred, even though a much more vigorous birth-control policy, the 'single-child policy' came into effect in 1979.

The fertility trends between selected periods are shown in Table 6.1. The fertility rates here are three-year averages and changes are compared with the previous period.

During the first decade from the mid-1950s to the mid-1960s, the fertility levels measured by the PTFR rose slightly in the overwhelming majority of provinces. The increase was about 20 per cent in Guangxi, Jiangxi, Anhui, Henan, and Gansu. Fertility rates in these provinces were all lower than the national average in the mid-1950s. By contrast, the initial fertility decline had taken place in the rural areas of the three big municipalities, in which the partial total fertility rate fell by 20 per cent during this decade.

As in the urban areas, fertility in the countryside was also affected by disturbances associated with the Cultural Revolution in the late 1960s. But the extent of this fluctuation was far smaller for the rural population than for the urban population. On the whole, China's rural fertility remained practically unchanged till the early 1970s.

By the early 1970s rural fertility began to decline, but the extent was rather small before the vigorous family-planning programme went into effect. The reduction in the total fertility rate was less than 10 per cent in about half of all provinces compared with the fertility of the mid-1960s. Nevertheless, the steep decline in the three large municipalities continued. In addition, fertility rates dropped by more than 20 per cent in Zhejiang and Jiangsu provinces.

China's rural fertility transition in the mid-1970s was very impressive. The sharp fertility decline can be seen in almost all provinces. On average, the total fertility rate declined by more than 40 per cent in this half decade. In 13 out of 28 provinces, the total fertility rate in the period 1976–8 was half that of the early 1970s. Although fertility did decline, the magnitude was much smaller in Jiangxi, Yunnan, Qinghai, and Xinjiang.

The downward tendency continued until the early 1980s, but the decline was tiny compared with the previous period. Among the top quarter, in which the decline exceeded 20 per cent, were Fujian, Jiangxi, Yunnan, Sichuan, and Tianjin.

The overall magnitude of the rural fertility decline from the mid-1960s to the early 1980s can also be seen in Table 6.1. During this one and a half decades, China's rural fertility declined by more than 55 per cent, taken as a whole. The reductions in 14 provinces exceeded 60 per cent. The total fertility rates in Tianjin, Jiangsu, and Sichuan in the early 1980s were only 30 per cent of those 15 years earlier. Qinghai,

TABLE 6.1. *Fertility trend in rural China by province*[a]

Province	Mid-1950s	1964–6			1970–2		1976–8		1979–81		Total Change
	PTFR	PTFR	Change	TFR	TFR	Change	TFR	Change	TFR	Change	1964–6/1979–81
CHINA (rural)	5.69	6.12	0.08	6.71	5.97	–0.11	3.22	–0.46	2.81	–0.13	–0.54
Guangdong	5.15	5.89	0.14	6.41	6.11	–0.05	4.02	–0.34	4.12	0.02	–0.36
Guangxi	5.14	6.41	0.25	7.17	5.89	–0.18	4.22	–0.28	4.53	0.007	–0.37
Hubei	6.03	6.53	0.08	7.09	6.17	–0.13	2.98	–0.52	2.64	–0.11	–0.63
Hunan	6.02	6.76	0.12	7.39	6.15	–0.17	2.90	–0.53	2.71	–0.07	–0.63
Fujian	5.97	6.59	0.10	7.21	6.52	–0.10	4.29	–0.34	2.78	–0.35	–0.61
Jiangxi	5.59	6.81	0.22	7.40	6.94	–0.06	5.72	–0.18	3.77	–0.34	–0.49
Zhejiang	6.11	6.56	0.07	6.98	4.52	–0.35	2.55	–0.44	2.23	–0.12	–0.68
Shanghai	6.09	4.75	–0.22	5.09	2.69	–0.47	1.83	–0.32	1.69	–0.08	–0.67
Jiangsu	5.46	5.44	–0.01	5.86	4.26	–0.27	2.14	–0.50	1.75	–0.18	–0.70
Anhui	5.14	6.20	0.21	6.80	6.47	–0.05	3.41	–0.47	3.18	–0.07	–0.53
Shandong	5.49	5.27	–0.04	5.75	5.37	–0.07	2.48	–0.54	2.13	–0.14	–0.63
Yunnan	6.03	6.33	0.05	6.93	6.33	–0.09	5.28	–0.17	4.14	–0.22	–0.40
Guizhou	6.25	6.61	0.06	7.31	7.43	0.02	5.04	–0.32	4.51	–0.11	–0.38
Sichuan	6.00	6.41	0.07	7.06	6.83	–0.03	2.83	–0.59	2.13	–0.25	–0.70
Shaanxi	6.07	5.91	0.03	6.40	5.85	–0.09	2.99	–0.49	2.62	–0.12	–0.59
Nei Monggol	6.82	6.93	0.02	7.68	6.63	–0.14	3.22	–0.51	2.94	–0.09	–0.62
Shanxi	5.20	5.53	0.06	6.00	5.95	–0.01	2.81	–0.53	2.28	–0.19	–0.62
Henan	5.18	6.03	0.17	6.63	6.36	–0.04	3.26	–0.49	2.85	–0.13	–0.57
Hebei	5.37	5.44	0.01	5.97	5.19	–0.13	2.48	–0.52	2.55	0.03	–0.57
Beijing	5.73	4.69	–0.18	5.32	4.45	–0.16	1.46	–0.67	1.96	0.34	–0.63
Tianjin	7.49	5.57	–0.26	6.19	4.36	–0.30	2.54	–0.42	1.82	–0.28	–0.71
Xinjiang	6.01	6.75	0.12	7.81	7.02	–0.10	5.61	–0.20	4.66	–0.17	–0.40
Gansu	5.76	6.77	0.18	7.52	7.29	–0.03	3.26	–0.55	3.31	0.02	–0.56
Qinghai	4.29	5.81	0.35	6.66	6.43	–0.04	6.01	–0.07	5.65	–0.06	–0.15
Ningxia	7.60	7.44	–0.02	8.51	7.67	–0.10	5.51	–0.28	5.51	–0.00	–0.35
Jilin	6.53	6.69	0.03	7.44	6.56	–0.12	2.54	–0.61	2.46	–0.03	–0.67
Heilongjiang	6.83	6.78	–0.01	7.50	6.61	–0.12	2.90	–0.56	2.82	–0.03	–0.62
Liaoning	6.83	6.45	–0.05	6.99	4.80	–0.31	2.32	–0.52	2.25	–0.03	–0.68
MEAN	5.93	6.19	0.05			–0.13		–0.43		–0.10	–0.55
ST. D.	0.74	0.68	0.14			0.11		0.15		0.14	0.14

[a] All changes are compared with the previous period. The total change refers to the TFR.

Ningxia, Guangdong, Guangxi, Guizhou, Yunnan, and Xinjiang constituted another group. The fertility decline in these provinces was less than 40 per cent over the entire period.

The Onset of Fertility Transition

The approximate onset date of China's rural fertility transition is estimated for each province. Two criteria are employed: the date at which the PTFR declined by 10 per cent from the initial level (defined as the PTFR in the mid-1950s), and the date at which the PTFR fell below 5, no matter what the initial fertility level was.

The criteria differ slightly from those used to analyse the urban transition. Annual fluctuations, except during the famine period, were much smaller in the rural areas. This is due in part to the relatively large sample size. In addition, it may be attributed to the fact that the reaction of the rural population to the country's political events was less dramatic. In the vast rural areas, therefore, a 10-per-cent decline is of sufficient magnitude to indicate that a substantial fertility decline is on the way. Because of regional variations in the original fertility level, the criterion of the PTFR lower than 5 marks the beginning of the sustained fertility decline at the national level, since the PTFR in the mid-1950s for China's rural population as a whole was about 5.7. Another constraint used in the urban analysis—that the above two criteria should be satisfied at least for three successive years—remains valid.

The massive fertility fluctuation which occurred during the period 1958–63 is obviously abnormal and should not be treated as the start of the genuine fertility decline. Almost all provinces experienced fertility compensation immediately following the massive deficit and high fertility remained until the early 1970s. Therefore, the possibility of the concealment of the real fertility limitation among the rural population is rather small, although it may still have happened in some places. We shall therefore, temporarily leave the period of the great fertility fluctuation out of the current analysis, and assume that the onset of the fertility transition is not earlier than 1964.

Estimates of the year when the PTFR declined by more than 10 per cent from the pre-decline level are given for each province in chronological order in Table 6.2. These are accompanied by estimates of the other important dates of China's rural fertility transition. It should be stressed that these figures are at best only rough estimates.

The regional variation is substantial. We can see that the starting date of the prolonged fertility decline, as indicated by the 10-per-cent

TABLE 6.2. *Important dates in China's rural fertility transition*

Province	PTFR		TFR	
	Decline > 10%	PTFR < 5	TFR < 4	TFR < 3
CHINA (rural)	1972	1973	1975	1980
Shanghai	1964	1967	1969	1971
Tianjin	1964	1966	1972	1973
Beijing	1965	1965	1971	1974
Liaoning	1967	1970	1974	1975
Jiangsu	1969	1969	1972	1973
Zhejiang	1969	1970	1972	1975
Shandong	1971	1971	1973	1976
Hebei	1971	1971	1974	1975
Jilin	1971	1973	1974	1975
Shaanxi	1971	1973	1975	1980
Nei Monggol	1971	1975	1976	—
Hubei	1972	1972	1975	1980
Hunan	1972	1973	1976	1977
Shanxi	1973	1973	1975	1977
Heilongjiang	1973	1974	1975	1980
Fujian	1973	1974	1978	—
Yunnan	1973	1977	—	—
Anhui	1974	1973	1975	—
Sichuan	1974	1975	1976	1977
Gansu	1974	1975	1975	—
Guangdong	1975	1974	—	—
Henan	1975	1973	1975	1980
Guangxi	1976	1976	—	—
Guizhou	1976	1977	—	—
Xinjiang	1977	1977	—	—
Jiangxi	1978	1978	1980	—

criterion, ranged from as early as 1964 in Shanghai to 1978 in Jiangxi: a remarkable 14-year gap. In 16 out of 26 provinces, the initial fertility decline began in the first half of the 1970s. In other words, the transition in most provinces started around the time of the launch of China's third family-planning campaign. In addition to Shanghai, another five provinces experienced a more than 10-per-cent decline in the PTFR before the end of the 1960s. By contrast, it was not until the second half of the 1970s that the 10-per-cent decline in the PTFR was achieved in the remaining six provinces.

Similar results are obtained on the basis of the second criterion. Because of diversities in the original fertility level, the relationship between these two criteria is different between provinces. In about half of the provinces, the date at which their PTFRs fell below 5 was later than the point at which the 10-per-cent fertility decline was reached. In another 9 provinces, the onset date of the fertility transition was the same on either criterion. On the other hand, the partial total fertility rate reached a level below 5 before the steep fertility decline occurred in Anhui, Guangdong, and Henan. This is due to the very low fertility level in these three provinces during the mid-1950s. On the whole, the provincial difference in the onset of the sustained fertility transition is conveniently illustrated by these two sets of dates.

It is worth drawing attention to some special cases. It was four years after the beginning of the sustained decline, that the PTFR in Nei Monggol and Yunnan province fell below 5. This was caused mainly by the high fertility for the pre-decline period and more importantly, resulted from the very slow but steady fertility decline at the early stage of the transition.

Table 6.2 also reveals some regional patterns with respect to the onset of the transition. Those provinces which experienced decline earliest were, no matter which criterion is applied, all located along China's eastern coast. This seems to confirm the impression that while the rural districts of some major cities and the eastern provinces had already experienced substantial rural fertility decline by the end of the 1960s, others lagged well behind. In general the western regions of China entered the transition later.

Moving on to consider two further important dates, it can be seen that the progress of the transition varied considerably between provinces. The total fertility rate in the three big municipalities, and in Jiangsu province, fell below 3 as early as in the early 1970s. But there were still ten provinces in which the TFR remained above this level at least in the early 1980s. In Yunnan, Guangdong, Guangxi, Guizhou, and Xinjiang, the total fertility rate was still above 4 in 1981.

Provincial Variation

The above analysis has shown the great diversity in the timing of the rural fertility transition between provinces. In addition, the provincial variations of the fertility level and the magnitude of the reduction are no less significant. We first look at some statistics of the provincial fertility levels over time.

For obvious reasons, we leave out the situation in the periods 1958–60 and 1961–3. For the other periods, it can be seen that the extent of provincial variability rose steadily during the first two decades of the People's Republic and reached a peak in the period 1973–5. The

TABLE 6.3. *Provincial variability in TFR,[a] rural China*

Period	Mean	Median	St.D.	Min.	Max.	Q1	Q3
1954–7	5.935	6.007	0.739	4.293	7.602	5.389	6.216
1958–60	4.569	4.575	0.950	2.553	6.420	3.884	5.173
1961–3	5.523	5.567	0.670	3.487	6.940	5.274	5.912
1964–6	6.825	6.988	0.789	5.087	8.508	6.243	7.396
1967–9	6.432	6.749	1.045	3.609	8.355	5.860	7.140
1970–2	5.959	6.250	1.137	2.693	7.667	5.231	6.622
1973–5	4.650	4.662	1.486	1.698	7.435	3.454	5.731
1976–8	3.451	2.984	1.277	1.461	6.007	2.543	4.277
1979–81	3.071	2.743	1.118	1.687	5.646	2.238	4.034

[a] Fertility rates before 1964 refer to the PTFR.

standard deviation in 1973–5 was just double that of the mid-1950s. Thereafter, the provincial variation declined slightly, but it was still greater than that in the mid-1950s. This shows clearly the heterogeneous nature of China's rural fertility transition.

The situation in Qinghai and Ningxia is of particular interest. The fertility level in Qinghai province was extremely low until the mid-1960s. Its PTFR was only 4.29 in 1954–7, (25 per cent lower than the national average). This may reflect the harshness of life in this province. Historically, population growth in Qinghai, especially in its minority areas, was very slow. This has been attributed to many factors, the tough nomadic life, local disease, polygamic custom, religious practice, and so on.[1] But the data may also reflect reporting and sampling errors. Since the mid-1960s, however, Qinghai's fertility has remained very high and almost constant up to the present. In the early 1980s the total fertility rate in Qinghai (about 6) was the highest in China. The fertility level in Ningxia, on the other hand, has been consistently among the highest in the country throughout the last three decades. In the early 1980s the total fertility rate in Ningxia (5.51) was only second to that in Qinghai. Because of the small sample size in these two provinces, the risk of the sampling error is much larger than in other provinces and caution is advisable in interpretation.

Apart from these two extremes, the highest provincial fertility rate in the mid-1950s was about 46 per cent higher than the lowest one. The difference in the mid-1960s increased to 53 per cent, and 176 per cent in the early 1970s, remaining at this level in the early 1980s.

The regional pattern is further illustrated by examining the ratios of provincial fertility rates, the PTFR in the mid-1950s (1954–7) and the TFR thereafter, to the national ones throughout the last thirty years.

These ratios are calculated on a three-year average basis and presented graphically in Figure 6.2.

The ratios for the period 1958–63 are affected by the massive fertility fluctuation of that era. Apart from that, provinces can be classified roughly into a few groups according to the trend of their ratios.

The first group is composed of Xinjiang, Guizhou, Yunnan, Gansu, and Ningxia. The fertility levels in these provinces were consistently higher than the national average, and the ratios increased as time passed. The second group consists of provinces like Guangdong, Guangxi, Anhui, Qinghai, and probably Henan as well. The common feature of this group is that the fertility levels of these provinces were lower than the national average in the mid-1950s, but higher during the 1970s. Bearing in mind the sharp fertility decline during the 1970s, the increased ratios indicate that the tempo of the fertility transition in those provinces was relatively slow and that they lagged behind the national trend.

Shanghai, Zhejiang, Beijing, Tianjin, Sichuan, Jilin, Liaoning, and Fujian comprise the third group. The fertility rates of these provinces were all above the national average in the mid-1950s, although some were only marginally higher. However, the fertility transition in this group was ahead of the rest, which led to the sharp falls in these ratios. By the early 1980s, ratios for these provinces were well below one. The fourth group includes Jiangsu, Shandong, and Hebei. The fertility levels in these three provinces were always among the national lowest. Finally, Nei Monggol and Heilongjiang had features in common. Although the fertility level was constantly above the national level, the reduced ratio seems to suggest that the fertility decline in these two provinces was faster than the national average.

Now, we have roughly two kinds of provinces: the first is the province in which the fertility transition lagged behind the national trend, and the second consists of provinces which led the transition process.

The case of Sichuan deserves some attention. The fertility decline there lagged behind the national trend until the mid-1970s, a pattern similar to that in Guizhou. The reverse trend, however, then emerged and a sudden and very sharp fertility decline occurred. Indeed, Sichuan's TFR declined by 67 per cent between 1975 and 1980, the sharpest fall nationally and probably the fastest decline anywhere for a sizeable population (in excess of 100 million).

The differences in relative fertility, as measured in the ratios, widened over time. Apart from Qinghai, as well as Tianjin and Ningxia, the ratios in the mid-1950s ranged from a high of 1.20 to a low

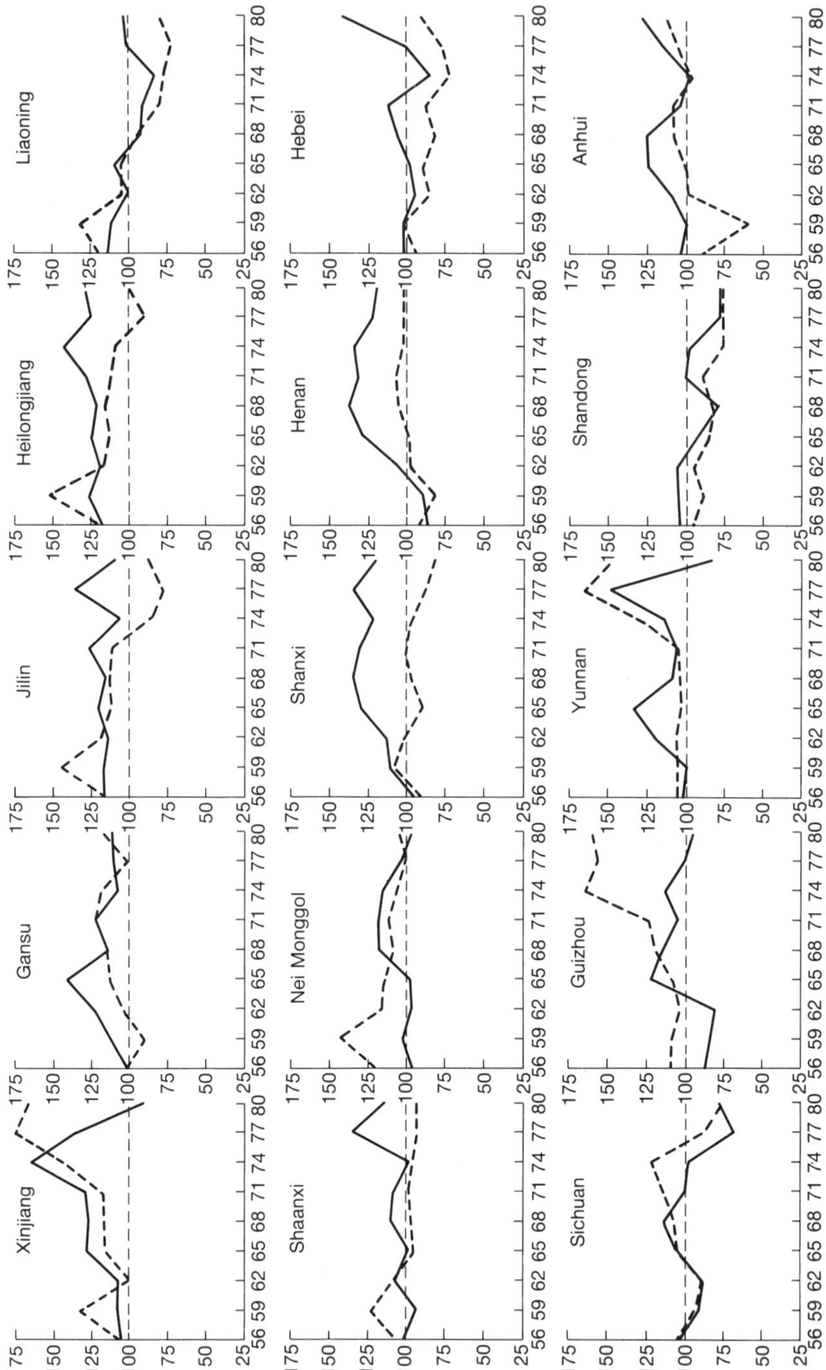
Xinjiang
Gansu
Jilin
Heilongjiang
Liaoning
Shaanxi
Nei Monggol
Shanxi
Henan
Hebei
Sichuan
Guizhou
Yunnan
Shandong
Anhui
175
150
125
100
75
50
25
56 59 62 65 68 71 74 77 80

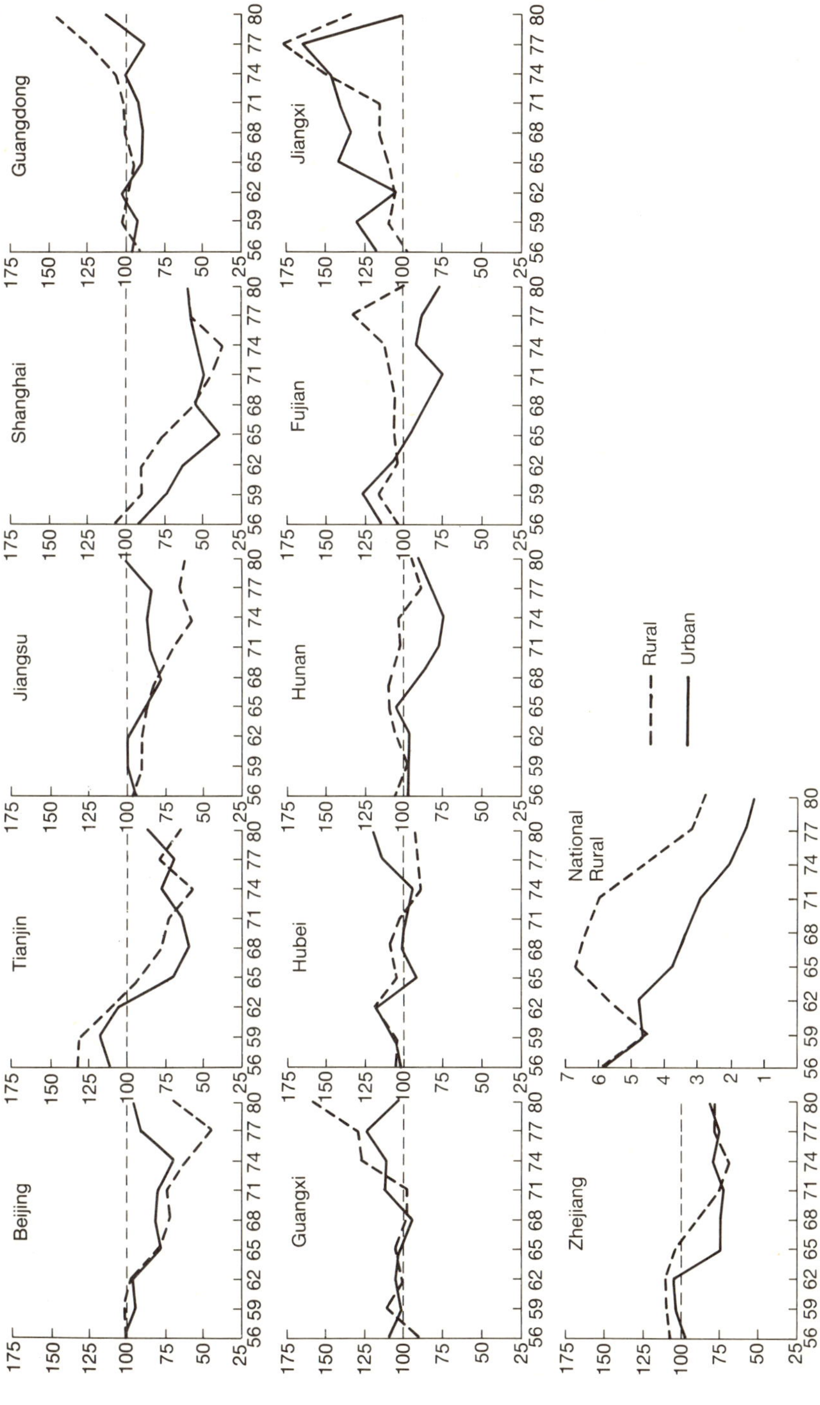

Fig. 6.2 Ratios of provincial fertility to national ones

of 0.90. In the early 1980s the highest ratio was 1.66, while the lowest was only 0.60. This confirms the uneven progress of the fertility transition.

Geographical generalizations may oversimplify the matter. It can be seen, nevertheless, that the eastern part of China was the advanced region in terms of fertility transition, with Shanghai leading the way. Then followed the northern provinces. On the other hand, the transition commenced much later in the western and some southern provinces. The fertility levels in the north were originally higher than in other regions, but this gap was eliminated as time passed.

Rural–Urban Comparison

We have seen from the analysis of the national pattern that the rural–urban differential in the fertility transition is considerable, not only in timing, but also in the magnitude of change. The differentials are even more striking at the provincial level. Comparisons have been made between the urban and rural fertility transition in each province. There are some similarities and great differences. The overall fertility reduction throughout the last three decades and the onset dates of the sustained fertility decline are examined first.

Table 6.4 reveals several important features of the rural–urban differences. First, the onset of China's rural fertility transition which generally started from the early 1970s was roughly one decade later than the urban transition. However, while the initial urban fertility decline started around the mid-1960s in almost all provinces, the onset dates for the vast rural area were more widely spread. With a few exceptions, such as Shanghai and Henan, a 15 per cent fertility decline in the urban areas had been achieved by 1967 in all provinces. The time difference in the onset of decline between provinces was only three years. By contrast, the sustained fertility transition began as early as 1964 for the rural population in some major municipalities, whereas this only took place in the late 1970s in Jiangxi, Xinjiang, Guizhou, and Guangxi. In other words, rural women in these four provinces began to use birth control extensively more than ten years after their counterparts in the rural districts of the major municipalities.

Secondly, the overall magnitude of the fertility decline in general is smaller in the rural areas than that in the urban. On average, the total fertility decline measured by the partial fertility rate over the period between the mid-1950s and the early 1980s was about 75 per cent for the urban population, but only 50 per cent for the rural population. This is not surprising since the fertility transition in China's rural areas

TABLE 6.4. *Rural–urban comparison of the fertility transition*

Province	Urban PTFR		Total	Rural PTFR		Total	Onset Date	
	1954–7	1979–81	decline %	1954–7	1979–81	decline %	Rural	Urban
CHINA	5.18	1.29	73.6	5.69	2.71	52.3	1972	1964
Shanghai	4.75	0.75	84.2	6.09	1.68	72.3	1964	1958
Tianjin	5.78	1.14	80.3	7.49	1.80	76.0	1964	1964
Beijing	5.26	1.26	76.1	5.72	1.94	66.1	1965	1964
Liaoning	5.88	1.34	77.2	6.83	2.23	67.3	1967	1964
Zhejiang	5.04	1.06	79.0	6.11	2.19	64.1	1969	1964
Jiangsu	4.82	1.30	73.0	5.46	1.73	68.3	1969	1964
Shandong	5.39	1.02	81.0	5.49	2.09	61.9	1971	1964
Jilin	6.02	1.40	76.7	6.53	2.40	63.2	1971	1964
Nei Monggol	4.98	1.25	75.0	6.82	2.83	58.6	1971	1964
Shaanxi	5.22	1.48	71.6	6.07	2.54	58.2	1971	1964
Hebei	5.27	1.84	64.9	5.36	2.50	53.4	1971	1964
Hunan	5.06	1.20	76.2	6.02	2.65	55.9	1972	1965
Hubei	5.35	1.57	70.7	6.03	2.59	57.1	1972	1964
Fujian	5.98	1.00	83.3	5.97	2.68	55.0	1973	1964
Yunnan	5.27	1.03	80.4	6.03	3.83	36.5	1973	1966
Heilongjiang	6.07	1.67	72.5	6.83	2.74	59.8	1973	1964
Shanxi	4.98	1.55	68.8	5.20	2.24	56.9	1973	1966
Sichuan	5.39	1.02	81.1	6.00	2.08	65.4	1974	1964
Gansu	5.24	1.44	72.4	5.76	3.21	44.3	1974	1967
Anhui	5.41	1.67	69.1	5.14	3.08	40.1	1974	1966
Guangdong	4.93	1.48	70.0	5.15	3.92	23.9	1975	1964
Henan	4.48	1.53	65.8	5.17	2.77	46.5	1975	1971
Guangxi	5.73	1.32	76.9	5.14	4.33	15.8	1976	1964
Guizhou	4.53	1.23	72.8	6.25	4.20	32.8	1976	1964
Xinjiang	5.42	1.17	78.4	6.01	4.40	26.8	1977	1965
Jiangxi	6.00	1.31	78.2	5.58	3.63	35.1	1978	1965
MEAN	5.32	1.31	75.2	5.93	2.79	52.4		
ST.D	0.45	0.25	5.2	0.61	0.83	15.9		

Note: Total percentage decline is calculated as ($PTFR_{1979-81}/PTFR_{1954-57} - 1) \times 100$.

is still progressing, while the transition from the high to low fertility has been virtually completed in the urban areas.

Thirdly, the provincial differences for the rural population are much larger than those for the urban. The urban differences with respect to the transition fell substantially over time. The regional differences in urban fertility level were within a very narrow range by the end of the 1970s.

By contrast, the rural variation was bigger and widened over time. For instance, the total fertility reduction in the urban areas ranged from 84 per cent in Shanghai to 65 per cent in Hebei province. The former is 1.3 times the latter. For the rural population, the sharpest decline of 76 per cent in Tianjin is 3.80 times greater than the smallest of 16 per cent in Guangxi. In addition, it seems that the provincial difference in fertility level for the rural population has always been larger than that of the urban population, as can be seen from the bigger standard deviation for rural fertility over time. On the whole, it can be said that the urban transition was more homogeneous between provinces compared with rural fertility changes, even though the variation in the urban areas was still very marked.

There are some other general observations about China's rural–urban fertility differentials that are worth noting. Perhaps the single most important point is that rural fertility was higher than urban fertility with very few exceptions over the entire period concerned. The ratios of the rural to urban fertility rate for the selected period have been calculated and are presented in Table 6.5. Since the numerator of the ratio is the rural total fertility rate, the larger the ratio, the higher the rural fertility is, compared with the urban fertility.

The size of the pre-decline differential was small, indicated by the ratios being close to unity in most provinces in the mid-1950s. On average, rural fertility was about 12 per cent higher than urban fertility. The largest rural–urban differences at that time were in Guizhou, Nei Monggol, and Tianjin, where the ratios were greater than 1.3. It can be seen that the rural partial total fertility rate was exceeded by urban fertility prior to the onset of the sustained decline only in Guangxi, Anhui, and Jiangxi provinces. Apart from these provinces, the ratios of the rural to the urban fertility rates were consistently greater than one.

The situation for the period 1958–63 is clearly special. Rural fertility in several provinces fell well below urban fertility, which suggests the more severe nature of the crisis in those rural areas. These ratios are not presented in Table 6.5 since we are interested here in the general pattern.

The uneven progress of the transition is evident. The first jump in

TABLE 6.5. *Ratios of the rural to urban fertility rate by province*

Province	Ratios in period						
	1954–7	1964–6	1967–9	1970–2	1973–5	1976–8	1979–81
NATIONAL	1.10	1.79	1.90	2.04	2.21	2.04	2.16
Guangdong	1.04	1.89	2.14	2.25	2.36	2.89	2.78
Guangxi	0.90	1.86	1.99	1.78	2.52	2.14	3.31
Hubei	1.13	2.04	2.05	2.10	2.10	1.64	1.67
Hunan	1.19	1.86	2.28	2.64	3.02	2.18	2.26
Fujian	1.00	1.99	2.31	2.92	2.68	3.07	2.78
Jiangxi	0.93	1.39	1.64	1.67	2.24	2.17	2.88
Zhejiang	1.21	2.47	2.31	2.11	1.94	2.12	2.10
Shanghai	1.28	3.44	1.95	1.86	1.55	1.99	2.19
Jiangsu	1.13	1.76	1.97	1.71	1.48	1.61	1.34
Anhui	0.95	1.46	1.65	2.13	2.19	1.89	1.90
Shandong	1.02	1.63	1.96	1.84	1.73	2.02	2.09
Yunnan	1.14	1.39	1.84	2.04	2.50	2.24	3.83
Guizhou	1.38	1.60	1.97	2.38	3.19	3.17	3.67
Sichuan	1.11	1.79	1.80	2.34	2.76	2.64	2.09
Shaanxi	1.16	1.72	1.67	1.85	2.17	1.40	1.77
Nei Monggol	1.37	2.08	1.75	1.91	2.04	1.98	2.35
Shanxi	1.04	1.24	1.35	1.57	1.74	1.33	1.47
Henan	1.16	1.38	1.46	1.65	1.68	1.69	1.84
Hebei	1.02	1.63	1.47	1.58	1.86	1.55	1.38
Beijing	1.09	1.82	1.67	1.90	1.95	1.00	1.56
Tianjin	1.30	2.34	2.47	2.28	1.64	2.31	1.60
Xinjiang	1.11	1.63	1.75	1.85	1.92	2.63	3.98
Gansu	1.10	1.42	1.90	2.04	2.43	1.87	2.30
Jilin	1.08	1.66	1.86	1.77	1.80	1.19	1.74
Heilongjiang	1.13	1.61	1.80	1.76	1.67	1.46	1.68
Liaoning	1.16	1.70	1.94	1.80	2.04	1.45	1.68
MEAN	1.12	1.80	1.88	1.99	2.12	1.98	2.24
MEDIAN	1.12	1.71	1.88	1.88	2.04	1.98	2.09
ST.D.	0.12	0.44	0.27	0.33	0.45	0.57	0.76
MIN.	0.90	1.24	1.35	1.57	1.48	1.00	1.34
MAX.	1.38	3.44	2.47	2.92	3.19	3.17	3.98
Q1.	1.04	1.57	1.67	1.77	1.74	1.53	1.68
Q3.	1.17	1.92	2.00	2.16	2.45	2.25	2.78
CORR. COEFFIC.	0.351	0.628	0.752	0.734	0.741	0.581	0.140

terms of these ratios was in the mid-1960s, while the steep fertility decline started in the urban areas. The average value of these ratios was 1.80 for that period. In Shanghai, Zhejiang, Tianjin, Nei Monggol, and Hubei, the rural fertility was more than twice as high as the urban fertility.

The rural–urban difference became bigger during the course of the transition as urban fertility declined more rapidly in the initial stages. This is a pattern which was observed in the European fertility transition, although change there took place over a longer period.[2] By the early 1980s the rural–urban difference in fertility was just double that of in the mid-1950s on average. The smallest difference was in Jiangsu and Hebei provinces with the ratio less than 1.4, which was the highest value in the mid-1950s. There were four provinces, Guangxi, Yunnan, Guizhou, and Xinjiang, in which rural fertility was more than 3 times as high as urban fertility.

Since urban fertility levels were similar in the early 1980s, regional differences in these ratios are mainly determined by the levels of and changes in rural fertility.

Another prominent feature is the relationship between urban and rural fertility. It can be seen from Table 6.5 that the trend of the correlation coefficients is a bell shape: from low in the mid-1950s to a peak in the late 1960s and dropping to the lowest level in the early 1980s. If rural and urban fertility for the period between the mid-1960s to the early 1970s were highly correlated, this was not the case for other periods. In the early 1980s, because there was almost no variability in urban fertility, rural and urban fertility were hardly associated, at least with respect to a linear relation.

II. Changes in Nuptiality

The traditional Chinese marriage pattern can be generalized as early and universal marriage. In addition, arranged marriage was practised widely across the country. This total neglect of the wishes of the parties concerned was almost without parallel in the world.[3] Since the founding of the People's Republic, social reform has changed this traditional pattern, not only in the cities, but also in the vast rural areas. The younger generation now have the legal right to select their own marriage partners. Marriage has been considerably postponed. The mean age at first marriage (MAFM) for China's rural female population as a whole rose from 18.5 in 1950 to 19.3 in 1965, a slow but steady increase over this fifteen-year period. Afterwards, the upward trend accelerated, especially during the 1970s. By 1970, a year before the official launch of the 'Later, Longer, Fewer' policy, the MAFM had reached 19.9, further jumping to 21.4 and 22.5 in 1975 and 1980 respectively.

Mean Age at First Marriage

The provincial trends are, generally speaking, similar to the national one (see Figure 6.3). The mean age at first marriage rose in all provinces. Nowadays, rural women get married much later than their mothers did. Nevertheless, the tempo and the quantum of this increase in MAFM varies somewhat among the provinces.

The statutory age at marriage for women set by the marriage law of 1950 was 18 years which was two years higher than that stated in the Family Law of 1931. However, Table 6.6 shows that by the end of the 1950s there were still seven provinces in which the average age at first marriage for rural females fell below the legal requirement. All seven were the northwest provinces. Women got married at very young ages especially in Ningxia and Xinjiang. A large proportion of the population in these provinces was composed of ethnic minorities, with Muslims as the main religious group. This very early marriage was to a certain extent associated with local custom and religious practice.[4]

During this decade the marriage age rose very slowly. In some southeastern provinces, such as Fujian and Zhejiang, it actually declined. Only Tianjin experienced a sizeable rise. The marriage age continued to rise quite rapidly during the great famine period, 1959–61. This can be partly viewed as the population's response to the disturbance at that time. During the recovery period, however, the marriage age declined slightly in about two-thirds of all provinces and returned to the level of the mid-1950s.

Since the mid-1960s the postponement of marriage has gathered momentum. The age at marriage rose sharply in most provinces around the mid-1970s. Social developments, such as improvements in mass education, should have contributed to ending very early marriages. However, it is more likely that this achievement was largely attributable to the success of the late-marriage campaign.

But the effects of the campaign differed from province to province. On the one hand, the target age for later marriage varied between localities. On the other hand, the efforts of the local authorities in enforcing this campaign also differed. By the early 1980s there were still four provinces, Xinjiang, Gansu, Ningxia, and Qinghai, in which women got married on average below the age of 20. These four adjacent provinces are located in the northwestern part of China. By contrast, the average age of brides in the rural sectors of the big municipalities and some eastern provinces was well above 23 years.

As a consequence of the implementation of the new marriage law of 1980, and also due in part to the relaxation of marriage control which

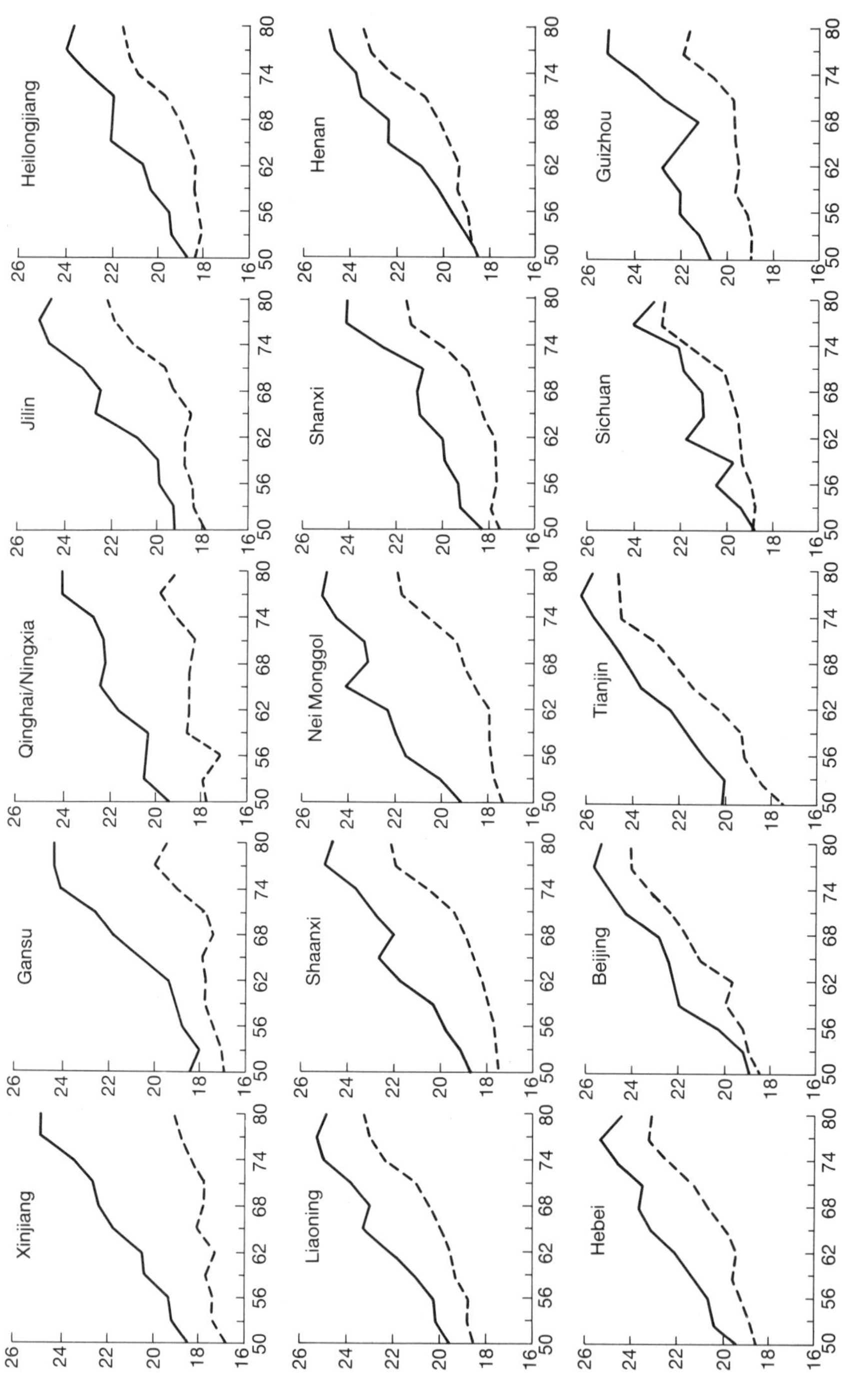
Xinjiang
Gansu
Qinghai/Ningxia
Jilin
Heilongjiang
Liaoning
Shaanxi
Nei Monggol
Shanxi
Henan
Hebei
Beijing
Tianjin
Sichuan
Guizhou

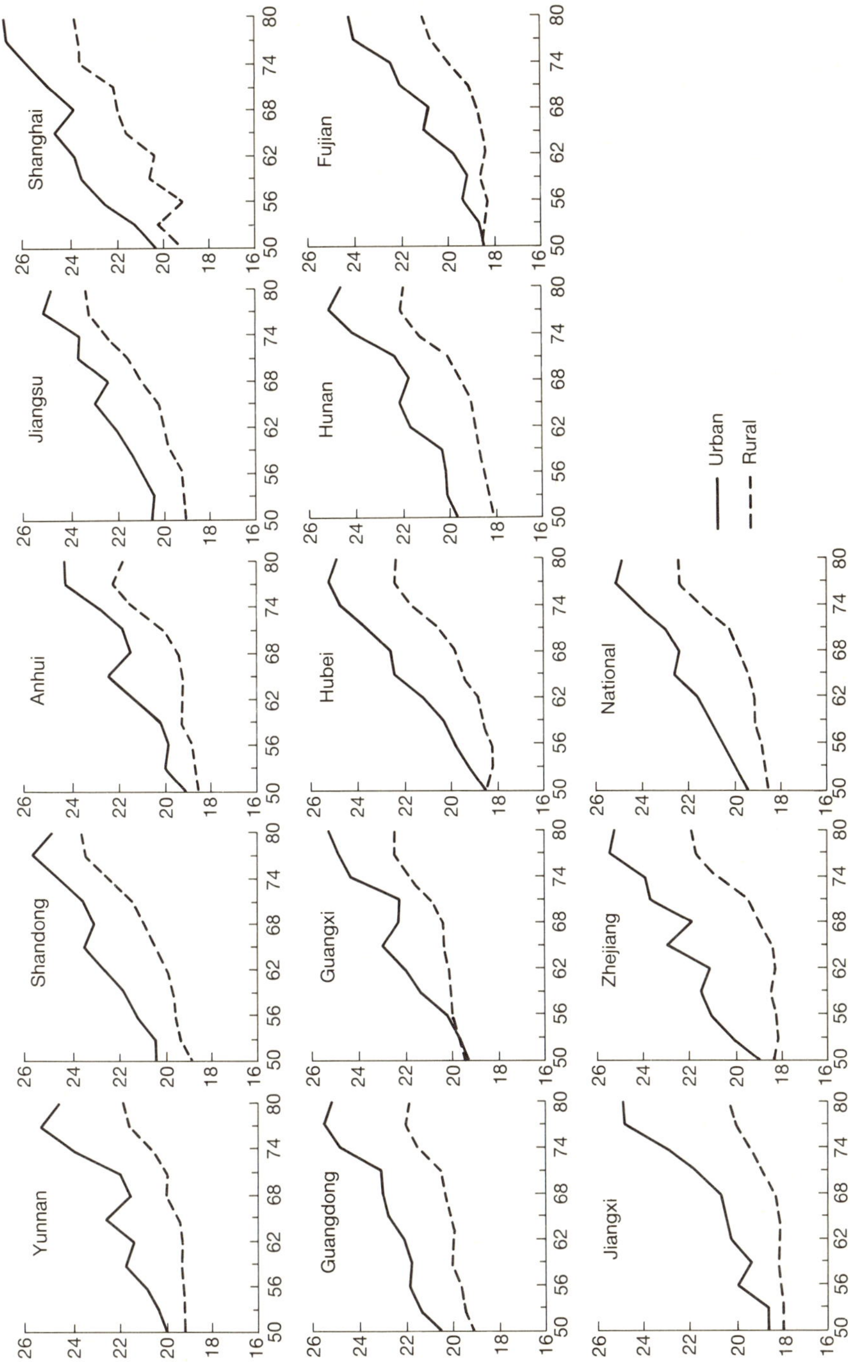

Fig. 6.3 Provincial mean age at first marriage, rural and urban 1950–1981

TABLE 6.6. *Mean age at first marriage, rural China 1950–1981*

Province	Mean age at the first marriage for the period										
	1950–2	1953–5	1956–8	1959–61	1962–4	1965–7	1968–70	1971–3	1974–6	1977–9	1980–1
CHINA (rural)	18.55	18.70	18.84	19.16	19.19	19.40	19.82	20.24	21.40	22.37	22.41
Guangdong	19.12	19.53	19.71	20.10	20.03	20.13	20.39	20.57	21.53	22.03	21.89
Guangxi	19.32	19.70	20.04	20.08	20.19	20.39	20.44	20.91	21.85	22.50	22.49
Hubei	18.50	18.28	18.37	18.71	18.88	19.56	19.88	20.61	21.73	22.44	22.36
Hunan	18.14	18.30	18.53	18.77	18.87	19.06	19.55	20.11	21.39	22.12	21.97
Fujian	18.55	18.42	18.36	18.68	18.44	18.55	18.80	19.17	20.05	20.80	21.13
Jiangxi	17.93	17.93	18.07	18.17	18.14	18.10	18.29	18.89	19.41	20.03	20.32
Zhejiang	18.39	18.20	18.26	18.52	18.33	18.43	18.99	19.45	20.80	21.75	21.93
Shanghai	19.28	20.29	19.22	20.63	20.42	21.68	22.07	22.25	23.62	23.72	23.91
Jiangsu	19.12	19.20	19.27	19.84	20.07	20.30	21.05	21.63	22.56	23.26	23.41
Anhui	18.62	18.74	18.88	19.38	19.30	19.31	19.55	20.14	21.42	22.31	21.87
Shandong	18.90	19.43	19.66	19.74	20.02	20.49	20.97	21.44	22.52	23.48	23.67
Yunnan	19.25	19.29	19.33	19.42	19.37	19.53	20.08	20.04	20.61	21.62	21.91
Guizhou	18.99	18.94	19.17	19.69	19.53	19.66	19.73	19.78	20.67	21.92	21.61
Sichuan	18.92	18.79	18.97	19.40	19.51	19.57	19.85	20.16	21.51	22.79	22.66
Shaanxi	17.45	17.56	17.67	17.89	18.17	18.53	18.92	19.38	20.50	21.89	22.10
Nei Monggol	17.28	17.65	17.82	17.93	17.90	18.57	19.06	19.37	20.51	21.70	21.88
Shanxi	17.46	17.89	17.63	17.65	17.71	18.23	18.55	18.99	19.96	21.34	21.54
Henan	18.44	18.77	18.89	19.33	19.24	19.64	20.13	20.73	22.09	23.06	23.36
Hebei	18.55	18.82	19.15	19.54	19.41	19.82	20.59	21.24	22.28	23.20	23.05
Beijing	18.38	18.91	19.18	19.88	19.56	21.03	21.56	22.26	23.21	24.03	24.06
Tianjin	17.45	18.49	19.14	19.27	20.19	21.39	22.23	23.04	24.52	24.64	24.67
Xinjiang	16.78	17.38	17.36	17.66	17.30	18.06	17.75	17.73	18.32	18.80	19.11
Gansu	16.93	17.06	17.41	17.79	17.74	17.91	17.44	17.75	19.05	20.04	19.47
Qinghai	18.69	18.99	17.61	20.41	19.27	19.02	19.23	17.95	18.96	19.09	18.12
Ningxia	16.71	16.76	16.60	16.75	17.70	18.00	17.64	18.55	19.33	20.63	19.94
Jilin	17.85	18.36	18.43	18.78	18.73	18.53	19.24	19.67	21.00	21.87	22.21
Heilongjiang	18.33	18.07	18.20	18.41	18.33	18.66	19.03	19.59	20.86	21.33	21.55
Liaoning	18.55	18.85	18.86	19.39	19.61	19.97	20.46	21.05	22.35	23.04	23.27
MEAN	18.28	18.52	18.56	18.99	19.00	19.36	19.70	20.09	21.17	21.98	21.98
MEDIAN	18.47	18.62	18.70	19.30	19.26	19.42	19.64	20.08	21.20	21.98	21.95
ST.D.	0.776	0.811	0.826	0.957	0.895	1.049	1.238	1.355	1.468	1.409	1.533

Note: All figures are 3-year averages.

was the by-product of the rural responsibility system, age at marriage declined slightly in the majority of provinces in the early 1980s. In some provinces the setback was considerable. In Anhui, for instance, women in rural areas on average got married in 1981 one year earlier than in 1979. Nevertheless, the mean age at first marriage for all provinces was still well above that of one decade earlier.

In Table 6.7, changes in the MAFM over different periods are estimated for each province. The MAFM has increased in all but Qinghai province over the last thirty years. But the amount of this increase differed enormously—from 7.22 years in Tianjin to only 2.33 in Xinjiang. It can be seen that the increase in the first twenty-year period was very modest with an annual rise of only about 0.07 years for China's rural population as a whole. Nevertheless, the increase in seven eastern provinces exceeded 0.1 years per annum. In Tianjin and Beijing, the marriage age rose one year in every four-year period.

The early 1970s can be viewed as a turning-point, from which the upward trend accelerated in almost all provinces. The marriage age increased at an annual rate of about 0.3 years. The exceptions to this general trend in the postponement of marriage were in the western provinces. While there were 14 provinces where the annual rise exceeded 0.3 years, the rise in Yunnan, Guizhou, Xinjiang, and Ningxia was less than 0.1 years. The opposite occurred in Qinghai. This may reflect the persistence of local marriage customs, but may also be caused by sampling errors. This uneven development widened the regional differences.

The trend towards later marriage slowed down in most provinces in the later 1970s. However, the major increase in the MAFM took place only during the second half of the 1970s in Shaanxi, Shanxi, Yunnan, and Guizhou. Those provinces had previously lagged behind the general trend of delaying marriage but now caught up.

Another broad generalization is that the regional marriage pattern measured by the MAFM had persisted throughout the past three decades. This can be seen from the changes in ratios of the provincial MAFM to the national one in Figure 6.4. Provinces in which the MAFM was higher than the national average in 1980 were largely the same as thirty years earlier. The marriage age in the eastern and far southern regions was commonly higher than other places. On the other hand, rural marriage in the far north and the southeastern parts of China generally occurred early. The lowest MAFM was found consistently in the northwest. Furthermore, provinces with an early marriage tradition seem to have lagged more and more behind the national progress, as is confirmed by the falls of the ratios. Despite strong government

TABLE 6.7. *Changes in MAFM and the proportion of women ever married by province, rural China*

Province	Changes in marriage age[a]				Proportion of ever married[b]
	Total increase	Annual rise			
	1950/2–1980/1	1950–70	1970–5	1975–80	1979–81 (%)
CHINA (rural)	3.86	0.069	0.296	0.238	99.73
Tianjin	7.22	0.250	0.316	0.154	100.00
Beijing	5.68	0.277	0.132	0.276	100.00
Henan	4.93	0.084	0.356	0.324	99.76
Shandong	4.77	0.113	0.316	0.244	100.00
Liaoning	4.72	0.118	0.352	0.194	99.58
Shaanxi	4.65	0.066	0.190	0.496	99.15
Shanghai	4.63	0.151	0.366	0.076	99.12
Nei Monggol	4.60	0.093	0.332	0.228	100.00
Hebei	4.50	0.110	0.308	0.182	99.83
Jilin	4.36	0.057	0.402	0.234	100.00
Jiangsu	4.29	0.113	0.248	0.212	99.84
Shanxi	4.08	0.054	0.198	0.376	100.00
Hubei	3.86	0.079	0.378	0.180	99.75
Hunan	3.82	0.078	0.326	0.174	99.91
Sichuan	3.74	0.041	0.376	0.282	99.64
Zhejiang	3.54	0.041	0.368	0.208	100.00
Anhui	3.25	0.051	0.360	0.144	99.78
Ningxia	3.22	0.164	0.054	0.116	99.00
Heilongjiang	3.22	0.026	0.364	0.118	100.00
Guangxi	3.17	0.064	0.332	0.094	98.98
Guangdong	2.76	0.072	0.278	0.036	99.77
Yunnan	2.65	0.052	0.094	0.250	99.14
Guizhou	2.62	0.057	0.092	0.312	100.00
Fujian	2.58	0.024	0.220	0.132	100.00
Gansu	2.54	0.032	0.296	0.132	100.00
Jiangxi	2.39	0.017	0.200	0.170	99.62
Xinjiang	2.33	0.048	0.086	0.108	98.64
Qinghai	–0.57	0.025	–0.204	–0.112	98.85
MEAN	3.698	0.0845	0.2549	0.1907	99.65
MEDIAN	3.780	0.0650	0.3120	0.1810	99.80
ST.D.	1.398	0.0635	0.1371	0.1144	0.44

[a] measured in years.
[b] for women at age 32.

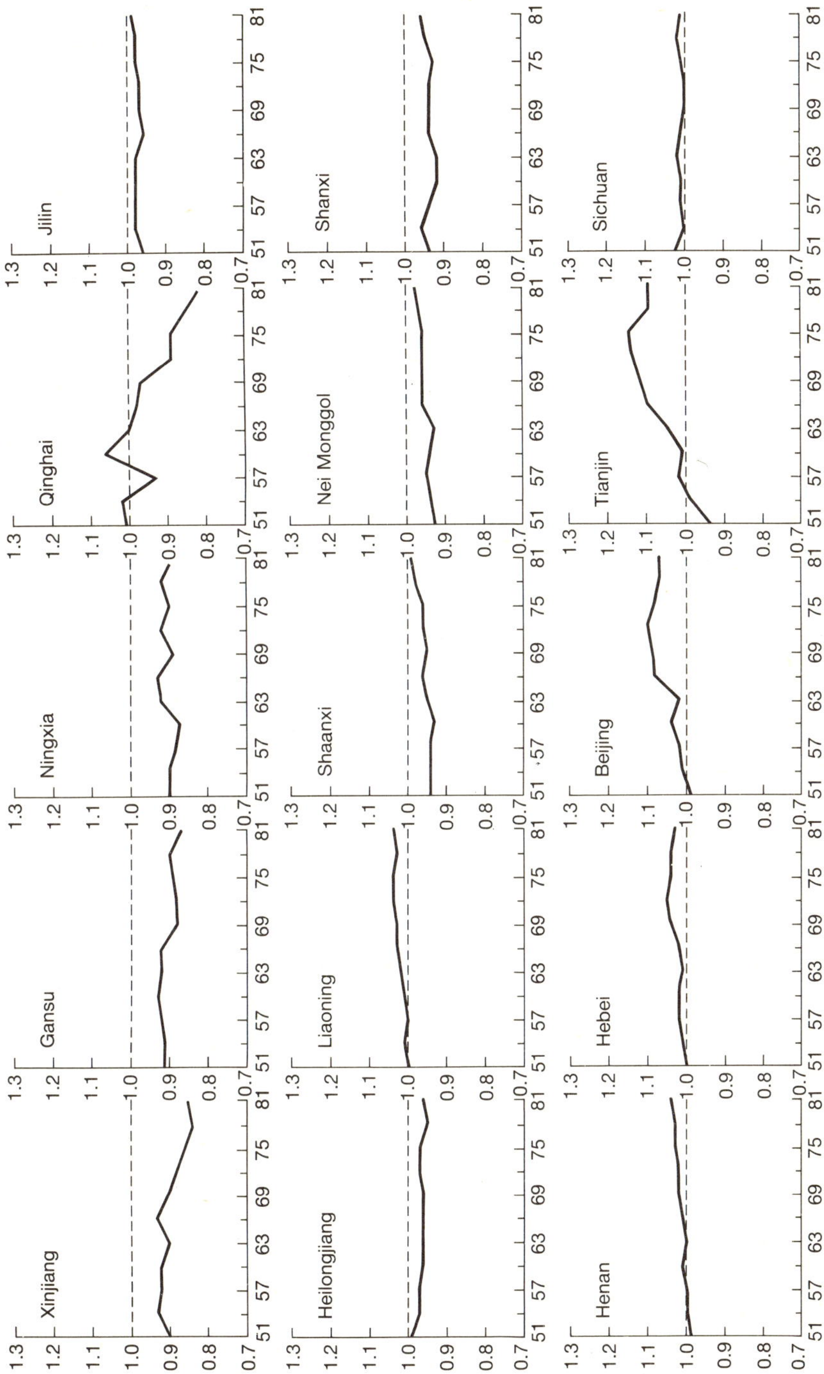
Xinjiang
Gansu
Ningxia
Qinghai
Jilin
Heilongjiang
Liaoning
Shaanxi
Nei Monggol
Shanxi
Henan
Hebei
Beijing
Tianjin
Sichuan

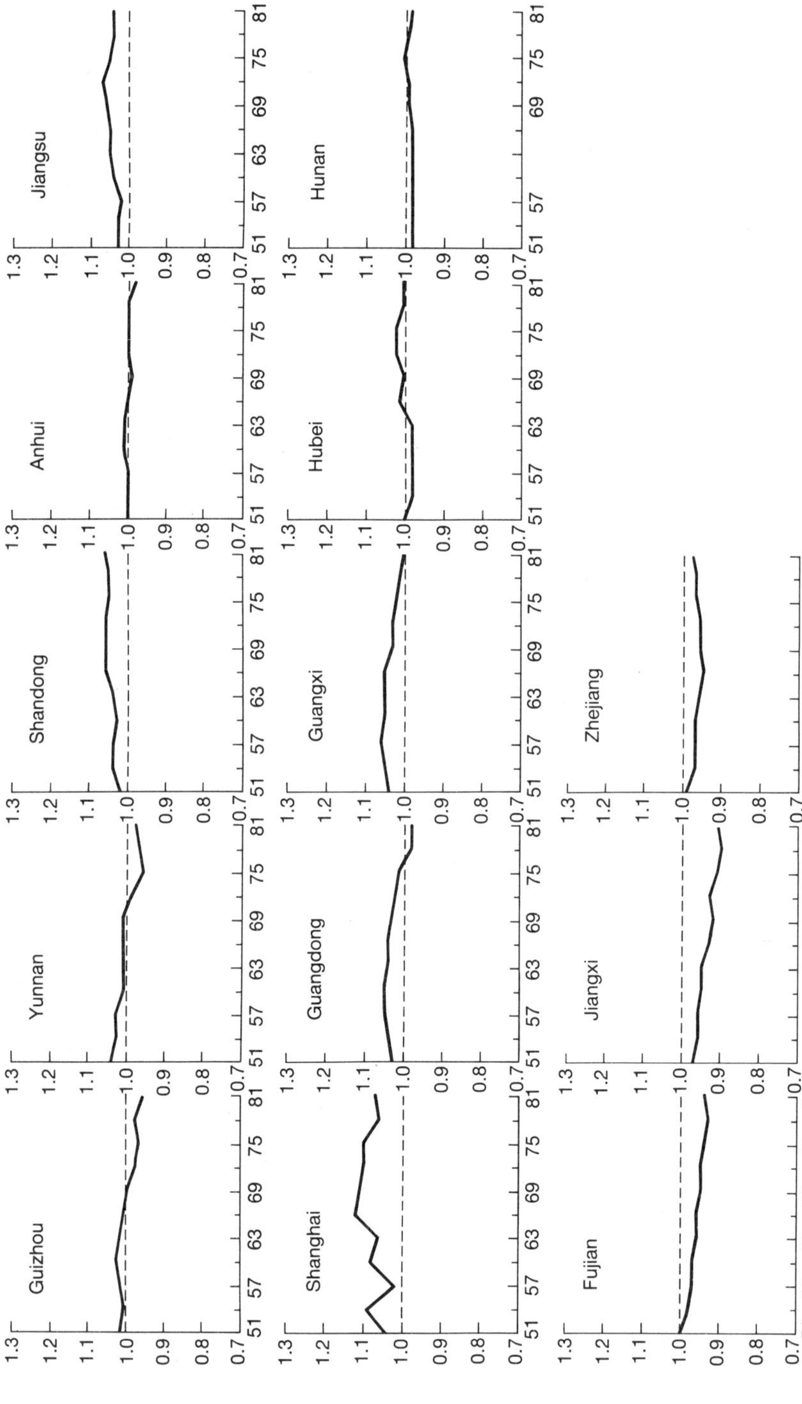

Fig. 6.4 Ratios of provincial MAFM to national ones, rural 1950–1981

intervention, this consistency suggests that local marriage tradition persists and plays a very important role in current marriage patterns.

There are many references on this subject. The story of Huian county in Fujian province has attracted much attention. Women in this region traditionally must be engaged around the age of 10 and get married in their teens. After marriage, couples can stay together only on special occasions and the wife stays with her own parents unless a child is born.[5] This case may be special, but it does provide evidence about the persistence of local tradition. Another example comes from Lintong county in Shaanxi province. Child marriage was common in some mountain areas, where a few teenagers became engaged even when they were studying in primary schools.[6] Since the negotiation of marriage in rural areas, especially in remote areas, is still largely the responsibility of the parents, the main resistance to later marriage came from the older generations.[7] It is worth noting that the MAFM for Beijing and Tianjin in the early 1950s was lower than in adjacent provinces. The reasons for this situation needs further study.

Universal Marriage

After three decades of marriage reform, universality is still one of the salient characteristics of the Chinese marriage pattern. If there is an increasing tendency for urban women to remain single, this is certainly not the case for the rural population. In 1981 only two in every thousand women in the countryside aged 50 and over reported that they had never been married. There are provincial variations (see Table 6.7), but the proportion of women remaining single is so small that it is unlikely to have any significant impact on fertility.

Analysis of the World Fertility Survey data reveals that universal marriage is common in all patrilineal societies.[8] Although the role of Chinese women in society has changed greatly in the past several decades, to remain permanently single is still not only socially unacceptable, but also exposes the person in question to pressure from public opinion and the family system. Consequently, marriage has been widely postponed, but still universally occurs. This suggests that the nuptiality changes which have occurred in rural China are to a great extent synonymous with delayed marriage. In other words, a widely divergent pattern of marriage timing is accompanied by a homogeneous pattern of universal marriage.[9] The regional variations in marriage have persisted and local tradition is one of the most important factors impinging on current provincial marriage patterns.

Rural–Urban Comparison

Marriage has been widely postponed in both rural and urban areas (see Figure 6.3). However, the timing and the extent of this change has varied. The rural–urban difference in marriage age has been calculated for each province for the last thirty years, and the results are shown in Table 6.8.

Urban women commonly get married later than their rural counterparts, no matter which province they live in and at what time the marriage takes place. This is commonly true in many other societies. Analysis based on WFS data shows that in most countries in both Asia and Latin America, rural women marry on average about two years before urban women.[10] Table 6.8 shows that in the early 1950s, the rural–urban differential in the mean age at first marriage was about one year, which was relatively small compared to that in the later periods. The age gap in Tianjin was extremely wide at 2.62 years. Tianjin is one of China's largest cities, as well as a major industrial centre. This large difference may be caused by the sharp contrast in life-style between rural and urban sectors. In addition to Tianjin, the top third of provinces, in which the rural–urban difference was larger than 1.45 years, were Nei Monggol, Guizhou, Xinjiang, Gansu, Qinghai, Ningxia, Hunan, Jiangsu, and Shandong. These provinces were relatively concentrated in the northwest, but scattered in eastern China.

The rural–urban difference gradually widened over time, and reached a peak in the period 1965–7. The age gap at that time was as high as 3 years on the average. This coincided with the implementation of the second family-planning programme which was focused on urban areas. After a slight decline in 1968–70, rural–urban differentials remained at a level of about 2.7 years with some fluctuations until the early 1980s. The age gaps in four northwestern provinces, Xinjiang, Gansu, Qinghai, and Ningxia, were consistently among the largest. Rural women in Xinjiang got married on average 6 years younger than those living in urban areas in the late 1970s. This indicates the difficulties in changing marriage behaviour in these remote rural areas with a large proportion of ethnic minority population. Apart from these extremes, there were seven more provinces where the age gap between the rural and urban population exceeded 3 years in the early 1980s. The three adjacent provinces, Fujian, Zhejiang, and Jiangxi constituted another group with relatively large rural–urban difference.

Results from WFS suggest that changes in mean age at marriage occurred at roughly the same level among both urban and rural women in all countries.[11] In this respect, China seems to be an exception. Although both the rural and the urban population experienced marriage postponement, the magnitude of this change is quite different.

The national figures show that, ignoring the original level, the urban marriage age increased 1.5 years more than the rural marriage age. Except for Tianjin and Shandong, the total increase in marriage age throughout the last three decades was consistently higher for the urban population. This firmly suggests that resistance to delaying marriage is much stronger in the rural areas.

Furthermore, this rural–urban difference varied substantially between provinces. As can be seen in Table 6.8, the absolute difference in the total increase over the last thirty years between the rural and the urban population ranged from the largest of 4.13 years in Xinjiang to the smallest of 0.06 years in Jiangsu (omitting negative differences). The provincial difference in the absolute increase in marriage age was smaller in the urban areas, so that the uneven progress in the rural areas must be the major cause of this phenomenon.

The point was made earlier that marriage postponement has been one of the main strands of the family-planning programme. The programme has been carried out more strictly in urban areas than in rural areas, and more efficiently in the eastern provinces than in the western region, and this has, in part, accounted for the regional and rural–urban differentials in marriage.

Two further general comments can be made from Table 6.9. The first is that the regional variation in marriage age in urban China has been smaller from the mid-1960s onwards. The regional differences in marriage ages widened gradually in both the urban and rural areas during the 1950s and reached the highest in the mid-1960s. While the regional variation in the rural areas continued to widen, the variation in the urban areas diminished. On the whole, we can say that the marriage age for China's urban female population is relatively similar across the country, but is significantly different among the rural population. In other words, later marriage has been widely accepted by the urban population, but less so in the rural areas. During the 1970s the recommended age for marriage was enforced by the local authorities. Since the urban population is well organized and controlled by various social and political organs, and also because of the impact of other relevant social policies, these stipulations were carried out much more thoroughly in the urban areas. By contrast, in addition to the strong resistance to change, regulations for the rural population were often ambiguous.

TABLE 6.8 *Urban–rural differences in the mean age at first marriage*[a]

Province	Difference in period											Total rise[b]		
	1950–2	1953–5	1956–8	1959–61	1962–4	1965–7	1968–70	1971–3	1974-6	1977–9	1980–1	Urban	Rural	Diff.
CHINA	0.91	1.28	1.66	1.85	2.38	3.22	2.59	2.78	2.70	2.75	2.46	5.41	3.86	1.55
Guangdong	1.33	1.88	2.19	1.73	2.10	2.66	2.66	2.53	3.33	3.52	3.34	4.78	2.76	2.02
Guangxi	0.16	0.07	0.27	1.35	1.89	2.64	1.89	1.38	2.52	2.41	2.83	5.84	3.17	2.67
Hubei	0.11	1.04	1.55	1.68	2.38	2.91	2.75	3.02	3.03	2.82	2.54	6.28	3.86	2.42
Hunan	1.55	1.86	1.68	1.60	2.86	3.10	2.21	2.28	2.79	3.07	2.69	4.97	3.82	1.15
Fujian	0.00	0.17	1.56	0.65	1.76	1.92	1.89	2.58	3.05	4.00	3.77	6.35	2.58	3.77
Jiangxi	0.58	0.77	1.32	1.02	1.65	2.97	2.53	3.22	3.10	4.05	3.97	5.78	2.39	3.39
Zhejiang	0.54	1.93	2.80	2.97	2.77	4.51	2.88	4.27	3.13	3.73	3.32	6.32	3.54	2.78
Shanghai	1.14	0.96	3.45	2.95	3.53	3.07	1.84	2.78	2.29	3.11	3.04	6.53	4.63	1.90
Jiangsu	1.45	1.28	1.77	1.72	2.11	2.72	1.39	2.09	1.12	1.96	1.52	4.35	4.29	0.06
Anhui	0.53	1.28	1.01	0.87	2.11	3.18	1.99	1.73	1.55	2.04	2.52	5.24	3.25	1.99
Shandong	1.58	1.08	1.65	2.08	2.57	3.03	2.12	2.14	2.09	2.27	1.27	4.46	4.77	–0.31
Yunnan	–0.47	0.13	1.12	0.27	2.41	1.45	0.94	1.84	1.49	2.37	1.22	4.34	2.65	1.69
Guizhou	1.73	2.21	2.90	2.34	3.28	2.39	1.49	2.95	3.17	3.25	3.49	4.38	2.62	1.76
Sichuan	1.09	1.60	1.97	2.43	1.94	3.09	1.79	1.93	2.56	2.68	2.01	4.66	3.74	0.92
Shaanxi	1.22	1.53	2.16	2.42	3.52	4.07	3.03	3.48	3.11	3.04	2.48	5.91	4.65	1.26
Nei Monggol	1.88	2.41	3.69	4.04	4.39	5.51	4.10	3.95	3.99	3.41	3.04	5.76	4.60	1.16
Shanxi	0.72	1.33	1.70	2.24	2.28	2.72	2.52	1.81	2.60	2.74	2.48	5.84	4.08	1.76
Henan	–0.06	0.12	0.66	0.81	1.61	2.63	2.11	2.70	1.55	1.52	1.45	6.43	4.93	1.50

Hebei	0.67	1.60	1.47	1.74	2.62	3.24	3.03	2.21	2.24	2.06	1.31	5.14	4.50	0.64
Beijing	0.49	0.26	1.08	2.04	2.60	1.38	1.23	1.96	1.72	1.59	1.25	6.43	5.68	0.75
Tianjin	2.62	1.50	1.72	2.34	2.12	2.28	2.07	1.92	1.21	1.67	1.13	5.73	7.22	−1.49
Xinjiang	1.70	1.81	1.94	2.73	3.21	3.72	4.66	4.91	5.21	6.16	5.83	6.46	2.33	4.13
Gansu	1.48	0.94	1.35	1.28	1.65	2.65	4.44	4.86	5.07	4.39	4.96	6.02	2.54	3.48
Qinghai/Ningxia[c]	1.69	2.64	3.34	1.76	3.22	3.94	3.79	4.07	3.59	4.22	5.05	4.68	1.32	3.36
Jilin	1.35	0.87	1.46	1.18	2.18	4.15	3.21	3.54	3.65	3.25	2.36	5.37	4.36	1.01
Heilongjiang	0.39	1.31	1.31	1.93	2.34	3.40	2.95	2.35	2.19	2.64	2.08	4.91	3.22	1.69
Liaoning	1.03	1.33	1.45	1.71	2.50	3.33	2.57	2.80	2.65	2.25	1.59	5.27	4.72	0.55
MEAN	0.981	1.256	1.799	1.847	2.504	3.061	2.521	2.789	2.741	2.971	2.687	5.49	3.79	1.70
MEDIAN	1.09	1.31	1.65	1.74	2.38	3.03	2.52	2.58	2.65	2.82	2.52			
ST.D.	0.720	0.703	0.824	0.815	0.674	0.888	0.940	0.966	1.028	1.030	1.254	0.73	1.21	1.28
MIN.	−0.47	0.07	0.27	0.27	1.61	1.38	0.94	1.38	1.12	1.52	1.13			
MAX.	2.62	2.64	3.69	4.04	4.39	5.51	4.66	4.91	5.21	6.16	5.83			
Q1	0.49	0.87	1.32	1.28	2.10	2.64	1.89	1.96	2.09	2.25	1.52			
Q3	1.55	1.81	2.16	2.34	2.86	3.40	3.03	3.48	3.17	3.52	3.34			

[a] Measured in years.
[b] Total increase in the mean age at the first marriage = $MAFM_{1980-1981} - MAFM_{1950-52}$
[c] Data for Qinghai and Ningxia are combined.

TABLE 6.9. *Standard deviations and the correlation coefficients for the provincial MAFM by the rural and urban population*

	1950–2	1953–5	1956–8	1959–61	1962–4	1965–7	1968–70	1971–3	1974–6	1977–9	1980–1
Standard Deviations											
Rural	0.78	0.81	0.83	0.96	0.89	1.05	1.24	1.35	1.47	1.41	1.53
Urban	0.77	0.84	0.93	1.07	1.01	1.03	0.92	1.00	0.96	0.70	0.70
Correlation coefficients	0.544	0.618	0.548	0.658	0.755	0.634	0.645	0.689	0.701	0.667	0.475

Secondly, age at marriage in rural and urban areas appears to be highly associated, as can be seen from the high value of the correlation coefficients. The strong influence of local traditions and institutions on marriage must be responsible for this relation, at least for the 1950s and 1960s. On top of the rural–urban differentials, nuptiality behaviour seems to be similar in regional groups with the same local cultural background. During the third family-planning campaign in the 1970s, the minimum age for marriage was proposed by provincial authorities in accordance with local conditions. The target age for rural women was commonly two or three years lower than for their urban counterparts. The strict implementation of these regulations would lead to the close relationship between the marriage age for the urban and the rural population, other things being equal.

III. Age Patterns

Age-Specific Fertility Rate

As in urban areas, the fertility transition in rural China did not occur simultaneously for all age groups. While the ASFR for other age groups remained unchanged or even increased, fertility decline was already under way for the 15–19 group. Table 6.10, where the age pattern of the fertility decline is examined, reveals some interesting findings.

The provincial PTFR in 1970 was in general similar to that in the mid-1950s; only six out of the twenty-six provinces had witnessed a more than 10 per cent fertility decline. However, the age-specific fertility rates of the 15–19 age group declined substantially, no matter what the PTFR was. Except for Fujian, Jiangxi, Gansu, and Xinjiang, the ASFR for the 15–19 age group in all provinces declined by more than 30 per cent. Rural Tianjin actually eliminated births to women younger than 20 years old. In Shanghai, the ASFR of teenagers decreased by more than 90 per cent. Among the top third of provinces where the ASFR for the 15–19 age group declined by more than 60 per cent were six other provinces, namely Beijing, Liaoning, Hebei, Shandong, Jiangsu, and Henan.

Although the ASFR for teenagers dropped sharply, because of the offsetting effects of an increase in fertility for women in their 20s and 30s, the PTFR in Shandong and Henan increased by 4 and 18 per cent respectively from the mid-1950s level. Higher ASFRs for the 20s and 30s groups were a common feature across the country. In some

TABLE 6.10. *Changes in rural fertility rates by age group (%)*

Province	Mid-50s–1970				1970–5					1975–80				
	PTFR (1)	−19 (2)	20s (3)	30s (4)	TFR (5)	−19 (6)	20s (7)	30s (8)	40s (9)	TFR (10)	19 (11)	20s (12)	30s (13)	40s (14)
CHINA (rural)	+3	−46	+7	+8	−38	−54	−27	−48	−50	−37	−38	−20	−61	−70
Shanghai	−45	−91	−25	−52	−56	−100	−52	−71	−11	−14	−5	+6	−100	−100
Tianjin	−42	−100	−31	−38	−48	—	−44	−49	−81	−28	—	−9	−66	−100
Beijing	−29	−78	−14	−35	−63	−100	−54	−72	−100	+7	—	+15	−27	−100
Liaoning	−28	−69	−16	−34	−49	−67	−35	−63	−71	−24	+25	−5	−67	−100
Zhejiang	−23	−36	−11	−37	−41	−63	−34	−51	−25	−33	−47	−16	−64	−82
Jiangsu	−15	−62	−6	−19	−53	−82	−41	−67	−75	−36	−63	−20	−74	−83
Shaanxi	−9	−53	0	−8	−42	−61	−33	−45	−66	−37	−76	−15	−66	−65
Heilongjiang	−9	−32	−3	−12	−42	−52	−25	−59	−62	−34	−36	−16	−69	−73
Yunnan	−4	−38	+11	−2	−10	−9	−7	−11	−24	−34	−53	−31	−35	−39
Hebei	−1	−75	+6	+6	−53	−69	−41	−66	−62	−11	−66	+5	−30	−78
Ningxia	−1	−39	+3	+7	−9	−40	−3	−23	38	−27	−77	−15	−33	−36
Hunan	0	−41	+4	+4	−36	−69	−17	−52	−53	−44	−66	−25	−76	−89
Hubei	+2	−56	+3	+14	−47	−61	−30	−61	−72	−36	−56	−22	−63	−58
Guangxi	+3	−51	−3	+19	−9	−23	+6	−13	−45	−5	−46	+31	−39	−67
Nei Monggol	+3	−50	+17	+4	−45	−69	−37	−58	−9	−32	−10	−14	−50	−93
Jilin	+3	−30	+13	−2	−63	−77	−52	−73	−76	−24	−33	−4	−67	−69
Fujian	+3	+4	+5	0	−32	−46	−12	−49	−60	−52	−43	−39	−80	−85
Shandong	+4	−63	+7	+10	−49	−77	−38	−61	−65	−43	−73	−25	−73	−80
Sichuan	+6	−52	+12	+10	−31	−59	−18	−41	−40	−67	−53	−52	−85	−92
Guangdong	+8	−34	+7	+13	−32	−52	−19	−39	−55	−8	−7	+2	−20	−32
Shanxi	+11	−36	+16	+22	−42	−71	−29	−58	−19	−38	−17	−17	−69	−93
Guizhou	+13	−32	+10	+23	−9	−22	−11	−6	−7	−43	−74	−27	−51	−67
Xinjiang	+16	+11	+32	+2	−22	−5	−20	−29	−29	−29	−20	−17	−42	−64
Henan	+18	−67	+14	+40	−48	−30	−35	−56	−71	−31	−83	−13	−52	−71
Jiangxi	+21	−18	+16	+37	−16	−42	−3	−30	−3	−47	−10	−26	−75	−80
Gansu	+22	− 9	+17	+40	−48	−40	−37	−68	−30	−26	−49	+7	−68	−80
Anhui	+23	−40	+27	+31	−45	−65	−31	−57	−60	−24	+4	−13	−41	−63
Qinghai	+43	+37	+33	+58	−13	−52	−4	−38	89	−21	−16	−23	−18	−24
MEAN	+2	−41	+6	+5	−37	−55	−26	−49	−39	−29	−39	−14	−57	−73
ST.D.	18	28	14	26	17	26	16	19	40	17	30	17	21	21

provinces, such as Henan and Gansu, the ASFR for the 30–9 group rose by 40 per cent from the mid-1950s level. Only about a quarter of provinces, all situated along the coast, witnessed some kind of decline in the ASFR of the 20–9 and 30–9 age groups during the period from the mid-1950s to 1970. Given the small contribution of the ASFR for the 15–19 to the total fertility rate, the PTFRs in a majority of provinces remained as high as, or even higher than, those in the mid-1950s.

Remarkable changes began to occur in the first half of the 1970s. It can be seen that fertility decline was experienced by virtually all age groups. The fertility reduction for China's rural population as a whole in the first part of the 1970s was about 50 per cent for all but the 20–9 age group. This pattern was followed by most provinces. It seems certain that the sharp fertility decline which occurred in this period was brought about by the adoption of birth control by women of all ages.

The age pattern of the later 1970s shows a different picture. The ASFR for the age group 15–19 continued to decline, but the most important reduction in the total fertility rate came from women aged 30–49. The national figure shows that while the total fertility declined by about 37 per cent, the ASFR for the 30–9 and 40–9 age groups dropped by more than 60 and 70 per cent respectively. This is true for two-thirds of all provinces. There were virtually no births to women in their 40s in Shanghai, Tianjin, Beijing, and Liaoning in 1980. The ASFR for the 15–19 group had already reached a very low level, making a further decline unlikely. In future, further fertility reduction will have to come from women in their later reproductive ages. This also indicates that the fertility decline over the later 1970s relied heavily on reducing births of higher orders. This aspect will be examined in detail later.

In Figure 6.5, the age-specific fertility rates in 1970, 1975, 1980, and the reference period, which is the average of the ASFR in 1964 and 1965, are presented. As may be seen, curves for the reference period and for 1970 were roughly parallel to, or even overlaid, one another for a majority of provinces. The curve for 1980, however, was quite different. This was not only because of the great decline of the ASFR of the most fertile ages (i.e. the 20s), but also because even more dramatic reductions of fertility occurred in the later 30s and 40s. The age patterns in 1975 in half of all provinces were close to that in 1980, but the ASFR for women in their late fertile ages was relatively higher. There was almost no change in the ASFR over the second half of the 1970s in three large municipalities. In Sichuan, changes in the age pattern were very impressive during the 1970s, especially the later

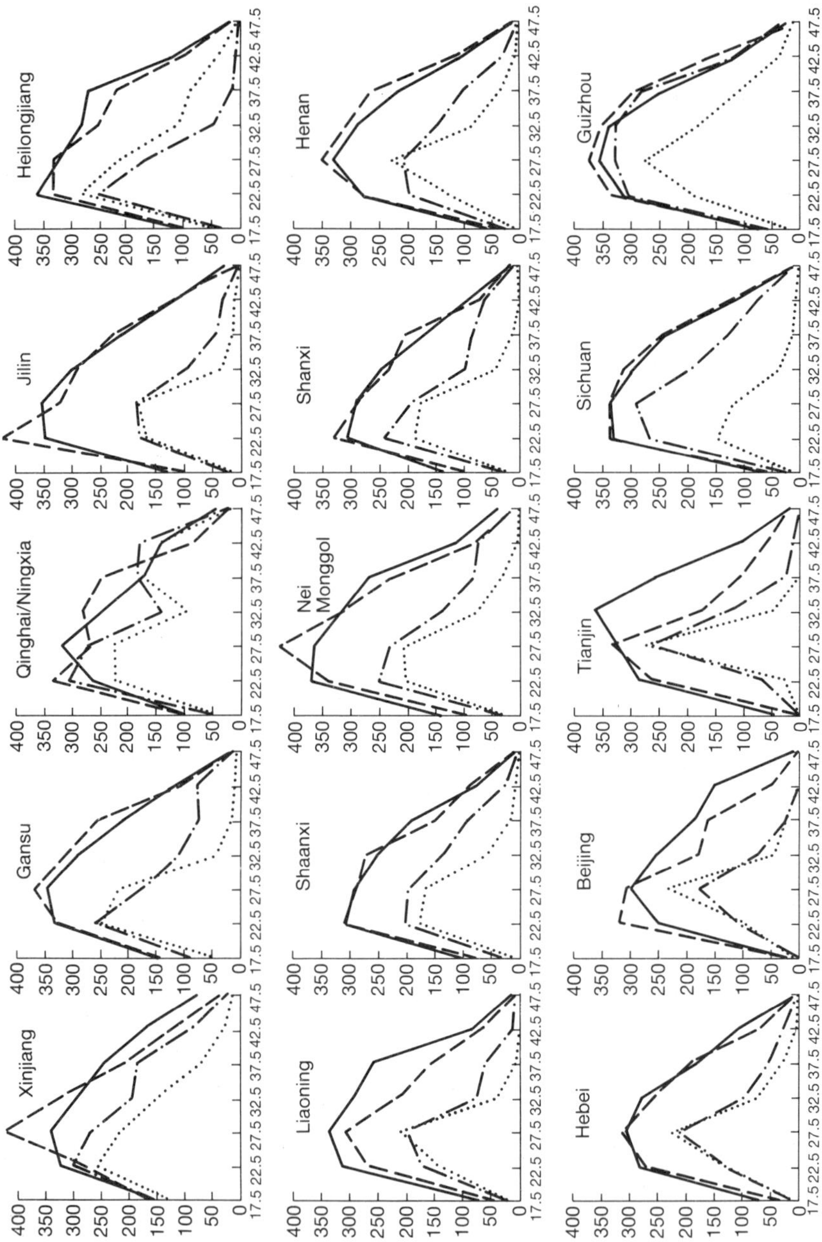
Xinjiang
Gansu
Qinghai/Ningxia
Jilin
Heilongjiang
Liaoning
Shaanxi
Nei Monggol
Shanxi
Henan
Hebei
Beijing
Tianjin
Sichuan
Guizhou
400 350 300 250 200 150 100 50 0
17.5 22.5 27.5 32.5 37.5 42.5 47.5

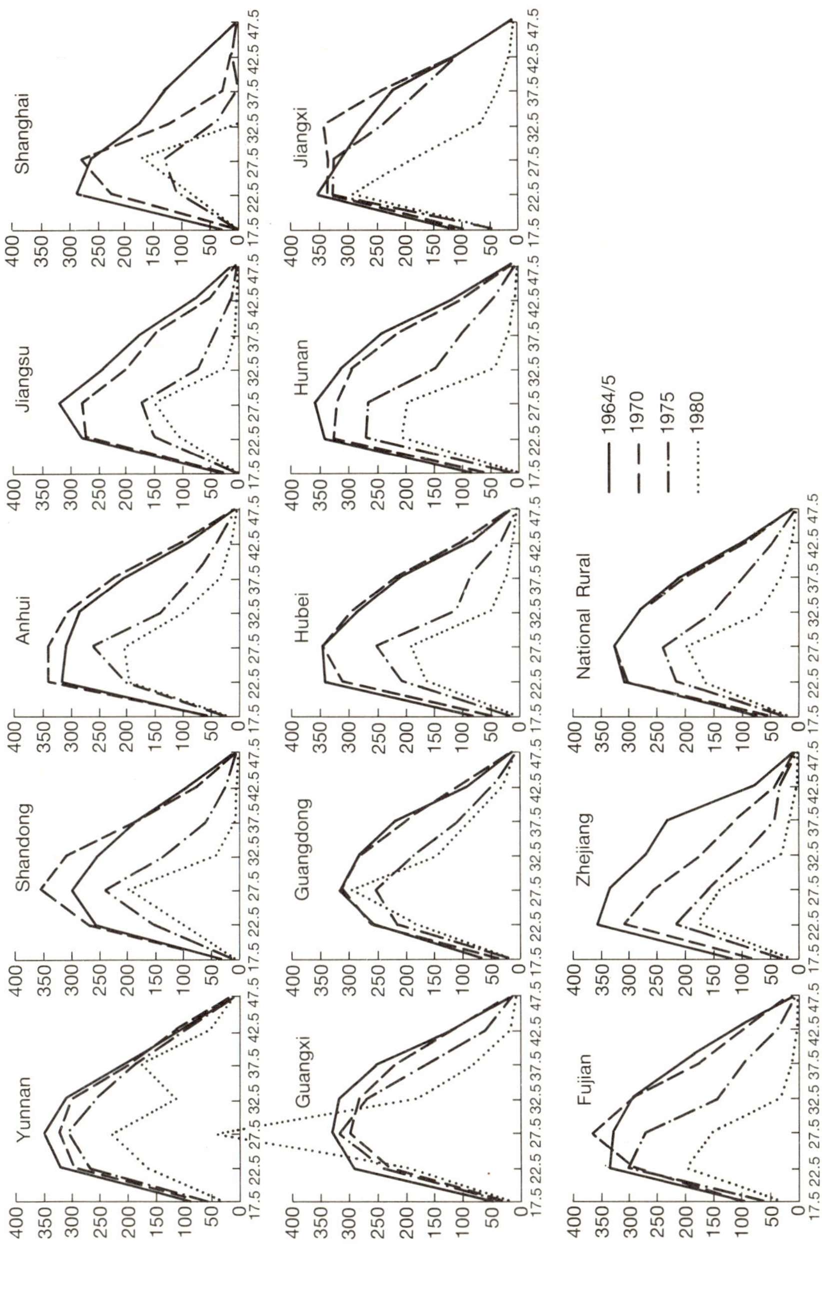

Fig. 6.5 Age-specific fertility rate for selected years by province, rural

1970s. It is likely that changes in age pattern of fertility were more gradual for some remaining provinces, such as Zhejiang, Shandong, Hunan, etc. We can see once again that there was little change in the age pattern of fertility over time in Yunnan, Guangxi, Guizhou, Xinjiang, and Guangdong, even though the overall level was in decline.

In conclusion, China's rural fertility transition started from the 15–19 age group—undoubtedly because of the postponement of marriage. In the first half of the 1970s fertility decline occurred for all ages to a roughly similar extent. With the progress of the transition, the major source of the fertility decline turned to the reduction of fertility for women aged 30 and over.

Cumulated Fertility Rate

The age pattern of China's rural fertility transition is further analysed by the examination of the trend in the cumulated period fertility rate. Indices of the A_{10} and A_{90}, which indicate the ages at which 10 and 90 per cent of the cumulated total period fertility rate is reached, are examined as for the urban population. The sequence of these indices from 1964 onwards is presented graphically in Figure 6.6.

It is interesting to discover that changes in the index of A_{10} were very small compared with changes in A_{90}. The national figures show that the index of A_{10} only rose one year from 21 to 22 over the past two decades in spite of the postponement of marriage. However, the A_{90} index fell substantially from 39 in 1964, to 34 in the early 1980s. The 80-per-cent interval, which was defined earlier, has declined from 18 years in 1964 to 13 years in 1981 for China's rural population as a whole. This means that the most active period of the reproduction cycle for Chinese rural females has shortened greatly over the past two decades.

So far as the regional patterns, we can see that the indices were very similar between provinces and remained relatively constant until the mid-1970s. The situation then changed and provincial diversity became marked. The 80-per-cent interval in a majority of provinces had fallen to about 10 years by the early 1980s. The interval for Shanghai in 1981 was only 5 years, compared to 17 and 12 years in 1964 and 1970 respectively. This means that women aged 23 to 28 were responsible for 80 per cent of Shanghai's total fertility in 1981. It is very interesting to see that the impressive fall of the A_{90} occurred mainly in the second half of the 1970s instead of the first half, as the TFR did. This provides further evidence that the great reduction of the ASFR for the old ages occurred mainly in the late 1970s.

In contrast, the indices for Guizhou, Yunnan, Guangdong, and

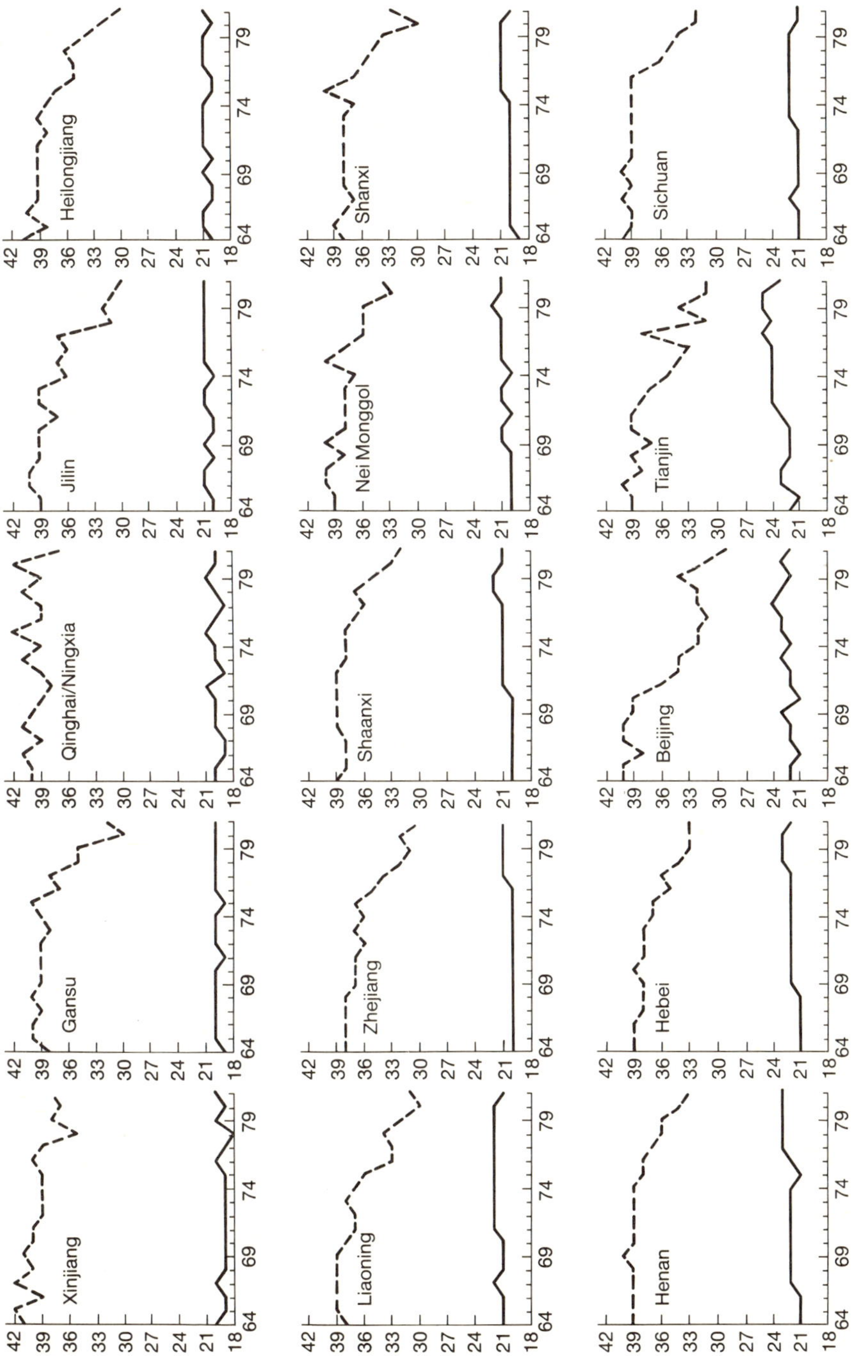
Heilongjiang
Jilin
Qinghai/Ningxia
Gansu
Xinjiang
Shanxi
Nei Monggol
Shaanxi
Zhejiang
Liaoning
Sichuan
Tianjin
Beijing
Hebei
Henan

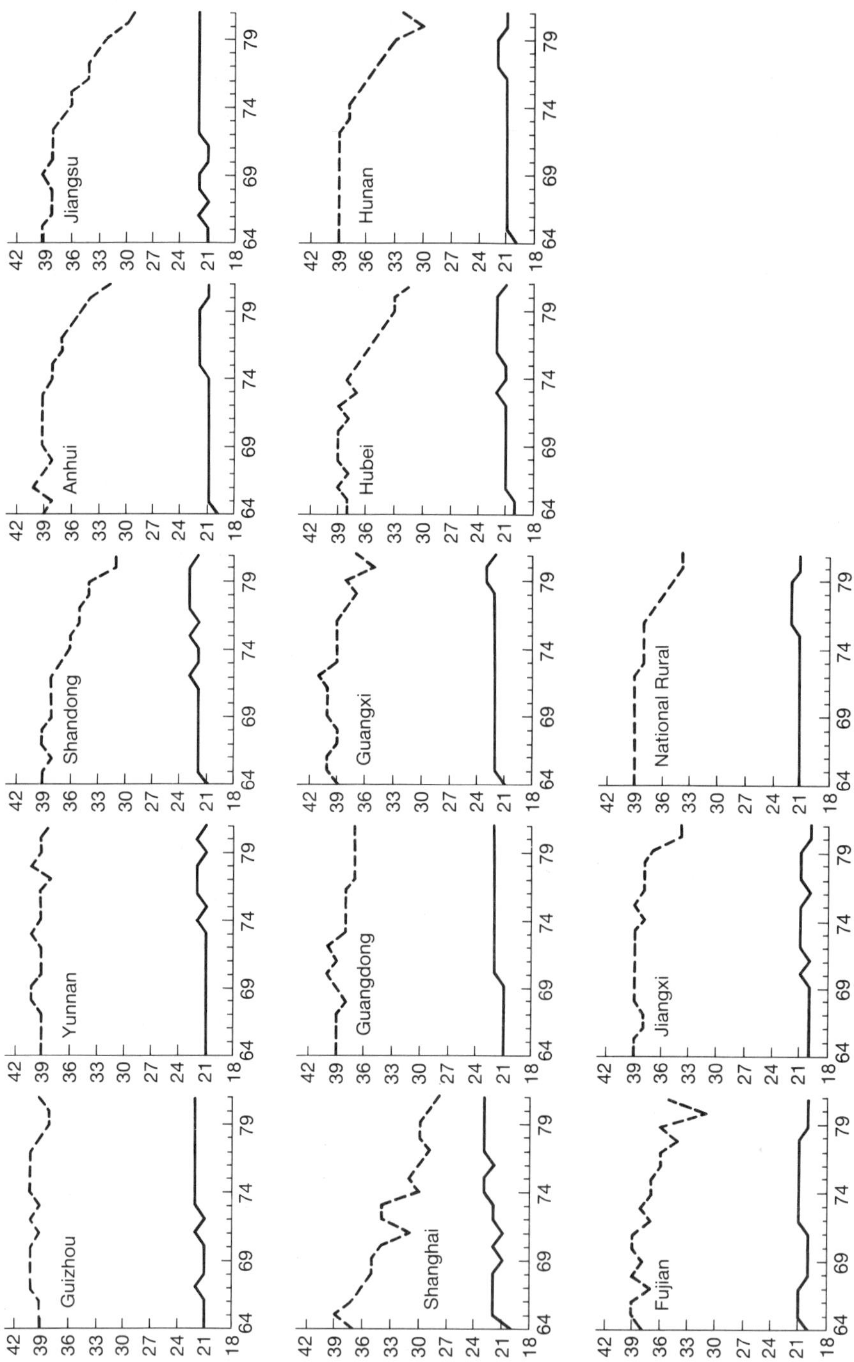

Fig. 6.6 Provincial indices of A_{10} and A_{90}, rural 1964–1981

Xinjiang, show hardly any change over the period under study. It is an interesting phenomenon that on the one hand, fertility reduction did occur across the country, but that on the other hand, the age pattern of fertility remained unchanged in a few provinces.

Some general points can be made from the comparison. First, the major fertility decline occurred in the first half of the 1970s, but births to women in the later 30s and 40s still accounted for a certain proportion of total births. Secondly, although the magnitude of the total fertility decline in the late 1970s was not as large as that in the previous period, the reduction of fertility for women in their later fertile ages was remarkable. This reflects the changing objectives of the family-planning programme over time. At the early stage of the programme, the principal target was later, longer, and fewer. With the progress of the campaign, direct efforts were made to reduce the ultimate number of children a woman would produce. Partly as a result, the great reduction of fertility in the early 1970s was mainly attributable to the birth control for all age groups, while the attempts to reduce births to women in their late reproductive ages were more successful in the late 1970s. Finally, as the decline in fertility of women at their most fertile ages was modest, the reduction of the ASFR for the old ages resulted in a moderate decline in total fertility rate. This is likely to answer the question of why the strict single-child policy had only a small impact in reducing the TFR.

Changes in Birth Orders

Analysis has shown that in China the first-birth interval became shorter with the increase in ages of marriage. In addition, very few Chinese advocate voluntary childlessness. Therefore, births to women in their later fertile ages are certainly births of higher orders. Figure 6.7 gives the distribution of births by birth orders for each province. Information for the calculations is only available for 1970, 1977, 1981, and 1984, but this is sufficient for the comparison and to show the general trend.

The share of first births in total births increased continually, while those of higher order, which is defined as births of the third and higher orders, declined. The changes in the share of the second births varied between provinces, but in general the proportion of the second births increased. It is worth drawing attention to the proportions of the higher orders. In 1981, 31 per cent of births were third or higher order for rural China as a whole. The provincial variation was great; higher-order births accounted for less than 4 per cent of the total births in the outskirts of the three major municipalities, and less than 20 per cent in

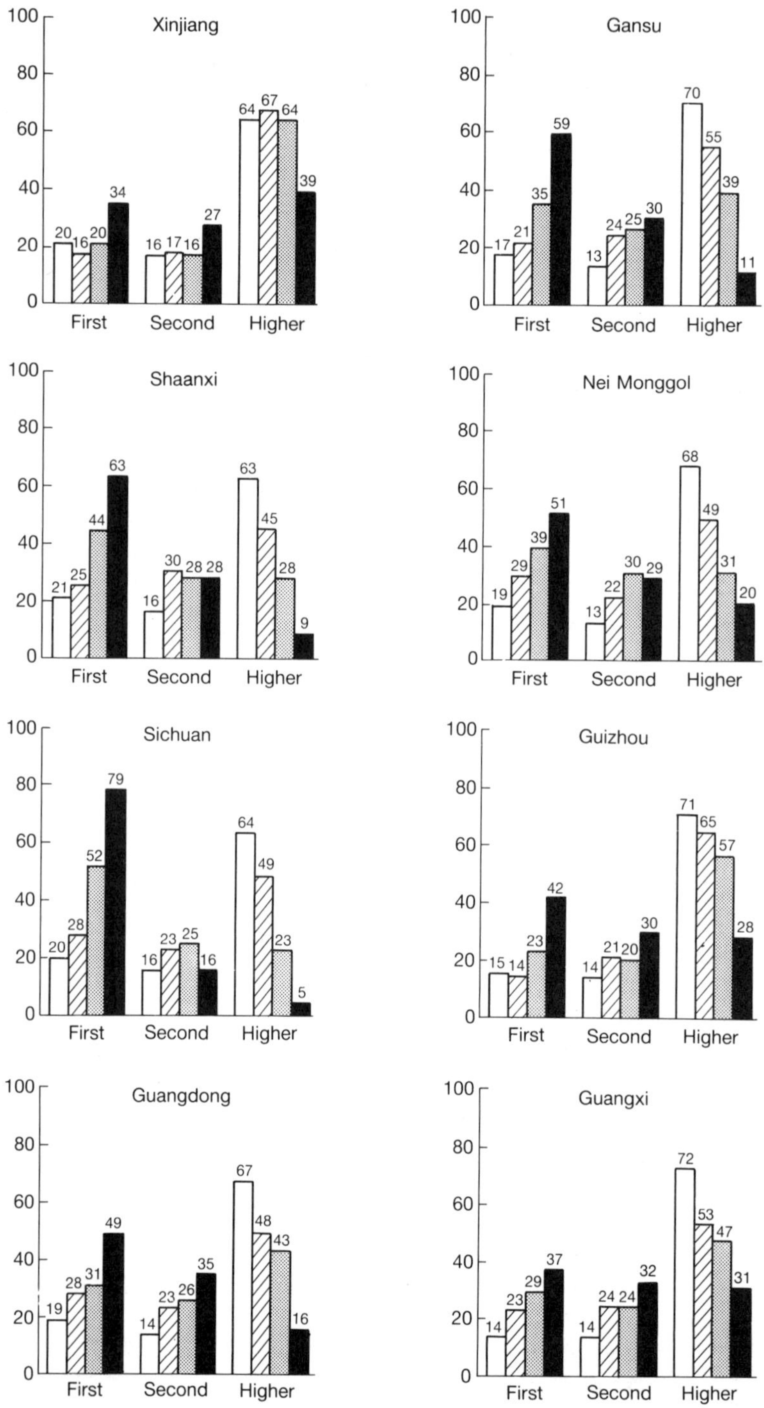
Xinjiang
100
80
60
40
20
0
20 16 20 34
16 17 16 27
64 67 64 39
First
Second
Higher
Gansu
17 21 35 59
13 24 25 30
70 55 39 11
First
Second
Higher
Shaanxi
21 25 44 63
16 30 28 28
63 45 28 9
First
Second
Higher
Nei Monggol
19 29 39 51
13 22 30 29
68 49 31 20
First
Second
Higher
Sichuan
20 28 52 79
16 23 25 16
64 49 23 5
First
Second
Higher
Guizhou
15 14 23 42
14 21 20 30
71 65 57 28
First
Second
Higher
Guangdong
19 28 31 49
14 23 26 35
67 48 43 16
First
Second
Higher
Guangxi
14 23 29 37
14 24 24 32
72 53 47 31
First
Second
Higher

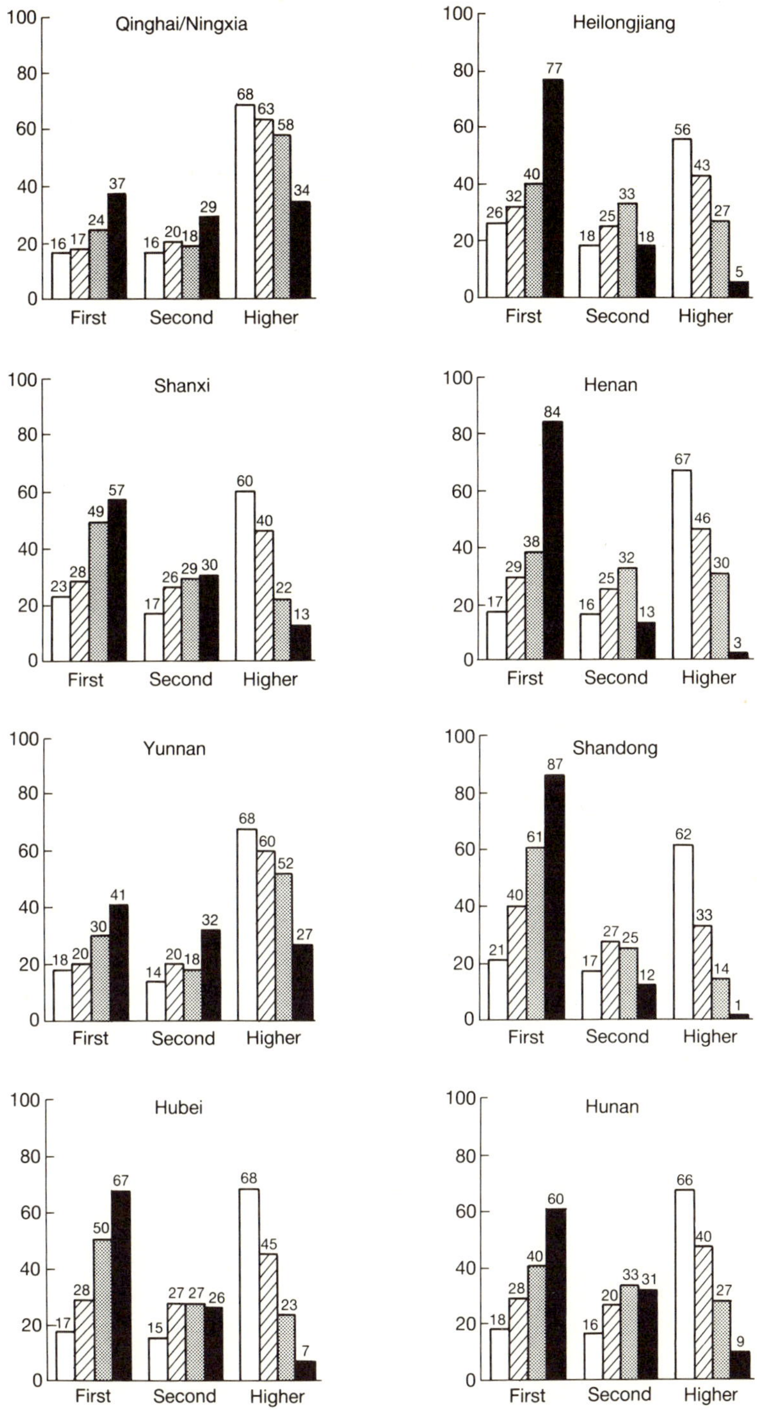
Qinghai/Ningxia
100
80
60
40
20
0
16 17 24 37
16 20 18 29
68 63 58 34
First Second Higher
Heilongjiang
100
80
60
40
20
0
26 32 40 77
18 25 33 18
56 43 27 5
First Second Higher
Shanxi
100
80
60
40
20
0
23 28 49 57
17 26 29 30
60 40 22 13
First Second Higher
Henan
100
80
60
40
20
0
17 29 38 84
16 25 32 13
67 46 30 3
First Second Higher
Yunnan
100
80
60
40
20
0
18 20 30 41
14 20 18 32
68 60 52 27
First Second Higher
Shandong
100
80
60
40
20
0
21 40 61 87
17 27 25 12
62 33 14 1
First Second Higher
Hubei
100
80
60
40
20
0
17 28 50 67
15 27 27 26
68 45 23 7
First Second Higher
Hunan
100
80
60
40
20
0
18 28 40 60
16 20 33 31
66 40 27 9
First Second Higher

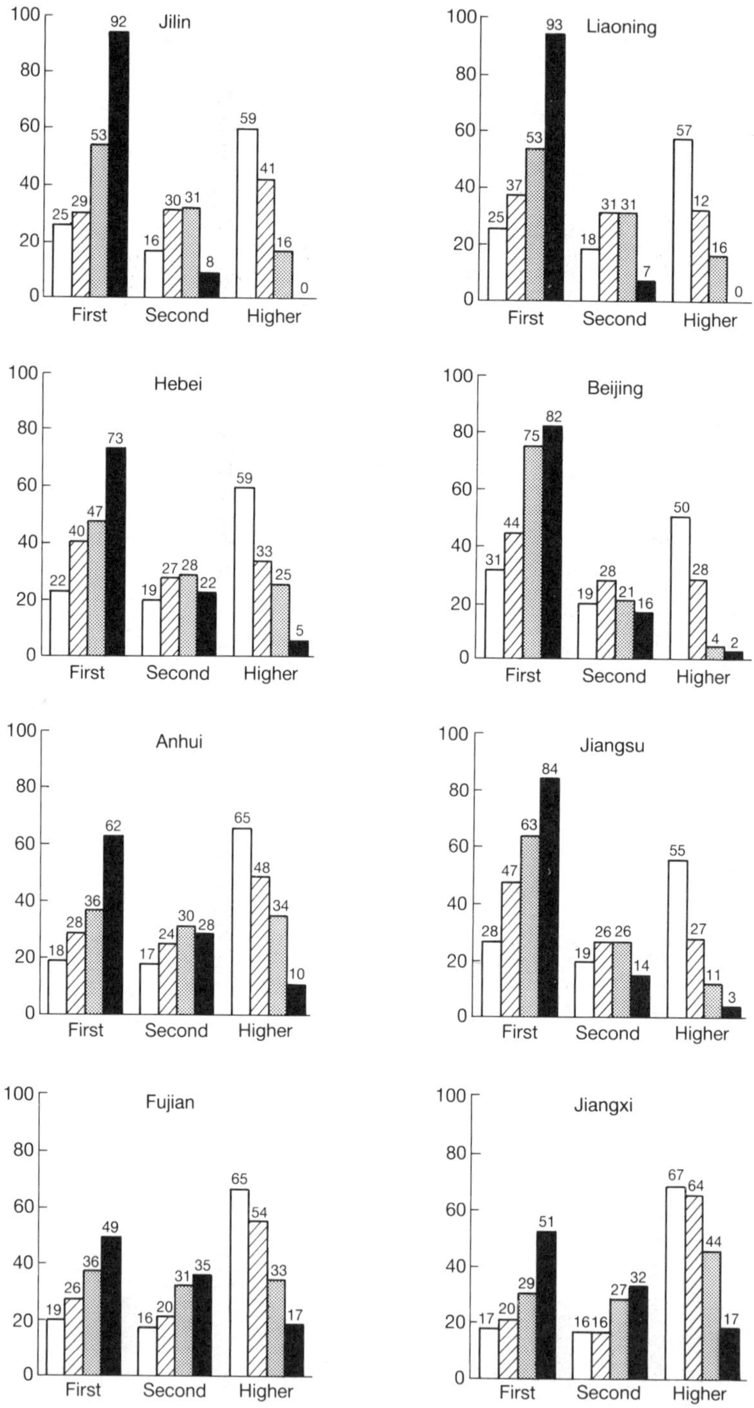
Jilin
Liaoning
Hebei
Beijing
Anhui
Jiangsu
Fujian
Jiangxi
First
Second
Higher

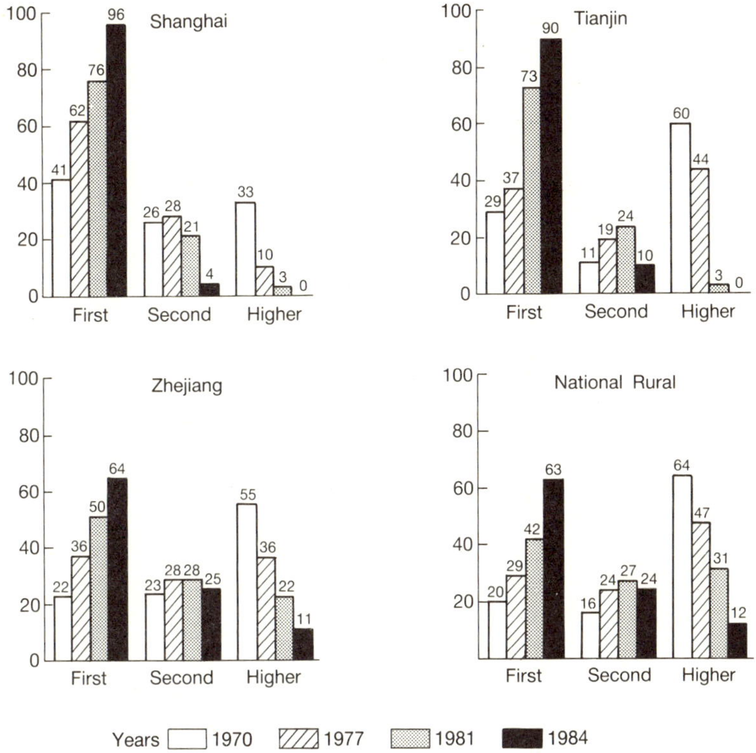

Fig. 6.7 Contribution to total births by birth order, rural

Jiangsu, Shandong, Liaoning, and Jilin province, but more than 50 per cent in Xinjiang, Yunnan, and Guizhou. This reflects the fact that the response to the one-child policy was quite different between provinces. The national figure shows that births of higher orders accounted for about only 12 per cent of total births in 1984, compared with 64 per cent in 1970. The regional diversity had narrowed by 1984 but was still considerable, even though five years had passed since the implementation of the one-child policy. There were about half of all provinces where the proportion of higher-order births was below 10 per cent. No higher-order births at all were reported in 1984 in Shanghai, Tianjin, Liaoning, and Jilin. In contrast, the births of higher order in Guangxi, Guizhou, Yunnan, Xinjiang, Nei Monggol, Qinghai and Ningxia, Jiangxi, and Fujian were still in excess of 20 per cent of the total births. Evidently the population living in the eastern provinces was more likely to accept the small family and respond positively to the single-child policy. On the other hand, changes in the vast interior, especially those western provinces, were less readily forthcoming.

Cohort Fertility Rate

It is obvious that the period fertility rate has undergone a dramatic decline during the 1970s. The question is whether this means the real change in the ultimate family size, or is just caused by women temporarily spacing their childbearing. In this section, changes in the cumulated cohort fertility up to the age of 39 are analysed. The age of 39 is chosen in order to extend our study as far as possible. Moreover, since women in their 30s were the major object of the various family-planning programmes, changes in the number of children they produced is one of the main indicators of the fertility transition.

Table 6.11 shows the cumulative cohort fertility up to the age of 39 in different periods and ratios between successive periods. These ratios are useful measures for comparisons of fertility levels for successive periods between cohorts at the same stage of the life cycle.[12]

It is interesting to note that the number of children ever borne for women up to age 39 increased steadily from the mid-1960s to the early 1970s with a few exceptions (Shanghai, Jiangsu, Zhejiang, Liaoning, and Ningxia). For China's rural population as a whole, the cohort fertility rate increased by 6 per cent over this period. In addition, analysis of the younger age cohorts suggests that the upward trend was common throughout the 1950s. This might result from the under-reporting in birth histories of older women, which was common in fertility surveys conducted in less developed societies.[13] Misreporting in some provinces may have been severe.[14] However, the data quality in China, on the whole, is not so bad and there are good reasons to accept the accuracy of China's 1982 Survey in most provinces. Therefore, the increase in the cohort fertility rate during the 1960s is believed to be genuine.

A similar trend has been observed in many other countries before the onset of the fertility transition.[15] Women aged 39 in the late 1960s started their childbearing in the early 1950s. Thus they were the cohort having experienced the general upward trend in the period fertility rate in the mid-1950s and the unprecedented fertility boom in the period 1962–3. Their reproductive behaviour was not significantly affected by efforts to promote birth control by the mid-1960s. Although the massive fertility crisis hit this age cohort during the Great Leap period 1958–61, it seems that they rapidly caught up and achieved their desired family size eventually. However, women in their late fertile ages were

TABLE 6.11. *Cumulative cohort fertility (CF) and ratios of successive CF by province, rural China*[a]

Province	1964–6	1967–9		1970–2		1973–5		1976–8		1979–81		Ratio
	CF	CF	Ratio	CF	Ratio	CF	Ratio	CF	Ratio	CF	Ratio	80/70[b]
CHINA (rural)	5.233	5.458	1.04	5.534	1.01	5.537	1.01	5.200	0.94	4.735	0.91	0.86
Guangdong	4.933	4.997	1.01	5.476	1.10	5.406	0.99	5.135	0.95	4.839	0.94	0.88
Guangxi	4.969	5.572	1.12	5.487	0.98	5.489	1.00	5.612	1.02	5.091	0.91	0.93
Hubei	5.556	6.025	1.08	5.987	0.99	5.996	1.00	5.542	0.92	5.022	0.91	0.84
Hunan	5.779	5.876	1.02	5.871	1.00	5.833	0.99	5.376	0.92	4.738	0.88	0.81
Fujian	5.573	5.761	1.03	5.877	1.02	5.798	0.99	5.415	0.93	5.254	0.97	0.89
Jiangxi	5.234	5.786	1.11	6.128	1.06	6.438	1.05	5.905	0.92	6.082	1.03	0.99
Zhejiang	5.644	5.840	1.03	5.274	0.90	5.179	0.98	4.697	0.91	4.322	0.92	0.82
Shanghai	4.883	4.963	1.02	4.385	0.88	3.672	0.84	3.705	1.01	2.996	0.81	0.68
Jiangsu	4.960	5.075	1.02	4.877	0.96	4.651	0.95	4.116	0.88	3.653	0.89	0.75
Anhui	4.940	4.982	1.01	5.343	1.07	5.396	1.01	4.897	0.91	4.666	0.95	0.87
Shandong	4.987	5.031	1.01	5.009	1.00	4.837	0.97	4.657	0.96	4.193	0.90	0.84
Yunnan	5.585	5.818	1.04	5.842	1.00	5.743	0.98	5.802	1.01	5.468	0.94	0.94
Guizhou	5.743	6.006	1.05	6.212	1.03	6.681	1.08	6.106	0.91	6.022	0.99	0.97
Sichuan	5.216	5.603	1.07	5.648	1.01	5.828	1.03	5.314	0.91	4.835	0.91	0.86
Shaanxi	5.533	5.813	1.05	5.718	0.98	5.679	0.99	5.476	0.96	5.137	0.94	0.90
Nei Monggol	6.361	6.134	0.96	6.485	1.05	6.473	1.00	5.904	0.91	5.647	0.96	0.87
Shanxi	4.468	4.787	1.07	5.286	1.10	5.485	1.04	5.416	0.99	4.679	0.86	0.89
Henan	4.958	5.158	1.04	5.495	1.07	5.539	1.01	5.249	0.95	4.756	0.91	0.87
Hebei	4.698	4.921	1.05	5.148	1.05	5.080	0.99	4.619	0.91	4.068	0.88	0.79
Beijing	5.058	5.110	1.01	5.145	1.01	4.823	0.94	4.194	0.87	3.841	0.92	0.75
Tianjin	6.698	6.337	0.95	6.875	1.08	5.737	0.83	4.623	0.81	3.928	0.85	0.57
Xinjiang	5.422	5.554	1.02	5.583	1.01	5.478	0.98	6.162	1.12	5.360	0.87	0.96
Gansu	5.604	5.873	1.05	5.618	0.96	6.212	1.11	5.915	0.95	4.957	0.84	0.88
Qinghai	3.479	3.723	1.07	4.788	1.29	4.221	0.88	5.691	1.35	4.838	0.85	1.01
Ningxia	7.593	6.282	0.83	6.804	1.09	6.927	1.02	6.095	0.88	7.509	1.23	1.10
Jilin	5.975	6.152	1.03	6.357	1.03	6.703	1.05	5.727	0.85	4.975	0.87	0.78
Heilongjiang	6.393	6.565	1.03	6.850	1.04	6.455	0.94	5.716	0.89	5.500	0.96	0.80
Liaoning	6.342	6.330	1.00	5.800	0.92	5.815	1.00	4.810	0.83	4.301	0.89	0.74
MEAN	5.449	5.574	1.03	5.692	1.03	5.628	0.99	5.281	0.94	4.881	0.92	0.86
ST.D.	0.786	0.626	0.05	0.625	0.08	0.754	0.06	0.65	0.10	0.870	0.08	0.11

[a] Cumulative cohort fertility rates (CF_i) are sums of age-specific fertility rates by single years of age for cohort aged 39 in period *i*. Ratios of successive CF = $CFbi_{+1}/CF_i$

[b] Ratio 80/70 = CF_{79-81}/CF_{70-72}.

hit more seriously by the fertility crisis,[16] and chances for them to catch up after the crisis were limited because of their ages. This might be one of the causes of the low cohort fertility rate for women aged 39 in the mid-1960s.

The cohort fertility fell in almost all provinces throughout the 1970s. However, the magnitude of the decline was moderate in contrast to the sharp reduction in the period fertility rate. In the period 1979–81, the average number of children ever born to women aged 39 was still as high as 4.8, which was only 15 per cent lower than the early 1970s' level. Only in Shanghai, Beijing, Tianjin, and Jiangsu were the cumulative cohort fertility rates lower than 4 for the rural population. In Jiangxi, Guizhou, Xinjiang, Qinghai, and Ningxia, there was hardly any change. Even in the eastern provinces, the reduction in cumulative cohort fertility rate up to age 39 was only slightly higher than 20 per cent during the 1970s. The decline of 43 per cent in Tianjin was the highest in the country, which was due in part to the very high fertility level of the early 1970s.

This suggests that while a steep decline in period fertility took place across the country during the 1970s, the cohort fertility did not follow the trend simultaneously. There is a time-lag. It seems likely that the old generation of China's rural population merely prolonged their birth intervals rather than attempting to reduce the ultimate family size in the previous three decades. The fertility behaviour of rural women in their 20s and early 30s in the early 1980s has been the most affected by the rigid implementation of the birth-control measures, especially the single-child policy. It is hard to say at the moment whether they will stop their childbearing permanently after they have had one or two children, or just wait for the relaxation of the control. It is certain that changing reproductive behaviour in China's rural areas will be an arduous and long-term task.

Comparison between Period and Cohort Fertility Rate

The general trend of China's fertility transition has already been shown clearly. Nevertheless, the conventional P/F ratio method is used to facilitate analyses of fertility levels and trends.[17] It is impossible to present all these comparisons for the entire period concerned because of limitation of space. The P/F ratios presented here are on a three-year basis for the period immediately prior to the survey, 1979–81.

These P/F ratios are plotted in Figure 6.8 for each province, separating rural from urban sector. The ratios for women below 20 are

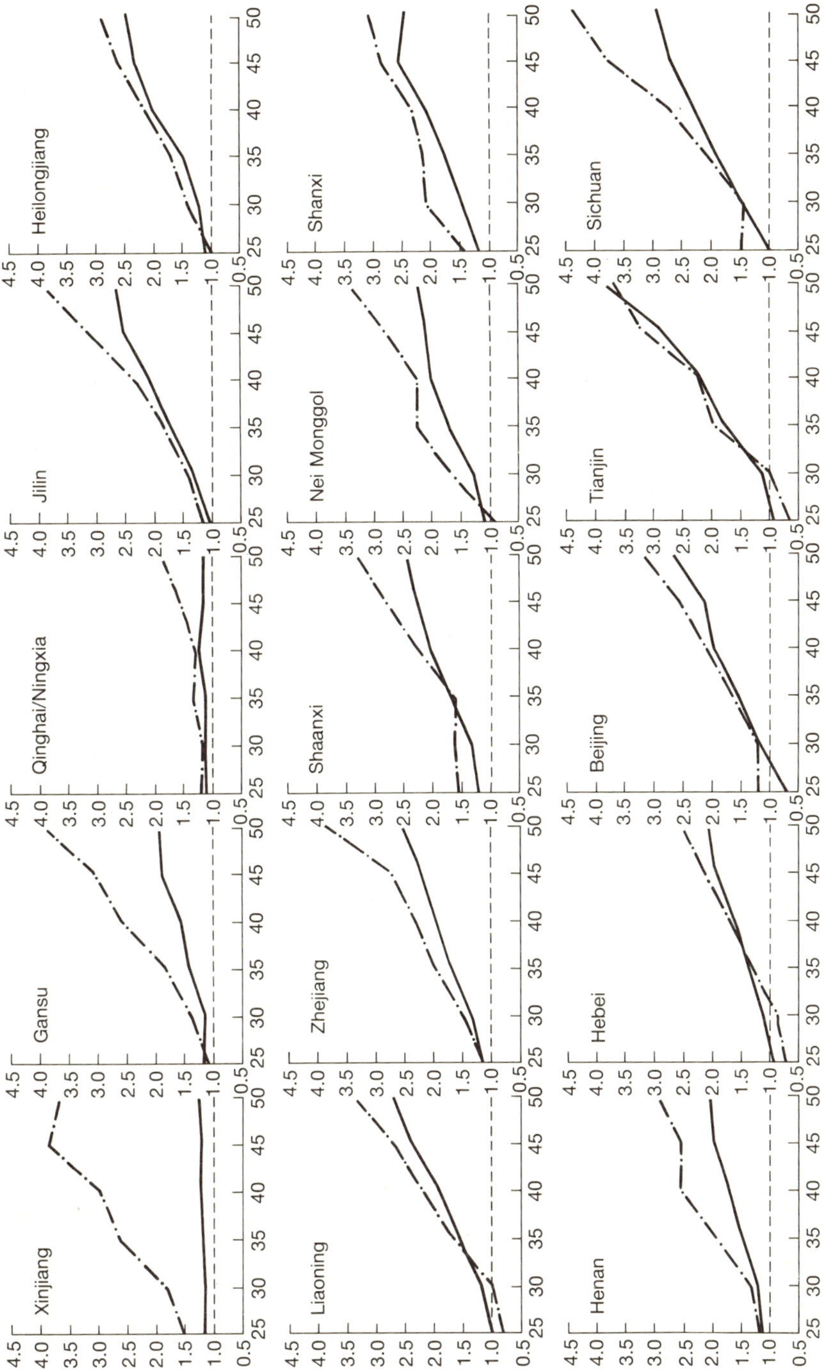

Xinjiang
Gansu
Qinghai/Ningxia
Jilin
Heilongjiang
Liaoning
Zhejiang
Shaanxi
Nei Monggol
Shanxi
Henan
Hebei
Beijing
Tianjin
Sichuan

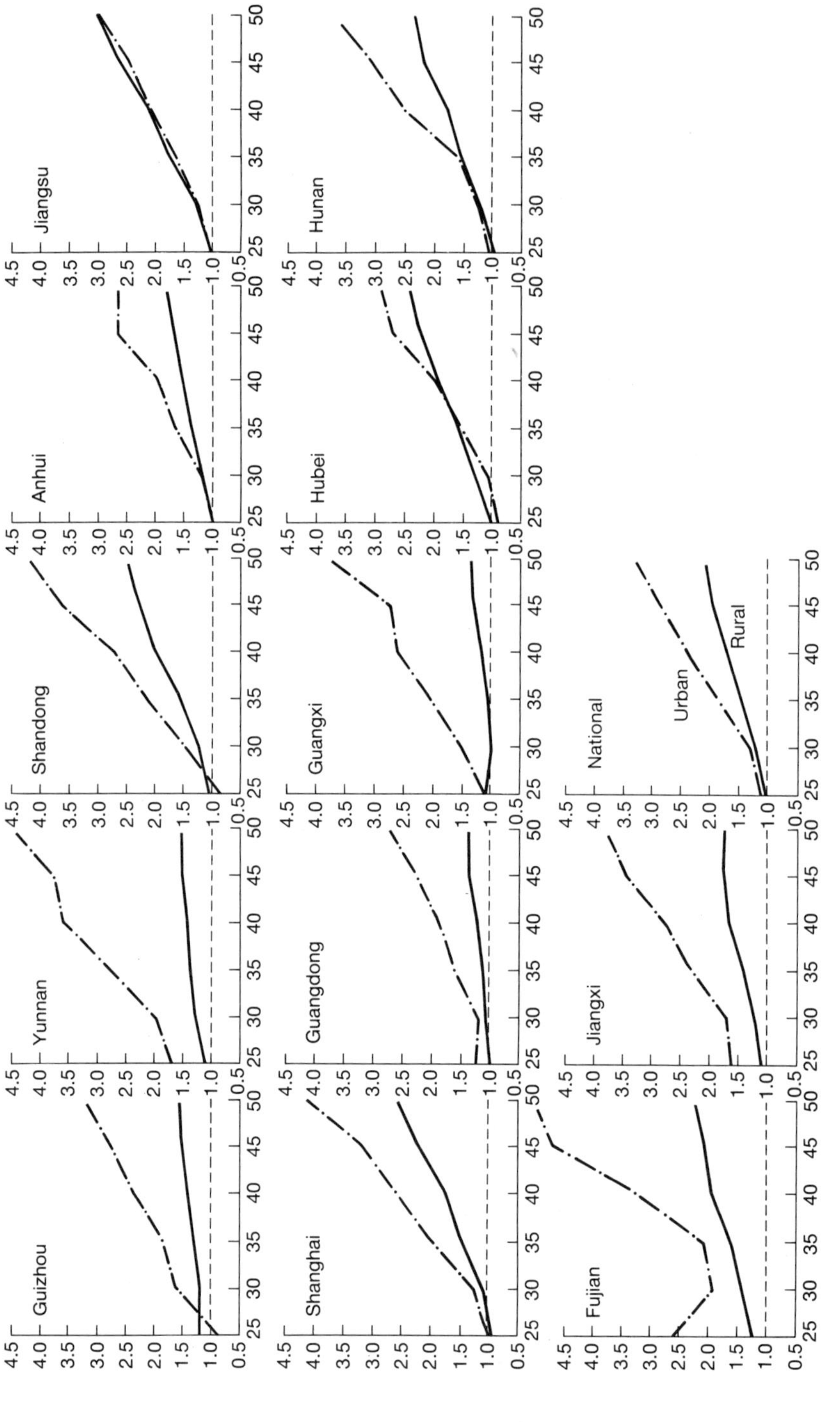

Fig. 6.8 Provincial P/F ratios for the rural and urban population, 1979–1981

not included, because the fertility rate of teens has been all but eliminated. The fertility changes in the past several decades is clearly demonstrated. The P/F ratios for women aged 50 are greater than unity in every province regardless of the rural and urban division. The ratios rise with increasing age, as expected, clearly indicating the elimination of childbearing to women in their late reproduction cycle. However, regional, as well as rural–urban, differences are considerable.

As can be seen the P/F ratios for the rural population were marginally above unity in Xinjiang, Qinghai and Ningxia, Guangxi, Guangdong, Yunnan, and Guizhou. This indicates that fertility decline in these provinces was very modest. On the other hand, the P/F ratios in the majority of eastern provinces exceeded 2.5. In other words, for women entering childbearing in the early 1980s, the ultimate family size would be only half of that achieved by women who had completed their childbearing at that time, assuming that the current period fertility level persists. The highest ratio of 4 for women aged 50 was recorded in Tianjin's rural sector.

The rural–urban comparison is of special interest. Generally speaking, the P/F ratios are higher for the urban than for the rural population. This is particularly true in provinces where the fertility change in rural areas was moderate, such as Xinjiang, Guangxi, Yunnan, and Jiangxi. By contrast, the gap between the ratios of the rural and urban sectors was very small in the eastern provinces. In Jiangsu and Tianjin, the two curves overlapped one another. This means that the magnitude of the fertility changes was similar between the rural and urban areas in these provinces.

Another common feature is that the regional differences in the P/F ratios are much smaller for the urban areas, in contrast to the considerable difference in rural areas. This confirms the relative similarity in China's urban fertility transition between provinces. However, since 80 per cent of China's total population live in the countryside, there is still a long way to go in order to complete the fertility transition in the vast rural areas.

IV. Nuptiality versus Marital Fertility Rate

In China, sexual activity outside marriage is a cultural taboo, and almost all births have taken place within marriage. Illegitimate births have little impact on fertility changes. Therefore, the marriage pattern and the marital fertility are the two decisive determinants of China's overall fertility level.

Marital Fertility Rate

The sequence of the total marital fertility rate (TMFR) is calculated for each province. As has been discussed in the previous chapters, the marital fertility estimated here is for ever married, rather than for currently married, women. Given the stability of Chinese marriage, combined with the sharp decline in mortality, this is reasonable. Ratios of the marital fertility in selected years to the reference are estimated in order to examine changes in marital fertility in the past. Because the sustained rural fertility decline began in the early 1970s, the average of the marital fertility rate in 1964 and 1965 is used as the reference value and set at 100 (see Table 6.12).

The general trend of marital fertility is similar to that of overall fertility. However, regional differences seem more considerable. During the mid-1960s, the national total marital fertility rate for China's rural population was about 7.4. Among the lowest quarter were 7 provinces in which the TMFR was below 7, with the lowest of 5.77 in Shanghai. There were 5 provinces where the TMFR was higher than 8. The highest marital fertility rate, 9.47, was in Nei Monggol. No clear geographic pattern can be found.

The marital fertility rate in 1970 was by and large similar to that of the mid-1960s, with some fluctuations. Only Shanghai, Tianjin, Zhejiang, and Liaoning witnessed a more than 15-per-cent decline. The steep decline in marital fertility took place in the first half of the 1970s, when regional differences reached their largest point. In 1975 the TMFR in Shanghai, Tianjin, Beijing, and Jilin fell below half of the level seen ten years earlier. On the other hand, no significant decline in marital fertility was recorded in Guizhou, Jiangxi, Guangxi, Xinjiang, and Yunnan provinces. On average, marital fertility for China's rural population declined by about 30 per cent in this period.

The transition process continued throughout the 1970s. By the early 1980s marital fertility had declined by about 50 per cent in about half of all provinces during the previous one and a half decades. The regional differential narrowed a little but remained remarkable. In Shanghai, Tianjin, and Jilin, the reduction was more than 60 per cent. In contrast, the decline in some provinces was very moderate. Guangdong and Guangxi were the two with the smallest decline, having less than half of the national average.

TABLE 6.12. *Trends in marital fertility rate by province, rural China*

Province	1964/5		1970		1975		1980/1	
	TMFR	Ratio	TMFR	Ratio	TMFR	Ratio	TMFR	Ratio
CHINA (rural)	7.34	100	7.29	99	5.38	73	4.04	55
Shanghai	5.77	100	4.40	76	2.05	36	2.08	36
Tianjin	7.83	100	5.75	73	3.18	41	2.58	33
Jiangsu	6.49	100	6.20	96	3.43	53	2.74	42
Sichuan	7.60	100	7.87	104	6.09	80	3.01	40
Jilin	8.93	100	8.02	90	3.59	40	3.14	35
Shandong	6.07	100	7.22	119	4.31	71	3.17	52
Shaanxi	6.70	100	6.57	98	4.31	64	3.22	48
Zhejiang	7.56	100	5.65	75	4.52	60	3.29	44
Liaoning	7.65	100	6.42	84	4.08	53	3.43	45
Beijing	6.86	100	6.73	98	3.05	44	3.59	52
Fujian	7.44	100	7.45	100	5.38	72	3.68	49
Hunan	7.87	100	7.24	92	5.73	73	3.68	47
Heilongjiang	8.18	100	7.55	92	5.08	62	3.68	45
Hebei	7.10	100	6.59	93	3.60	51	3.74	53
Shanxi	6.65	100	6.88	103	4.20	63	3.76	56
Gansu	8.00	100	8.24	103	5.03	63	3.86	48
Hubei	7.87	100	7.57	96	5.24	67	3.95	50
Henan	6.84	100	7.48	109	5.31	78	4.09	60
Nei Monggol	9.47	100	8.01	85	4.96	52	4.21	44
Jiangxi	7.38	100	7.66	104	6.69	91	4.35	59
Anhui	7.01	100	7.59	108	4.65	66	4.81	69
Yunnan	7.95	100	7.40	93	7.10	89	5.14	65
Guizhou	7.95	100	8.84	112	8.47	107	5.31	67
Guangdong	7.00	100	7.07	101	5.53	79	5.34	76
Xinjiang	8.68	100	8.45	97	6.99	81	5.57	64
Guangxi	7.63	100	7.28	95	7.12	93	6.04	79
MEAN	7.48		7.16	96	4.99	67	3.90	52
ST.D.	0.84		0.96		1.48		0.97	12

Decomposition

As was discussed earlier, China's rural fertility transition was led by the great decline of the ASFR for the 15–19 age group, which is obviously connected with the changes in the nuptiality pattern. In this section, the impact of the changes in nuptiality and marital fertility on the total fertility transition is examined. The decomposition procedure is employed once again. The equation has been defined and discussed earlier in Chapter 4.

Although marriage has been widely postponed and births consequently delayed, the major source of the fertility reduction are changes in marital fertility rate. As can be seen in Table 6.13, changes in nuptiality pattern on the whole accounted for only one-fifth of the total fertility decline over the period concerned. On the other hand, 80 per cent of the fertility decline between the mid-1960s and the early 1980s is attributable to the decline in marital fertility.

The importance of delayed marriage on overall fertility change declined over time. In the first half of the 1970s, the marriage changes alone accounted for about 32 per cent of the total fertility reduction. This fell to 21 per cent in the second part of the 1970s and dropped further to only 17 per cent in the early 1980s. This is evidence that the fertility decline in China's rural areas mainly resulted from a decline in fertility within marriage. The marriage pattern itself did change. But the effect of postponing marriage was offset by the shortened first-birth interval.

Moreover, the near universal entry into marriage well before the end of the reproductive ages remained unchanged throughout the entire period. Consequently, the decline in marital fertility is the decisive cause of the rapid and sharp decline in overall fertility. This replicates the pattern we have found in China's urban fertility transition.

V. Recent Trends

Rapid fertility transition has been taking place in China's rural area. However, regional variations widened with the progress of the transition. It is certain that both marital fertility and nuptiality work together in the same direction to create relatively large differences in overall fertility. The uneven progress of the provincial family-planning programme and the local institutional settings are the major determinants of this trend.

Such a trend continues in the 1980s. As a result of differences in the

TABLE 6.13. *Changes in TFR and the net effects of component changes, rural China*[a]

Province	1965–9				1970–4				1975–9				1980–1				
	TFR (1)	F[b] (2)	M[c] (3)	DF[d] (4)	TFR (5)	F[b] (6)	M[c] (7)	DF[d] (8)	TFR (9)	F[b] (10)	M[c] (11)	DF[d] (12)	TFR (13)	F[b] (14)	M[c] (15)	DF[d] (16)	DM[e] (17)
CHINA (rural)	−0.01	+0.01	−0.02	—	−0.16	−0.11	−0.05	66	−0.49	−0.38	−0.11	77	−0.59	−0.48	−0.11	81	19
Tianjin	−0.23	−0.23	0.00	99	−0.46	−0.43	−0.04	94	−0.65	−0.59	−0.08	91	−0.76	−0.68	−0.08	90	10
Jiangsu	−0.05	−0.02	−0.03	40	−0.36	−0.28	−0.08	79	−0.63	−0.50	−0.13	80	−0.71	−0.58	−0.13	82	18
Jilin	−0.01	+0.01	−0.02	—	−0.23	−0.19	−0.03	86	−0.63	−0.56	−0.07	89	−0.71	−0.67	−0.04	94	6
Shanghai	−0.11	−0.06	−0.05	51	−0.52	−0.43	−0.08	83	−0.63	−0.48	−0.14	76	−0.69	−0.61	−0.07	89	11
Zhejiang	−0.10	−0.09	−0.01	85	−0.42	−0.36	−0.06	86	−0.63	−0.51	−0.12	81	−0.69	−0.56	−0.14	81	19
Sichuan	0.00	+0.02	−0.02	—	−0.07	−0.03	−0.04	40	−0.55	−0.45	−0.10	82	−0.69	−0.61	−0.08	88	12
Liaoning	−0.07	−0.04	−0.03	61	−0.36	−0.28	−0.08	78	−0.64	−0.52	−0.13	80	−0.69	−0.57	−0.13	82	18
Shandong	0.00	+0.03	−0.03	—	−0.16	−0.10	−0.07	59	−0.53	−0.40	−0.13	75	−0.65	−0.54	−0.12	82	18
Hubei	+0.04	+0.06	−0.02	—	−0.21	−0.13	−0.07	65	−0.55	−0.42	−0.13	77	−0.65	−0.52	−0.13	81	19
Heilongjiang	0.00	+0.02	−0.01	—	−0.17	−0.13	−0.05	74	−0.57	−0.48	−0.09	85	−0.65	−0.56	−0.09	86	14
Beijing	−0.20	−0.17	−0.03	86	−0.33	−0.30	−0.02	93	−0.73	−0.64	−0.09	88	−0.64	−0.54	−0.10	84	16
Nei Monggol	−0.13	−0.12	−0.01	92	−0.26	−0.22	−0.04	85	−0.59	−0.52	−0.06	89	−0.64	−0.56	−0.08	87	13
Shanxi	−0.03	−0.01	−0.02	33	−0.13	−0.08	−0.05	62	−0.54	−0.42	−0.12	77	−0.64	−0.49	−0.14	78	22
Hunan	−0.02	−0.01	−0.01	45	−0.22	−0.17	−0.05	77	−0.57	−0.47	−0.10	82	−0.63	−0.54	−0.09	85	15
Fujian	+0.01	+0.02	−0.01	—	−0.13	−0.10	−0.03	78	−0.41	−0.34	−0.07	83	−0.63	−0.53	−0.10	85	15
Shaanxi	0.00	+0.02	−0.02	—	−0.13	−0.08	−0.05	63	−0.50	−0.38	−0.12	76	−0.61	−0.49	−0.12	80	20
Henan	+0.06	+0.08	−0.02	—	−0.07	−0.01	−0.06	15	−0.48	−0.35	−0.13	73	−0.59	−0.45	−0.13	77	23
Gansu	+0.01	+0.01	0.00	—	−0.06	−0.05	−0.02	75	−0.51	−0.44	−0.08	85	−0.58	−0.51	−0.08	87	13
Hebei	−0.09	−0.07	−0.03	70	−0.26	−0.19	−0.07	73	−0.59	−0.46	−0.13	78	−0.57	−0.46	−0.11	81	19
Anhui	+0.10	+0.11	−0.01	—	−0.10	−0.05	−0.05	46	−0.45	−0.35	−0.10	78	−0.53	−0.42	−0.11	79	21
Jiangxi	+0.07	+0.08	−0.01	—	+0.01	+0.03	−0.03	—	−0.21	−0.14	−0.06	70	−0.50	−0.43	−0.08	84	16
Yunnan	−0.02	0.00	−0.02	10	−0.11	−0.07	−0.04	68	−0.24	−0.16	−0.08	67	−0.43	−0.34	−0.09	80	20
Xinjiang	−0.05	−0.05	0.00	99	−0.14	−0.13	0.00	97	−0.31	−0.28	−0.02	92	−0.42	−0.38	−0.05	89	11
Guangxi	−0.03	−0.01	−0.02	37	−0.15	−0.09	−0.05	63	−0.34	−0.24	−0.11	69	−0.36	−0.24	−0.11	68	32
Guangdong	+0.03	+0.05	−0.02	—	−0.08	−0.03	−0.05	34	−0.34	−0.25	−0.09	74	−0.35	−0.25	−0.09	73	27
Ningxia	+0.05	+0.05	−0.01	—	−0.07	−0.02	−0.05	29	−0.26	−0.18	−0.09	67	−0.32	−0.25	−0.08	75	25
Qinghai	+0.05	+0.02	+0.02	—	+0.02	−0.04	+0.05	—	−0.07	−0.12	+0.04	160	−0.15	−0.19	+0.03	123	−23
MEAN	−0.03				−0.19			68	−0.49			79	−0.57			83	
ST.D.	0.08				0.14			21	0.16			7.1	0.15			5.7	

Note: [a] The reference is the average of 1964 and 1965.
All changes are period averages and compared to the reference.
[b] F indicates the net effect of marital fertility change on TFR.
[c] M indicates the net effect of nuptiality change on TFR.
[d] DF indicates the contribution of F to total TFR changes, in percentage.
[e] DM indicates the contribution of M to total TFR changes, in percentage.
— means either TFR or Marital fertility, or both, is higher than reference.

interpretation of recent modification of population policies, and in the degree of relaxation of control over reproduction, the regional diversity in childbearing remains considerable. In Table 6.14, contributions to total births by birth order for China's rural population are estimated for each province.

For the countryside as a whole, about 61 per cent of new-born babies in 1986 were first children, 2.5 percentage points lower than in 1984. The regional differences are enormous. In Shanghai's rural area, the first child accounted for 93.44 per cent of total births in 1986, and there were almost no higher-order births at all. By contrast, only 27.41 per cent of total births in Xinjiang were first children, and the third and higher-order births accounted for about half of its total births.

Among those provinces where the numbers of higher-order births constituted more than 20 per cent of their annual total births in 1986, were Xinjiang, Ningxia, Qinghai, Guangxi, Guizhou, and Yunnan. These are provinces with a high proportion of minority populations, where the family-planning programme has been carried out later and less effectively. The higher proportion of higher-order births is readily understandable. The minority population in Guangdong, Jiangxi, and Fujian accounts for a very small proportion of their combined total. However, the proportion of third and higher parities in these three provinces was around 10 per cent, although this was already an improved record. Even after the adjustment of the one-child policy, the third child in China's rural areas for Han population is still not allowed. Therefore, these rates indicate clearly that the performance of birth control in these provinces was very poor.

Generally speaking, the incidence of third and higher parities has diminished over time. The key for China's rural fertility transition is the second birth. Since the relaxation of the one-child campaign in 1984, the second child has virtually been allowed for a large proportion of Chinese peasants in an overwhelmingly majority of provinces. Consequently, the proportion of second births has increased in almost all provinces. Such a rise was very sharp in Sichuan, Henan, and Liaoning provinces. There is no doubt that the magnitude of the increase is closely associated with the degree of relaxation of control over the second births. Shanghai and Jiangsu remained the best nationally, which is largely owing to continuous commitment to family planning and strict control over childbearing. It also reflects public support for population programmes in these regions.[18]

The regional difference for the rural population is larger than for the city inhabitants. However, there is a close relationship between the two. The correlation coefficients between the rural and urban populations in 1986 are 0.852, 0.832, and 0.855 for proportions of the first-, second-, and higher-order births. These coefficients are more or less constant during the period 1984–6. It is plausible to suggest that differentials are not only a rural–urban phenomenon, but rather a regional one.

Trends in the provincial implementation of the family-planning programme in the recent past are illustrated in Table 6.15. It is clear that women in China's countryside at present get married at younger ages than a few years ago. In 1986 only 48 per cent of rural women got married at the age of 23 years or more, in contrast to at least 82.5 per cent in 1979. It should be noted that there was no nation-wide standard for late marriage in 1979, although the common criterion in the rural areas was set at 23 years—and higher in some individual regions. Thus, the direct comparison of the late-marriage rate between 1979 and the 1980s may slightly underestimate the real changes.

The late-marriage rate in 1986 varies widely from 73.55 per cent in Henan to 18.41 in Ningxia. It is worthwhile to note that the highest late-marriage rates are to be found not in the three big municipalities, but in Henan and Guangdong where the family-planning work has been less effective. The quality of data reporting may also be partly responsible for that. Nevertheless, we can say that very late marriage in these two provinces is mainly associated with local marriage custom and other institutional factors.

Another interesting case is Sichuan province. During 1979–86 the late-marriage rate for Sichuan's rural population dropped by more than 68 percentage points and Sichuan is now in the lowest quarter nationally. Bearing in mind developments in Sichuan's urban areas, it would seem that this province has witnessed a major relaxation of control over the age of marriage.

The trend of contraceptive practice is relatively promising. About 85 per cent of ever married women at fertile ages in China's rural areas practised contraception in 1986. This is a figure 6 percentage points higher than that of 1979. The improvement in 11 provinces exceeds 10 points. Even in remote provinces, birth control is practised by two-thirds of all women at risk of childbearing. The apparent decline in Xinjiang's contraceptive prevalence rate from 76 per cent (1979) to only 44 per cent (1986) is likely to reflect a reporting error.

The rural–urban difference in contraceptive practice is very small and has fallen over time. For the country as a whole, the contraceptive-prevalence rate for the rural population was only 5 per cent lower than that for the urban population in 1986, compared with 12 per cent in 1979. In some provinces, such as Shanghai and Jilin, the proportion of

TABLE 6.14. *Contribution to total births by birth order, rural China 1986*

Province	First birth (%)				Second birth (%)				Third and higher (%)			
	1986	Change[a]	Ratio[b]	R/U[c]	1986	Change[a]	Ratio[b]	R/U[c]	1986	Change[a]	Ratio[b]	R/U[c]
CHINA (rural)	60.82	−2.49	1.00	0.76	30.22	5.79	1.00		8.96	−3.29	1.00	
Beijing	76.63	−5.22	1.26	0.78	22.00	5.63	0.73	13.50	1.37	−0.41	0.15	68.49
Tianjin	80.10	−9.94	1.32	0.81	19.59	10.09	0.65	15.19	0.31	−0.15	0.03	30.99
Hebei	67.58	−5.18	1.11	0.81	30.15	8.32	1.00	1.88	2.27	−3.14	0.25	2.91
Shanxi	60.07	3.20	0.99	0.77	31.76	1.41	1.05	1.62	8.17	−4.61	0.91	3.14
Nei Monggol	57.40	6.85	0.94	0.70	33.00	3.58	1.09	2.01	9.60	−10.43	1.07	6.76
Liaoning	71.76	−20.79	1.18	0.79	27.71	20.55	0.92	2.99	0.53	0.24	0.06	3.31
Jilin	84.36	−7.82	1.39	0.94	15.25	7.77	0.50	1.55	0.39	0.05	0.04	2.60
Heilongjiang	73.30	−4.16	1.21	0.85	22.95	5.46	0.76	1.83	3.75	−1.30	0.42	2.39
Shanghai	93.64	−2.77	1.54	0.94	6.31	2.78	0.21	7.25	0.05	−0.01	0.01	2.50
Jiangsu	82.77	−0.84	1.36	0.91	16.17	2.56	0.54	1.93	1.06	−1.72	0.12	2.94
Zhejiang	65.96	1.84	1.08	0.87	31.41	6.50	1.04	1.38	2.63	−8.34	0.29	1.79
Anhui	62.57	0.49	1.03	0.80	29.79	1.68	0.99	1.63	7.64	−2.17	0.85	2.12
Fujian	56.86	8.38	0.93	0.81	34.08	−0.72	1.13	1.38	9.06	−7.66	1.01	1.90
Jiangxi	53.64	2.51	0.88	0.84	34.71	2.49	1.15	1.33	11.65	−5.00	1.30	1.19
Shandong	76.00	−10.48	1.25	0.93	23.01	10.71	0.76	1.29	0.99	−0.23	0.11	1.77

Henan	64.73	−19.23	1.06	0.75	30.06	16.86	0.99	2.35	5.21	2.37	0.58	7.89
Hubei	63.39	−3.50	1.04	0.85	31.41	5.72	1.04	1.46	5.20	−2.22	0.58	1.41
Hunan	59.04	−0.65	0.97	0.85	32.90	2.19	1.09	1.28	8.06	−1.54	0.90	1.58
Guangdong	53.45	4.30	0.88	0.79	35.60	0.98	1.18	1.40	10.95	−5.28	1.22	1.59
Guangxi	40.06	3.37	0.66	0.63	33.80	1.90	1.12	1.51	26.14	−5.27	2.92	1.80
Sichuan	64.33	−14.80	1.06	0.82	31.80	16.06	1.05	1.56	3.87	−1.26	0.43	3.34
Guizhou	42.68	1.04	0.70	0.79	33.44	3.10	1.11	1.21	23.88	−4.14	2.67	1.31
Yunnan	42.45	1.32	0.70	0.67	34.31	1.94	1.14	1.27	23.24	−3.26	2.59	2.48
Shaanxi	58.33	−5.09	0.96	0.78	34.10	6.32	1.13	1.54	7.57	−1.23	0.84	2.23
Gansu	58.33	−0.78	0.96	0.78	34.16	4.61	1.13	1.53	7.51	−3.83	0.84	2.97
Qinghai	42.70	7.11	0.70	0.53	30.50	4.47	1.01	2.05	26.80	−11.58	2.99	5.69
Ningxia	38.83	0.06	0.64	0.60	33.06	1.26	1.09	1.24	28.11	−1.32	3.14	3.38
Xinjiang	27.41	−6.54	0.45	0.42	22.84	−4.02	0.76	1.27	49.75	10.56	5.55	3.01
MEAN	61.37	−2.76		0.78	28.42	5.36		2.73	10.21	−2.60		6.20
ST.D.	15.54	7.35		0.12	7.24	5.45		3.48	11.70	4.192		13.41

[a] Change = $Percentage_{1986}$–$Percentage_{1984}$
[b] The national figure is taken as reference value.
[c] R/U refers to ratios of proportion for rural population to that for urban residents.

TABLE 6.15. *Provincial performance of family-planning programmes, rural China 1986*

Province	Late marriage rate				Contraceptive prevalence				One-child certificate		
	1986	Ratio[a]	Change 1[b]	Change 2[c]	1986	Ratio[a]	Change 1[b]	Change 2[c]	1986	Change 1[b]	Ratio[a]
CHINA (rural)	47.78	1.00	−5.42	−34.92	84.58	1.00	−0.71	5.88	11.12	−1.75	1.00
Beijing	51.55	1.08	−5.12	−31.85	86.01	1.02	3.24	2.71	32.74	1.33	2.94
Tianjin	53.11	1.11	−3.04	−44.39	88.04	1.04	0.10	5.24	26.10	2.71	2.35
Hebei	49.88	1.04	−6.35	−45.62	86.73	1.03	1.80	2.43	11.40	−2.77	1.03
Shanxi	53.84	1.13	2.01	−28.16	86.46	1.02	−0.14	8.46	5.81	−2.26	0.52
Nei Monggol	56.27	1.18	3.79	−13.73	86.45	1.02	3.52	15.95	5.21	−2.12	0.47
Liaoning	45.67	0.96	4.15	−40.53	85.17	1.01	−3.98	0.27	17.94	−8.52	1.61
Jilin	48.68	1.02	−5.24	−28.12	89.35	1.06	0.01	10.05	19.38	−1.02	1.74
Heilongjiang	50.21	1.05	−11.16	−25.69	89.08	1.05	−2.37	5.98	13.72	−1.89	1.23
Shanghai	47.88	1.00	−3.83	−48.62	90.81	1.07	−3.52	−4.19	44.89	−0.01	4.04
Jiangsu	60.68	1.27	−12.86	−30.82	89.54	1.06	−1.22	1.54	26.00	−0.55	2.34
Zhejiang	48.28	1.01	−0.68	−28.42	89.69	1.06	0.12	10.89	12.21	−2.08	1.10
Anhui	63.73	1.33	0.23	−23.17	86.59	1.02	−1.80	10.19	3.32	−1.42	0.30
Fujian	32.65	0.68	−3.96	−30.85	86.20	1.02	0.16	5.10	2.23	−0.16	0.20
Jiangxi	31.09	0.65	−0.69	−31.41	79.59	0.94	0.71	3.19	1.14	−0.21	0.10
Shandong	61.10	1.28	−4.70	−33.50	89.40	1.06	−2.70	4.30	20.94	−2.46	1.88

Henan	73.55	1.54	−8.73	−21.45	88.01	1.04	−2.92	13.11	12.10	−3.66	1.09
Hubei	50.60	1.06	−10.84	−32.50	85.86	1.02	−0.99	8.36	6.91	−1.20	0.62
Hunan	38.35	0.80	−4.86	−45.85	87.17	1.03	−0.16	5.57	5.78	1.58	0.52
Guangdong	63.74	1.33	−0.47	−3.26	84.39	1.00	−5.53	12.49	2.46	1.19	0.22
Guangxi	37.53	0.79	−0.46	—	73.85	0.87	5.72	16.05	0.73	−0.28	0.07
Sichuan	26.13	0.55	−13.17	−68.27	87.13	1.03	−0.79	−1.27	19.52	−2.56	1.76
Guizhou	43.34	0.91	0.22	−25.76	76.24	0.90	1.74	10.04	1.43	0.10	0.13
Yunnan	28.95	0.61	−1.77	−46.45	66.24	0.78	2.89	11.64	1.49	−0.02	0.13
Shaanxi	45.17	0.95	−9.59	−36.73	83.84	0.99	−0.47	−0.26	6.97	−3.04	0.63
Gansu	20.26	0.42	3.46	−66.74	83.03	0.98	2.81	2.03	5.98	1.66	0.54
Qinghai	19.35	0.40	−10.95	8.35	65.58	0.78	−7.29	27.08	1.64	−0.35	0.15
Ningxia	18.41	0.39	2.86	−37.99	73.36	0.87	−0.24	17.36	0.09	−0.29	0.01
Xinjiang	32.37	0.68	−3.78	−53.93	44.42	0.53	6.79	−31.58	2.89	−1.11	0.26
MEAN	44.73		−3.77	−31.35	82.44		−0.16	6.17	11.11	−1.05	
ST.D.	14.46		5.18	21.15	0.06		3.13	9.99	11.20	2.15	

[a] The national figure is taken as 1.00.
[b] Change 1 = Rate_{1986}–Rate_{1984}
[c] Change 2 = Rate_{1986}–Rate_{1979}

women in the countryside who practise birth control is even higher than that of urban residents. The accuracy of those figures may suffer from reporting error, especially from exaggeration of the achievement. Nevertheless, easy access to family-planning services and wide availability of contraceptive methods do provide a solid basis for birth control in China's rural areas.

Finally, we can see that the one-child certificate rate declined during 1984–6. This is certainly related to the relaxation of control over the second child. However, about 45 per cent of couples at fertile ages in Shanghai's rural area pledged to have only one child and were issued with certificates in 1986. In Beijing, Tianjin, Jiangsu, and Shandong, more than 20 per cent of eligible couples did so. As already mentioned, in Sichuan's countryside, the age at marriage declined and the number of second children rose markedly in the recent past. Nevertheless, many more couples hold the one-child certificate in Sichuan than in other provinces. Combined with the relatively low proportion of the higher-order births, this may suggest that the one-child campaign in Sichuan has worked reasonably well. Except for those who were given express permission to have the second child, others have followed the government call to control their family size. On the other hand, there are almost no couples in Ningxia's rural areas who have been issued with one-child certificates. The certificate rates in the majority of southern and western provinces in 1986 were also very low. This regional diversity reflects the local resistance to the policy, and may also result from different degrees of lessening administrative control over childbearing.

NOTES

1. See Population Association of Qinghai, *Qinghai shaoshu minzu renkou wenti tansuo (Exploration of Qinghai's Minority Population Problems)* (Xining, 1984), 107–8.
2. A. Sharlin, 'Urban–Rural Differences in Fertility in Europe during the Demographic Transition', in A. J. Coale and S. C. Watkins (eds.), *The Decline of Fertility in Europe* (Princeton, NJ: Princeton University Press, 1986), 234–60.
3. O. Lang, *Chinese Family and Society* (New York: Archon Books, 1968), 35.
4. Hu Huanyong and Zhang Shanyu, *Population Geography of China* (Shanghai: Eastern Normal University Press, 1986), 401.
5. *Falu yu shenghuo (Law and Life)*, Mar. 1986.
6. See *Zhongguo qinanian Bao (Youth of China)*, 31 Dec. 1987.
7. See E. J. Croll, 'A Conflict for Control of Marriage Patterns: Primary Groups versus Political Organizations', in S. L. Greenblatt *et al.* (eds.), *Organizational Behavior in Chinese Society* (New York: Praeger Publishers, 1981), 231–55.
8. P. McDonald, 'Social Organization and Nuptiality in Developing Societies', in

J. Cleland and J. Hobcraft (eds.), *Reproductive Change in Developing Countries* (Oxford: Oxford University Press, 1985), 87–114.

9. This is also the picture presented by Asia and the Pacific region. See P. C. Smith, M. Shahidullah, and A. Alcantara, 'Cohort Nuptiality in Asia and the Pacific: An Analysis of WFS Surveys', *WFS Comparative Studies*, No. 22 (Apr. 1983).
10. J. McCarthy, 'Differentials in Age at First Marriage', *WFS Comparative Studies*, No. 19 (June 1982).
11. Ibid.
12. J. Hobcraft *et al.*, 'Advances in the P/F Ratio Method for the Analysis of Birth Histories', *Population Studies*, 36 (2), 291–316 (1982).
13. W. Brass, *Methods for Estimating Fertility and Mortality from Limited and Defective Data*, (Chapel Hill: Laboratories for Population Statistics, 1975).
14. Such as age misreporting in Xinjiang, personal communication.
15. T. Dyson and M. Murphy, 'The Onset of the Fertility Transition', *Population and Development Review*, 11 (3), 399–440 (1985).
16. See Xizhe Peng, 'Fertility Transition in China and its Provinces since 1949', Ph.D. diss. (London School of Economics, 1988), ch. 7.
17. See N. Goldman and J. Hobcraft, 'Birth Histories', *WFS Comparative Studies*, No. 17 (June 1982).
18. Personal communication.

7

Conclusion

I. Trends in Fertility and Nuptiality

During the last four decades, China has experienced a dramatic fertility transition. After a steady fertility increase in the early years of the People's Republic, its national total fertility rate (TFR) was around 6 in the mid-1950s and remained so until the end of the 1960s, except during the crisis period around 1959–63. Since the early 1970s the fertility transition has accelerated. The national TFR declined from 5.7 in 1970 to 3.6 in 1975 and fell further to 2.31 in 1980. In other words, China's fertility decreased by more than 50 per cent in only one decade. Since the early 1980s China's fertility level has fluctuated, and a slightly upward trend has emerged most recently. This is mainly due to relaxations of birth-control efforts and a marriage boom. Nevertheless, China's fertility remains at a relatively low level.

However, China is a country with enormous population, vast territory, and considerable regional differentials in terms of socio-economic development and cultural tradition. Fertility changes did not occur homogeneously across the country, and the timing and pace of the transition varied greatly between localities.

China's fertility transition is a process of diffusion. There have always been regional differentials in fertility and nuptiality behaviour. These became more marked during the 1960s, and widened further during the 1970s, thereafter changing little. Sustained fertility decline started in a few large municipalities and some eastern provinces, with Shanghai leading the way. They were then followed by the northern provinces, and the transition gradually spread to the interior. By the end of the 1970s fertility in those eastern provinces had already been red- ced to around replacement level. By contrast, the vast areas ng the northwest and some parts of southern China entered the n much later and have maintained relatively high fertility to the ay. Fertility levels in the north were originally higher than but this gap was gradually eliminated.

ansition in China's urban areas began much earlier and

progressed faster than in the rural areas. With a few exceptions, the onset of China's urban fertility transition occurred around the mid-1960s in all provinces. The provincial differences in urban fertility have been substantially reduced as time has passed, and already fell within a very narrow range by the end of the 1970s. It seems that the urban population is more willing, in some cases perhaps under pressure, to practise family limitation.

On the other hand, the uneven progress of the transition in China's rural areas is also evident, and the fertility variation has widened over time. The sustained fertility transition began as early as 1964 for the rural population in some major municipalities (such as Shanghai and Tianjin), whereas this only took place in the late 1970s in Jiangxi, Xinjiang, Guizhou, and Guangxi: a 14-year gap. The initial fertility decline began, in the rural areas of most provinces, around the time of the launch of China's third family-planning campaign ('Later, Longer, and Fewer') in the early 1970s, roughly one decade later than the urban transition.

Rural fertility was higher than urban fertility, with only very few exceptions, over the entire period concerned. The rural–urban difference became bigger during the course of the transition as urban fertility declined more rapidly in the initial stages. Moreover, the variations in the fertility level and the magnitude of the reduction are considerable for the rural population.

Roughly speaking, fertility levels in Xinjiang, Gansu, Guizhou, Yunnan, Ningxia, Fujian, and Jiangxi were consistently higher than the national average. Guangdong and Guangxi can also be classified into this group. The tempo of the fertility transition in these provinces was much slower and they have lagged further and further behind the national trend. Shanghai, Beijing, Tianjin, Hebei, Jiangsu, Shandong, and Liaoning comprise another group. Fertility rates in these provinces have been much lower than the national average since the mid-1960s. Changes in reproduction in this group have always been ahead of other provinces.

The transition from high to low fertility in Sichuan province was behind the national level until the mid-1970s. However, a sudden and very sharp fertility reduction has occurred since then. Its TFR fell by 67 per cent between 1975 and 1980, which was the sharpest fall in China and probably the fastest decline anywhere for a sizeable population (in excess of 100 million).

The fertility decline did not occur simultaneously in all age groups. While the age-specific fertility rate for all other ages remained unchanged or even increased, births to women in their teens fell steadily. This is closely associated with changes in the nuptiality patterns. Fertility decline had already occurred to an extent for the 15–19 age group by the 1960s, but this was offset by the increased fertility of women in their 20s. During that period, the fertility level for China as a whole and for the rural population remained more or less constant except for the famine period. By the end of the 1970s, births to women in their teens had been largely eliminated in both the rural and urban areas. This was followed by fertility reduction for women in their late reproductive ages. The national pattern has been repeated at the provincial level.

Voluntary childlessness is out of favour with Chinese society. The proportion of married women who progressed to a first child has been high and stable (close to 100 per cent) throughout the last few decades.[1] During the course of the fertility transition, childbearing of Chinese women in both urban and rural areas has been more and more concentrated in a compressed age range. At present, births are clustered to women in their late 20s for the urban population, but extend to the early 30s for their rural counterparts. Birth intervals for the first two parities have been shortened. The contribution of first births to total births increased continuously, while the proportion of higher-order births has fallen over time. However, regional variations were great, especially for the rural population.

In 1981, 31 per cent of births were of third or higher order, for rural China as a whole. The proportion of such births by then had already been reduced to less than 5 per cent of the total births in the outskirts of the three leading municipalities, and to less than 20 per cent of all births in Jiangsu, Shandong, Liaoning, and Jilin provinces, but remained more than 50 per cent of all births in Xinjiang, Yunnan, and Guizhou. This reflects the fact that the initial response to the one-child policy was quite different between provinces.

The regional differences had narrowed gradually, but were still considerable, even though a few years had passed since the launch of the one-child policy. The population living in the eastern provinces was more likely to accept the norm of small family and responded to the single-child policy positively. On the other hand, changes in the vast interior, especially those western provinces with a high proportion of people from groups with minority status, were more difficult and slower. Partly as a result of adjustment of local regulations on population control, regional variations have become marked most recently.

For the urban population, births of third and higher orders were eliminated rapidly. In 1970 over half of all births were at higher parities in 10 provinces. The figure fell to below 5 per cent in all but Henan province by 1981. There was a backlash in some provinces thereafter. In 1984 more than 20 per cent of births in Xinjiang, Guizhou, and Guangxi were births of higher orders. Nevertheless, the single-child policy was more successful in the urban areas.

By the early 1980s the transition in eastern provinces, for both the urban and rural areas, was nearing completion, but it still has a long way to go for these interior provinces.

However, although the period total fertility rate has been below 2 since 1974 for China's urban population as a whole, the average number of children ever borne to urban women aged 35 in the period 1979–81 in an overwhelming majority of provinces was above this level. Only three provinces, Shanghai, Beijing, and Hunan, reported the number below 2. This finding is supported by Feeney and Yu using parity progression measurement. They claim that 96 per cent of all women were proceeding from first to second births in 1979.[2] The figure for the more recent period is not available yet.

The decline in cohort fertility for the rural population is more moderate. The average number of children ever borne to women aged 35 in the period 1979–81 was still as high as 3.8 for China's rural population as a whole, which was only 10 per cent lower than that in the mid-1950s, or a 20 per cent fall from the early 1970s' level. There were 10 provinces where the cumulated cohort fertility rate up to the age of 35 in the early 1980s was as high as it had been two decades earlier. In Jiangxi, Xinjiang, and Guizhou, the average family size for rural women at the age of 35 was above 4.5.

Changes in nuptiality patterns—one of the proximate variables in determining fertility—in the last four decades have been examined. The traditional Chinese marriage pattern can be generalized as early and universal marriage. Since the founding of the People's Republic, social reform has changed this traditional pattern, not only in the urban areas, but also in the vast rural areas. Marriage has been considerably postponed, but still occurs almost universally.

The mean age at first marriage (MAFM) for China's rural female population as a whole rose from 18.5 in 1950 to 19.3 in 1965, a slow but steady increase. Afterwards, the upward trend accelerated, especially during the 1970s. By 1970 the MAFM had reached 19.9, and further rose to 21.4 and 22.5 in 1975 and 1980 respectively.

The situation in the urban areas is more striking. Increasing from about 19.5 in the early 1950s to 24.9 in the early 1980s, the mean age at first marriage for China's urban female population rose by 5.4 years throughout the last three decades.

The provincial trends are, generally speaking, similar to the national one. Nowadays, Chinese women get married much later than their mothers did several decades ago. Nevertheless, the tempo and the quantum of this change varied remarkably among the provinces.

The upward trend in age of marriage started from different levels. The mean age at first marriage rose slowly in the 1950s, due in part to the implementation of the 1950 marriage law. While the slow but steady increase in the age at marriage continued in the rural areas, a steep rise occurred in almost all urban areas during the mid-1960s. This should be partly attributed to the success of the second family-planning programme which started in the early 1960s. There was a set-back in the late 1960s, which is believed to be associated with the social disturbances caused by the Cultural Revolution. This in turn brought about a temporary increase in fertility.

A sharp increase in marriage ages took place throughout the 1970s and reached a peak at the end of this decade. The increase in almost all provinces exceeded 1.5 years, and the MAFM rose by 2.7 years during this decade for the urban areas as a whole, and by about 2.5 years for the rural population. This is no doubt owing to the vigorous implementation of the late-marriage campaign.

During the 1970s the age target for marriage was set by local authorities and varied between provinces. The difference in these target ages was minor, but it does account to some extent for the provincial variation in the mean age at marriage. Since the urban population is well organized and controlled by various social and political organs, but also because of other social policies, these stipulations were carried out much more thoroughly in the urban areas. By contrast, in addition to the strong resistance to change, regulations for the rural population were often ambiguous.

Urban women commonly get married later than their rural counterparts, no matter which province they inhabit, nor when the marriage takes place. In the early 1950s the rural–urban differential in mean age at first marriage was about one year, gradually widened to 3 years in the mid-1960s, and remained at a level of about 2.7 years with some fluctuations until the early 1980s. The age gaps in four northwestern provinces, Xinjiang, Gansu, Qinghai, and Ningxia, were consistently among the largest. The three adjacent provinces, Fujian, Zhejiang, and Jiangxi, composed another group with relatively large rural–urban difference.

The provincial difference in terms of marriage age seems to be closely associated with geographical locations. This is particularly true for the rural population. Provinces in which the MAFM was higher than the national average in 1980 were by and large those with the same feature 30 years before. The marriage age in the eastern and far southern regions was commonly higher than in other places. On the other hand, rural marriage in the far north and the southeastern parts of China generally occurred early. The lowest MAFM can be found consistently in these northwestern provinces.

Despite strong government intervention, the spatial pattern of age at marriage has persisted. This consistency not only reflects the local performance of the late-marriage campaign, but is also related to the persistence of local marriage traditions. The change to late marriage seems to be much more difficult to achieve in rural areas and places where early marriage prevailed in the past. Provinces with early marriage tradition seem to lag more and more behind the national progress.

In 1981 only two in every thousand women aged 50 and over among the rural female population reported that they had never been married. There are provincial variations, but the proportion of women remaining single is so small that it is unlikely to have any significant impact on fertility. Nearly 100 per cent entry into marriage was common across the country. The nuptiality changes in China, at least for the rural population, are to a great extent synonymous with delayed marriages. The age at marriage in rural and urban areas are highly associated, as indicated by high values of the correlation coefficients over time.

China has achieved a relatively low fertility accompanied by virtually universal marriage and motherhood. Both changes in nuptiality and fertility within marriage contributed to the decline in total fertility rate. Although marriage has been widely postponed and births consequently delayed too, the reduction of fertility within marriage, especially at longer durations, played a much more important role in reducing the total fertility level.

II. Major Determinants of China's Fertility Transition

The fertility transition in China seems to provide one exception to the classical theory of demographic transition. The Chinese experience suggests that initial fertility transition can occur in a society at a relatively low level of modernization, but with strong government commitment and an effective family-planning programme.

China's transition has been, by and large, not a natural process, but rather an induced one. Spontaneous fertility limitation was practised in some urban areas among certain social strata before the implementation of birth-control policies. The overall fertility decline, however, was brought about, or at least speeded up, by the government's determined efforts on population control. For a large proportion of Chinese couples, especially those in the countryside, the motivation for birth control in the first instance came from the government rather than couples themselves. This conscious motivation became stronger with the progress of the family-planning programme. Government intervention has played a prominent role, especially in later programmes. The cost of fertility regulation has long been covered by the government. Free contraceptive services made birth control much easier to accept. The evolution of the programme can be traced back to the mid-1950s and has been marked by fluctuations, which were largely due to political upheavals. Nevertheless, since the early 1960s, population control has been strongly advocated by the Chinese leadership, no matter who was in power. With the shift of the Party's priority from political struggle to economic construction, more and more efforts have been made to bring down the birth-rate and modernize reproduction.

The success of the Chinese family-planning programme relies largely on China's unique social structure and value system, which had been established by the Chinese revolution, but are also partly a heritage of the Chinese culture. Chinese civilization was shaped by a peculiar political system and based on a humanistic ideology.[3] Where other traditions have placed their final hope in Heaven, the Chinese ideal society was very much of this world. The perfectly ordered and controlled society was believed to be attainable and this idealism has been a central theme of Chinese political thought for centuries.[4]

Since the founding of the People's Republic of China in October 1949, every effort has been made to inculcate the belief that man will in the end remove all obstacles to creating a better society. The participation of millions of people in mass campaigns has been regarded as one of the most powerful weapons in establishing this new society,[5] and become one of the most dramatic aspects of the contemporary Chinese political scene. Mobilizing millions of people, these campaigns have greatly affected China's political and socio-economic development. Normal social life and institutional functions were frequently disrupted, which inevitably made imprints on the fertility transition. Roughly speaking, the movement of China's fertility rate—allowing for a lag between conception and birth—corresponds to different phases of these campaigns.[6]

Mass mobilization has also been a crucial factor in carrying out China's family-planning programme. The well-built network for birth-control services has penetrated every corner of the country. People, no matter how old they are nor where they live, have been organized to participate in the programme. Almost every facility used in other mass campaigns, such as propaganda and group education, has been employed by the programme. The success or failure of the programme has to a great extent been determined by the extent of this mass participation. In addition, the family-planning programme would not have been so successful without other reforms which have been carried out in all aspects of social life in China since 1949.

In general, Chinese people are more group-minded and less individualistic than those in the West. Therefore, the organizational behaviour of the Chinese people, the emphasis on mass participation, and effective government control have allowed the Chinese programme to be carried out relatively easily.

One of the distinctive features of China's family-planning programme is its decentralized policy implementation. Although the policy initiatives begin in the central government, their implementation is largely reliant on local accomplishment. Special regulations regarding family planning have been issued by the provincial authorities in order to adapt to local conditions. The regional differentials in the timing and pace of the transition have, to a great extent, resulted from the differentials in the formulation and conduct of the local family-planning programmes. On the one hand, differentials in the local programme testify to the importance attached to them. On the other hand, the implementation of these programmes is largely affected by local political atmosphere and stability.

Furthermore, the local regulations on family planning have varied between provinces, and even within province, and changed over time. The government's policy towards minority populations has led to different treatment in terms of birth control towards the majority Han population and minority groups. The marriage law does not apply equally to all races. Local marriage customs are respected and controls for early marriage are flexible. Restrictions on family size are waived altogether for minorities with exceptionally small populations. For those more populous minority groups, the policy places emphasis on voluntary rather than compulsory compliance. The extent to which policies are relaxed varies between regions. This has significantly contributed to the slow progress of the fertility transition in those provinces with a large proportion of minority population.

The first two Chinese family-planning campaigns were largely urban-orientated and left the rural areas almost untouched. In China's rural areas, contraceptives became easily accessible only after the establishment of the rural co-operative health system during the Cultural Revolution period. This is one of the major causes of the later onset of the fertility transition in China's rural areas.

The financial input of the programme also varied between provinces. Expenditure on birth control was usually above the national average in those northern provinces. However, high inputs do not necessarily secure better achievements. The Chinese revolution created a favourable network of social organizations for implementing family-planning programmes. The integration of the family-planning network with the health-care system has made China's contraceptive delivery system the largest community-based system in the world. Ideological education was supplemented by a well-built family-planning network designed to implement birth control with effective contraceptives. The achievement of the local family-planning programme has been closely associated with the efficiency of these organizations. It seems likely that the family-planning programme is a process of accumulation. The longer the programme is carried out, the better the outcome, other things being equal.

The Chinese experience indicates that fertility decline can to some extent be independent of development. However, fertility transition did occur along with socio-economic development. Socio-economic conditions vary substantially between China's provinces. What is more significant is that such differences have widened over time, reflecting the uneven process of development in the last thirty or more years. The government's programme, although important, has not operated in a vacuum. Population programmes appear to have been more effective where social and economic conditions were better, but less so in backward areas. Socio-economic structures are closely associated with fertility transition, but their impact differs over time. On the whole, socio-economic factors are more relevant to China's regional fertility differentials in the pre- and early period of fertility transition, but less so after the government's strong intervention, at least in terms of a linear relationship.

Over time contraceptive services have improved and the cost of fertility regulation to individual couples has fallen to close to zero. But motivation remains a dominant factor in fertility control. Chinese women's individual reproductive behaviour has been greatly affected by their educational and occupational background, and their place of residence. Women who received higher education tend to have had smaller families than those with less education. Peasant women bear more children than women classified as workers and cadre members. Women's status both in and out of household, considerations of old-age security, and many other factors all have an input in the decision-making process for childbearing. Consequently, the fertility differential among different social strata is a result of many different elements. However, with the same educational level, same occupation, and same rural–urban identity, fertility levels have also varied substantially between provinces, especially between the eastern and western parts of China. This difference has widened as time passed.

On top of the uneven progress of the family-planning programme among localities and at different levels of development, a variety of other forces has combined to create regional fertility diversity. At the start of the transition, the fertility differentials amongst social strata and localities were the combined products of birth-control diffusion and development factors. As the transition progressed and birth-control services became easily accessible, the reproductive decision became more clearly determined by social factors other than the availability of birth-control methods. At this stage, the institutional variables may play more important roles in determining the pattern of the transition.

China is such a large and heterogeneous country that various local 'little traditions' exist. It is probable that China's regional differentials in fertility transition are partly an outcome of the decision-making environment facing individual couples, as set by local institutional settings and cultural patterns. In other words, the mechanisms by which communities reduced fertility depended upon largely existing societal institutions.

Rooted deeply in the feudal tradition, preference for sons over daughters can be found almost everywhere in China, especially in rural areas. There is clear evidence of strong preference for boys over girls in Anhui, Guangdong, and some other provinces. This is closely related to cultural tradition in general and women's societal status in particular. It is not surprising that the fertility level in all these provinces was above the national average.

Regional fertility levels are also associated with structures of the local community and kinship system. Mainly owing to the diversities in cultural, social, political, ecological, and economic conditions, strong family lineages were traditionally more prevalent in central and southern parts of China than in the north. The sizes of family followed a similar pattern. Chinese family structure underwent a tremendous transformation after the Chinese revolution in 1949, but regional differences have by and large remained. The proportion of families with three or more generations is commonly high in southern coastal provinces and areas around Shaanxi province, whereas extended families in the eastern and the northeastern provinces are relatively infrequent.

In a society like China, people's thinking and action has always been strongly influenced by public opinion, especially pressures from these primary groups. Many social policies have weakened traditional values of family and kinship over the last several decades. However, they are still frequently regarded as real obstacles to social change and as active forces affecting marriage and childbearing. Economic dependency of youngsters in China, especially in the countryside, reduces their freedom of choice considerably. Reproductive behaviour of young couples living with their parents is often affected by older generations. In contrast, young couples who make their own decisions are more easily able and willing to accept and practise fertility limitation. With a few exceptions, there is a very close relationship between the provincial fertility level and the proportion of extended families there.

The linkage with overseas Chinese is particularly strong in the southern coastal provinces. The family-planning programme here has been less rigid. They have enjoyed certain privileges in childbearing. On the other hand, their reproductive behaviour was to a large extent determined by their relatives abroad. The stronger traditional mentality, better economic well-being, and less exposure to the pressure of birth control made their desires for children much higher than the government's requirement. Consequently, the implementation of family-planning programmes was more difficult, and fertility levels were relatively higher in those regions with a large proportion of overseas relatives.

By way of conclusion, it can be said that the regional diversity in China's fertility transition is the consequence of a variety of factors. For the country as a whole, the success of population control was mainly brought about by a strong and effective family-planning programme and overall development. At the regional level, the achievement of the programme has largely depended upon the efforts made by local governments to control population growth, and the local political and social environment. In addition, cultural influences and socio-economic development of the local community have combined to shape the pattern of fertility transition. While some policies have worked successfully in certain areas during certain periods of time, they have not done so in some other places and times.

It seems the role of development and culture is more fundamental in long-term fertility transition. Institutional factors may directly influence reproductive behaviour through sex roles, family structure, and kinship system. Socio-economic development will ultimately change people's attitude towards family and childbearing, and lead to the completion of the fertility transition.

III. The Impact of Current Reform

A new era of Chinese modern history has started since the Third Plenum of the Central Committee of the Communist Party in December 1978. Beginning with the introduction of the 'Production Responsibility System' in the countryside, subsequent economic reform has since then accelerated and extended to the cities. The reforms have also touched China's political structure.

The general goal of the reform is to speed up China's economic development, realize the 'four modernizations', and successfully build socialism with Chinese characteristics. To these ends, various measures have been adopted in the last several years, which have boosted China's economy considerably. The reform has also brought about profound changes in Chinese society, which have been striking in depth and rapidity.

Equally important is the impact of current reform on China's population growth. The Chinese government still seeks to control its rapid population growth so as to keep the pace of growth in line with social and economic development, ecological conditions, and resource endowment.[7] The stringent one-child policy was originally posited on this basis. However, China's demographic performance in the 1980s has not been promising: the age at marriage has declined, the fertility level fluctuated, and the birth-rate increased. This reversal of trend is most serious in the rural areas as was shown in the previous chapters, and is closely associated with political and economic reform.

It would be foolhardy to predict the ultimate effect of the reform of China's population issue. That reform is, after all, still continuing. Nevertheless some immediate demographic consequences of the rapid social change brought about by the changes can be briefly assessed.

The rural responsibility system was first introduced in late 1978 in order to increase farmers' enthusiasm for production and revitalize the rural economy. Incentives were offered to peasants to boost agricultural production. Peasants have been encouraged to diversify their productive activities and engage in private business. The policy permitted some peasants to get rich first. On balance, this policy has been a success and China's rural economy has certainly grown rapidly since 1979.

In addition, rural reform has had far-reaching implications for the form and content of rural social institutions. The commune system has been dismantled and the peasant household has become a complex unit of operation demonstrating a new and increasing degree of independence and autonomy. The household has once again assumed responsibility for production, consumption, and welfare.[8] But national and collective interests seem to be far away from the household interest. The expansion of the household economy, under the current labour-intensive agricultural system, primarily depends on the accumulation and distribution of family labour rather than material resources. The rural reform has brought the relationship between labour and family income even closer. A large family is still regarded as an asset. The perceived economic value of children has now become higher than when communes existed and this may have stimulated the desire for more children, especially sons, in order to get rich.

However, this causal linkage between rural reform and fertility should not be oversimplified. With the implementation of rural reform, peasant households have diversified their economic activities and undertaken a variety of domestic sidelines. Women have been offered more opportunities, such as cultivating private plots, raising livestock, making handicrafts, and providing services to the community. Their income-earning capacity has improved greatly. The opportunity cost of an extra child has therefore increased and bearing children inevitably implies a loss of a current household income. Peasants have to choose between children as potential income generators but net consumers when they are young and women as current contributors to the household well-being.[9] A peasant would be unlikely to sacrifice short-term, actual benefit for long-term, expected returns if the reproductive decision is made on purely economic grounds.

More importantly the introduction of rural reform has removed one of the major constraints of childbearing: authority control. As the reform has progressed the administrative function of the Party apparatus (which is one of the most important supporting powers of the birth-control campaign) has diminished. The rural communes have been reorganized and no longer assume political authority for administrative affairs. The power of local cadres has been undermined. Family-planning work has, however, not kept pace with this dramatic organizational change. In many rural areas, there has been no one in charge of birth control, and the office for family planning has even been abolished. The rural co-operative health care system, which was mingled with the family-planning network, has also been seriously affected. The result has been the deterioration of contraceptive services in many rural areas. Furthermore, as the rural collective economy has been declining, local family-planning personnel in many instances have no longer been able to receive financial subsidies from the collectives. Their activities have inevitably been affected, and some of them have taken a 'wait and see' attitude prefering not to carry out this difficult work. This has been a major factor undermining the family-planning statistical system. In short, the early advantage of combining the family-planning programme with administrative authority has tended to disappear. The direct authoritative regulations and political control over individual households have been loosened, as has the degree of control over childbearing.

Moreover, as a result of the reform, central control is dissipated and local authority has more autonomy than ever before to interpret and implement government policies. Since 1984 China's overall population policy has become more realistic and reasonable. More attention has been paid to overcoming commandism, and to perfecting the campaign in accordance with local conditions. Local regulations on birth control have undergone a gradual change towards the loosening of restrictions and become more flexible. A large proportion of rural couples are now allowed to have a second child. Paradoxically, the strictness of the one-child policy during the early 1980s has exacerbated the incidence of second children, as more and more couples have become eligible to have a second child. This may be the case in Sichuan and Shandong, as discussed in the previous chapters. In many places, however, there has simply been an acquiescence in public pressure for large families. Local authorities have influenced, even competed with, each other in relaxation of the family-planning effort.[10] Consequently, there has been not only a surge in births of second children, but also a marked increase in higher parities.

On the other hand, in spite of prolonged education and propaganda, the ideal family size in China's countryside has never been less than two children per family.[11] The perceived security benefit of children, especially sons, has remained both high and stable throughout the last four decades.[12] In the absence of a rural pension system and under the patriarchal structure, sons are essential not only for family continuity, but more crucially for old-age security. Although new options and promises have emerged, they have not been guaranteed. Many remain unconvinced by these social changes and children are still viewed as the best insurance against risk. This is a Chinese reality and should not simply be attributed to feudal remnants. There have always been contradictions between the government's population target and individuals' reproductive desires. The motivation for more children is not new but rather a persistent traditional desire. The reform may have increased the motivation. But more plausible is that rural institutional change has created an environment in which peasants' reproductive aspirations can be fulfilled. In other words, even without any economic stimulus, the removal of control itself could lead to the emergence of a temporary baby boom.

In practical terms, the weakened rural collective economy greatly reduces the pressure that the government can exert on rural families, since economic incentives for the one-child policy are largely reliant on a collective economy. For instance, the fixed and stable contract for land use, which is mainly aimed at reducing peasants' fear of policy change, means that preferential treatment in allocating private plots and contracting land to one-child families is no longer enforceable and only an incentive that exists on paper. Many other incentives cannot be realized under current rural conditions.[13]

The majority of Chinese peasant households have benefited economically from rural reform and have improved their standard of living in the last few years. During 1979–87, farmers' net income reportedly went up by 150 per cent.[14] While improvement of family welfare may in the long run lead to low fertility, in the short term it greatly reduces the importance of economic incentives and disincentives for birth control. Many peasant households now are increasingly willing, and can afford, to pay the financial penalty imposed for extra births. The economic incentive for a small family is outweighed by the newly revived household economy. Hence, the early regulations on birth control have lost their restrictive power. It is also probable that when women's labour becomes less crucial to family survival, peasant women may benefit more from having children, especially sons. As the original level of per capita income is very low, a limited improvement in family well-being may stimulate more births.

As government authoritarian control is loosened, there has been a revival of traditional culture in China's countryside. Clan organizations have been reinvigorated in some parts of China, especially in southern provinces. In some places, peasants, particularly those who have become rich recently, need clan organization to provide security and enrich social life.[15] It is widely reported that wealthy peasants have raised funds for restoring demolished temples and building new tombs rather than improving productive capacity or undertaking collective welfare activities.[16] While many early policy measures transformed China's traditional family structure, recent rural reform not only strengthens the economic and security role of family, but also increases the interdependency between household members. As discussed earlier, the stronger the family and kinship system is, the more difficult it is for the young generation to practise birth control. Traditional behaviour is an enduring feature of Chinese society. The revival of tradition will certainly make its mark on changing public attitudes towards childbearing and may delay the process of modernizing reproduction.

Rural reform allows peasants to pursue non-farm economic activities. Consequently, a large number of peasants leave their homeland, travelling between provinces or entering big cities to search for opportunities. This so-called 'floating population' has become a marked social phenomenon and has attracted considerable attention. In Beijing it is reported that the floating population amounts to 1 million, about one-sixth of the city's ordinary residents. The figure in Shanghai reaches 2 million and 1.2 million in Guangzhou.[17] At the height of the family-planning campaign, some peasants fled their villages to avoid local pressure on birth control. The majority of the current floating population moving into cities may not be these, but they do become a dead corner of the family-planning programme. They are not registered by administrative departments and are not covered by the contraceptive delivery network. They are frequently responsible for many births, which are almost certainly not registered.

Last but not least is the impact of people's psychological reaction to uncertainty. In the past, policies adopted by the Chinese government changed very often, so reducing the government's credibility. This has remained the case during the reform period since everything is new and policies have to be modified in order to match changing conditions. Although the government has repeatedly reiterated its firm commitment to rural reform, old fears are difficult to remove. Population control is regarded as one of the principal national policies of the Chinese government. The degree of control, however, varies widely between time periods and regions. For grass-root family-planning workers, such uncertainty makes them reluctant to take any positive or aggressive actions, as they live with their working target all the time. For the couples concerned, they rush into childbearing as regulations are relaxed for fear that controls may be strengthened at any time in the near future. The upsurge of second children in the last few years, to a great extent, reflects this factor. Many births may not occur, or will at least be postponed, if such births are rationally planned by couples themselves.

This is not to say, however, that the effects of reform on China's population control are all negative. But the positive effect of the reform does seem to be outweighed by these negative factors for the time being. This will remain true for a few years to come.

Reform has not only boosted China's economy, but also introduced many new concepts and ideas. Authoritarian control will probably be loosened further if the proposed political reform proceeds. The people's democratic consciousness has been awakened and this trend will certainly continue. People may be influenced more by Western ideas, such as individualism. They are now more concerned about the quality of their own spiritual and material lives, and ready to take a more rational attitude in determining their personal lives. Living standards have improved sharply in the last few years, albeit in many instances ahead of people's capacity. Meanwhile, young couples have much higher expectations for their children than ever before. They are increasingly willing to invest in raising and educating their only children, sometimes to an extraordinary extent. On the one hand, small family size makes this possible. On the other, it is partly a result of the introduction of competition in opportunities for better education and employment. This undoubtedly leads to a great increase in the cost of children and reduction in the economic benefits from them, which may reduce parents' demand for children.

There are large variations among different population groups in terms of economic benefits of the reforms. A high inflation rate, which is mainly a result of the current price reform, actually worsens the financial conditions of many urban families and puts another constraint on people's reproductive decisions.

The process of urbanization has accelerated during the reform period. The proportion of urban population has increased by 1 per cent annually since the reform started in 1979. More and more people are exposed to influences of modern urban life and are less affected by traditional attitudes towards family and childbearing. They have better access to contraceptive services than they had in the countryside. Their desires for family size are also affected by the increased opportunity cost of children for working women.

There is also a greater openness about human sexuality in China, which is helpful in the dissemination of birth-control knowledge, although some are worried about the destructive impact of excessive sexual freedom.[18] Reform has accelerated the socialization process in China and people are now better informed than ever before. This may speed up the diffusion of changes in attitudes and tastes relating to desired family size, age at marriage and childbearing, etc.

Many more points might be made. The general conclusion seems to be that modernization will in the long run reduce the demand for children, break the cultural barriers for birth control, and promote high motivation for fertility regulation.

IV. Looking into the Future

In 1979 China's population target was set *at* 1.2 billion by the year 2000. Thereafter, such a target has been quietly modified without wide notice to *around* 1.2 billion. However, the recent population trend seems to call into question even this revision. By the end of 1987 China's total population had already reached 1.08 billion[19] and it will continue to rise by an annual increment of about 22 million for the next decade.[20] In the next few years annual births may exceed 30 million, due partly to the fact that the large cohort born in the late 1960s will reach the age of marriage and childbearing. It is believed that the recent upsurge in period fertility rate is mainly a phenomenon of compensation, and that the fertility level will never return to the level prevailing in the early 1970s because there does exist strong motivation for birth control. This temporary trend will therefore probably disappear quite soon. The total fertility rate will probably remain at a level of 2.5 for a while, unless tough action is taken to strengthen the family-planning programme. A further significant reduction in the death-rate is unlikely due in part to the effect of population ageing, although the age-specific mortality rate may continue to decline. It seems certain that China's total population will exceed the 1.2 billion mark in the year 2000. Whether it will reach 1.3 billion, as the World Bank has suggested,[21] or an even higher figure, will largely depend on the government's commitment to birth control and the process of reform in the next few years. Under current conditions, China's total population will most likely be between 1.25 to 1.3 billion by the year 2000. Population control remains, today and for many years to come, one of the vital policy issues for China's development.

Future population policy has to consider two basic problems: the ageing population and rapid population growth. There has been wide concern about population ageing in China in recent years. This is one of the major criticisms of the one-child policy. However, ageing population is probably a universal process accompanying rapid declines in fertility and mortality. In addition, statistics have shown that in 1987, people aged 65 and over only accounted for 5.46 per cent of China's total population, only 0.6 per cent higher than in 1982.[22] It will take about 25 years, at the present rate, for China to reach an age composition in which 8.6 per cent of total population is aged 65 years or older, which is Shanghai's current level. The government must take population ageing into account in future development planning. The crucial question, however, is how to control China's population growth. What the optimal population should be in China is a topic of academic debate. Nevertheless, to approach zero-growth rate will no doubt be beneficial to China's modernization process.

Due to the large population base and the tremendous size of young cohorts already built into the age structure, China has to take every reasonable action, sometimes stringent, urgently to control its population growth. In an ideal world, the motivation for birth control would come spontaneously. However, this cannot be achieved in the short run. China cannot wait for people to make explicit their own wish to have small families. Rather, positive measures can and should be taken to promote this process, based on fundamental social and institutional change. Unless the desired values become the norm rather than progressive options, there will always be resistance to changes. Population policy should take cultural factors and the degree of public acceptance into account, but in the knowledge that concessions to culture can undermine programme success. As pointed by Warwick, if countries met criticism and resistance by drawing back from family planning, few would ever institute such programmes.[23]

Nevertheless, the future programme needs to be implemented on the basis of voluntary co-operation rather than coercion. The programme should not only ask people to follow the regulations, but even more should be done to provide better and safer contraceptive services, in order to enhance people's willingness to use such services. The future programme should place more emphasis on promoting people's motivation for birth control by creating a positive social and institutional environment. It is difficult for the family-planning programme alone to achieve this goal. To this end, population policy should be included in a comprehensive, overall development strategy rather than as a single, isolated policy. While many reform measures are aimed at speeding up economic growth, they sometimes serve to undermine the efforts for birth control. Policy measures should therefore complement one another. This in turn requires much more scientific research and wide democratic participation in the policy-making process.

Population policy should be stabilized, without any rash changes, for a fixed period. This is particularly important for reducing the impact of psychological uncertainty on reproduction. The one-child campaign has been launched in haste with a lack of solid theoretical and empirical research. There are alternatives. The option of two children plus a longer birth interval may fit Chinese conditions better. In any case, the relaxation of the one-child policy should be carried out very carefully. A relatively stable policy will not only make the policy easier to implement, but will also reduce people's fear of uncertainty in the future.

Regional differences in fertility transition will certainly persist in the near future. Since the contraceptive-prevalence rate is already very high and high parities have been reduced to a very low level in China's urban areas and many eastern regions, the marginal gain of birth control there would be very small. Therefore, the cost-effectiveness of extra investment and effort would be lower than in interior provinces. The services and existing network in these advanced areas must certainly be maintained. But greater attention should be paid to family planning in more backward regions. The final message must be that China's population problem can only be solved by the Chinese themselves.

NOTES

1. G. Feeney and Jingyuan Yu, 'Period Parity Progression Measures of Fertility in China', *Population Studies*, 41 (1), 77–102 (1987).
2. Ibid.
3. L. W. Pye, *China: An Introduction* (Boston: Little, Brown & Company, 1984).
4. T. Bary, *Sources of Chinese Tradition* (New York: Columbia University Press, 1960), p. 944.
5. The leadership of the Communist Party, the mass line, and a practical and realistic working style were praised as three 'magic weapons'.
6. A. P. Wolf, 'The Preeminent Role of Government Intervention in China's Family Revolution', *Population and Development Review*, 12 (1); 101–16 (1986).
7. *Beijing Review*, 30 (29), 5 (20 July 1987).
8. E. J. Croll, 'New Peasant Family Forms in Rural China', *The Journal of Peasant Studies*, 14 (4), 469–99 (1987).
9. There are reports on the increased use of child labour in small industry. However, this does not affect our argument here.
10. Qu Yibin, 'Woguo renkou chushenglu mingxian huisheng de yuanying ji duiche tantao (Exploring the Cause of the Increase in Birth-Rate and the Measures to deal with it in China), *Renkou Yanjiu (Population Research)*, No. 1 (1988).
11. This point is supported by many surveys. For example, a survey conducted in Shandong province shows that 70% of rural couples want two children, 26% want 3 or more, and only 4.3 per cent accept one-child-per-family norm. Zhou Qing, 'Woguo xiandaihua guocheng zhong nongcun jiating guimo yu leixing jiegou (The Size, Type, and Structure of Rural Families in the Course of Modernization in China)', *Renkou Yanjiu (Population Research)*, No. 2 (1988).
12. S. Greenhalgh, 'Fertility as Mobility: Sinitic Transitions', paper prepared for a Seminar on Societal Influences on Family Planning Programme Performance, Ocho Rios, Jamaica, 10–13 Apr. 1985.
13. Xie Cheng, 'Youguan Youdai dusheng zinu jiqi jiating zhengce wengti de tantao he jianyi (Remarks on Policies for Preferential Treatment Given to Only Children and their Parents)', *Renkou Yu Jingji (Population and Economy)*, No. 1 (1988).
14. *Beijing Review*, 30 (29), 4 (20 July 1987).
15. J. Baum, 'Religion's "Blank Slate" is Crowded with Beliefs', *The Christian Science Monitor*, 15–21 Aug. 1988.

16. See e.g. *Hongqi (Red Flag)*, No. 14 (1986).
17. Dun Songting, 'Dachengshi liudong renkou duiche chutan (Explore the Measures towards Floating Population in Big Cities)', *Zhongguo Chengshi Daobao*, 14 Jan. 1988. It should be noted, however, that the concept of 'Floating Population' needs to be defined scientifically and not all of these people are immigrant-like.
18. See e.g. *China Daily*, 12 July 1986.
19. See *Statistical Yearbook of China, 1988.*
20. Cheng Gang, 'China Faces Another Baby Boom', *Beijing Review*, 31 (27), 25–6 (4–10 July 1988).
21. 'Chinese Population "Still on Target" ', *People*, 14 (2), 24.
22. Li Rongshi, '1987 woguo renkou zhuangkuang fengxi (Analysis of China's Population Situation in 1987)', *Renkou Yanjiu (Population Research)*, No. 1 (1988).
23. D. Warwick, 'Culture and the Management of Family Planning Programme', *Studies in Family Planning*, 19 (1), 1–18 (1988).

Appendix

LOG-LINEAR MODELS

I. MODELS FOR EDUCATION, TYPE OF RESIDENCE AND PROVINCE LOCATION

Model: $M = Y \times Y_{1L} \times Y_{2E} \times Y_{3R}$

Where: M = Mean Parity; L = Province Location; E = Education; R = Type of Residence

Categories of Educational Level: 1. Illiteracy 2. Primary School 3. Junior Middle School 4. Higher

Categories of Province Location: 1. Municipalities 2. East Coast 3. South 4. North 5. Southwest 6. Northwest

For the 35 age cohort:

$Y = 2.69$

$Y_{12} = 1.17$ $Y_{13} = 1.44$ $Y_{14} = 1.46$ $Y_{15} = 1.65$ $Y_{16} = 1.71$

$Y_{22} = 0.95$ $Y_{23} = 0.87$ $Y_{24} = 0.71$

$Y_{32} = 0.696$ [$Y_{11} = 1$ $Y_{21} = 1$ $Y_{31} = 1$]

Deviance: $X^2 = 190$ on 196 degree of freedom

For the 40 age cohort:

$Y = 3.52$

$Y_{12} = 1.145$ $Y_{13} = 1.37$ $Y_{14} = 1.42$ $Y_{15} = 1.53$ $Y_{16} = 1.476$

$Y_{22} = 0.93$ $Y_{23} = 0.84$ $Y_{24} = 0.72$

$Y_{32} = 0.72$ [$Y_{11} = 1$ $Y_{21} = 1$ $Y_{31} = 1$]

Deviance: $X^2 = 163$ on 190 degree of freedom

For the 45 age cohort:

$Y = 4.39$

$Y_{12} = 1.10$ $Y_{13} = 1.276$ $Y_{14} = 1.32$ $Y_{15} = 1.44$ $Y_{16} = 1.40$

$Y_{22} = 0.91$ $Y_{23} = 0.80$ $Y_{24} = 0.64$

$Y_{32} = 0.75$ [$Y_{11} = 1$ $Y_{21} = 1$ $Y_{31} = 1$]

Deviance: $X^2 = 170$ on 175 degree of freedom

For the 50 + age cohort:

$Y = 5.307$

$Y_{12} = 1.02$ $Y_{13} = 1.119$ $Y_{14} = 1.115$ $Y_{15} = 1.126$ $Y_{16} = 1.025$

$Y_{22} = 0.923$ $Y_{23} = 0.795$ $Y_{24} = 0.618$

$Y_{32} = 0.837$ [$Y_{11} = 1$ $Y_{21} = 1$ $Y_{31} = 1$]

Deviance: $X^2 = 565$ on 179 degree of freedom

Fitted Values of Mean Parity (from Education Models)

	Municipality		*East Coast*		*South*		*North*		*Southwest*		*Northwest*	
	Urban	Rural	Urban	Rural	Urban	Rural	Urban	Rural	Urban	Rural	Urban	Rural
35 Age cohort												
Illiteracy	1.87	2.69	2.19	3.15	2.70	3.87	2.73	3.93	3.09	4.44	3.20	4.60
Primary	1.78	2.56	2.08	2.99	2.56	3.68	2.60	3.73	2.94	4.22	3.04	4.37
Junior-mid	1.63	2.34	1.91	2.74	2.35	3.37	2.38	3.42	2.69	3.86	2.78	4.00
Higher	1.33	1.91	1.55	2.23	1.91	2.75	1.94	2.79	2.19	3.15	2.27	3.27
40 Age cohort												
Illiteracy	2.53	3.52	2.90	4.03	3.47	4.82	3.60	5.00	3.88	5.39	3.74	5.20
Primary	2.36	3.27	2.70	3.75	3.23	4.48	3.35	4.65	3.61	5.01	3.48	4.83
Junior-mid	2.13	2.96	2.44	3.39	2.92	4.05	3.02	4.20	3.26	4.52	3.14	4.36
Higher	1.82	2.53	2.09	2.90	2.50	3.47	2.59	3.60	2.79	3.88	2.69	3.74
45 age cohort												
Illiteracy	3.29	4.39	3.62	4.83	4.20	5.60	4.35	5.79	4.74	6.32	4.61	6.15
Primary	3.06	4.08	3.30	4.39	3.82	5.10	3.95	5.27	4.31	5.75	4.19	5.59
Junior-mid	2.63	3.51	2.90	3.86	3.36	4.48	3.48	4.64	3.79	5.06	3.69	4.92
Higher	2.11	2.81	2.32	3.09	2.69	3.58	2.78	3.71	3.03	4.05	2.95	3.93
50+ age cohort												
Illiteracy	4.44	5.31	4.53	5.41	4.97	5.94	4.95	5.92	5.00	5.98	4.55	5.44
Primary	4.10	4.90	4.18	5.00	4.59	5.48	4.57	5.46	4.62	5.52	4.20	5.02
Junior-mid	3.53	4.22	3.60	4.30	3.95	4.72	3.94	4.70	3.98	4.75	3.62	4.32
Higher	2.74	3.28	2.80	3.34	3.07	3.67	3.06	3.66	3.09	3.69	2.81	3.36

II. Models for Occupation, Type of Residence and Province Location

Model: $M = Y \times Y_{1L} \times Y_{2O} \times Y_{3R}$

Where: M = Mean Parity; L = Province Location; O = Occupation
R = Type of Residence

Categories of Occupation are: 1. Peasant 2. Worker 3. Cadre 4. Housewife

Categories of Province Location: 1. Municipalities 2. East Coast 3. South 4. North 5. Southwest 6. Northwest

For the 35 age group:

$Y = 2.535$

$Y_{12} = 1.211$ $Y_{13} = 1.481$ $Y_{14} = 1.483$ $Y_{15} = 1.706$ $Y_{16} = 1.779$

$Y_{22} = 0.890$ $Y_{23} = 0.737$ $Y_{24} = 1.032$

$Y_{32} = 0.714$ [$Y_{11} = 1$ $Y_{21} = 1$ $Y_{31} = 1$]

Deviance: $X^2 = 152.22$ on 146 degree of freedom

For the 40 age group:

$Y = 3.421$

$Y_{12} = 1.138$ $Y_{13} = 1.374$ $Y_{14} = 1.405$ $Y_{15} = 1.543$ $Y_{16} = 1.494$

$Y_{22} = 0.882$ $Y_{23} = 0.723$ $Y_{24} = 0.957$

$Y_{32} = 0.758$ [$Y_{11} = 1$ $Y_{21} = 1$ $Y_{31} = 1$]

Deviance: $X^2 = 140.21$ on 136 degree of freedom

For the 45 age group:

$Y = 4.191$

$Y_{12} = 1.134$ $Y_{13} = 1.316$ $Y_{14} = 1.350$ $Y_{15} = 1.495$ $Y_{16} = 1.451$

$Y_{22} = 0.863$ $Y_{23} = 0.631$ $Y_{24} = 0.995$

$Y_{32} = 0.803$ [$Y_{11} = 1$ $Y_{21} = 1$ $Y_{31} = 1$]

Deviance: $X^2 = 144.87$ on 129 degree of freedom

For the 50+ age group:

$Y = 5.233$

$Y_{12} = 1.031$ $Y_{13} = 1.130$ $Y_{14} = 1.124$ $Y_{15} = 1.138$ $Y_{16} = 1.036$

$Y_{22} = 0.894$ $Y_{23} = 0.672$ $Y_{24} = 0.978$

$Y_{32} = 0.837$ [$Y_{11} = 1$ $Y_{21} = 1$ $Y_{31} = 1$]

Deviance: $X^2 = 525.03$ on 132 degree of freedom

Fitted Values of Mean Parity (from Occupation Models)

35 Age cohort	*Municipality*		*East Coast*		*South*		*North*		*Southwest*		*Northwest*	
	Urban	Rural	Urban	Rural	Urban	Rural	Urban	Rural	Urban	Rural	Urban	Rural
Peasants	1.81	2.53	2.19	3.07	2.68	3.75	2.68	3.76	3.09	4.23	3.22	4.51
Workers	1.61	2.26	1.95	2.73	2.39	3.34	2.39	3.35	2.75	3.85	2.87	4.01
Cadres	1.33	1.87	1.61	2.26	1.98	2.77	1.92	2.77	2.28	3.19	2.37	3.32
House-wife	1.87	2.62	2.26	3.17	2.77	3.87	2.77	3.88	3.19	4.46	3.32	4.65
40 age cohort												
Peasants	2.59	3.42	2.95	3.89	3.56	4.70	3.64	4.81	4.00	5.28	3.87	5.11
Workers	2.29	3.02	2.60	3.43	3.14	4.15	3.21	4.24	3.53	4.66	3.42	4.51
Cadres	1.87	2.47	2.13	2.81	2.58	3.40	2.63	3.48	2.89	3.82	2.80	3.70
House-wife	2.48	3.27	2.82	3.73	3.41	4.50	3.49	4.60	3.83	5.05	3.71	4.89
45 age cohort												
Peasants	3.37	4.19	3.82	4.75	4.43	5.52	4.54	5.66	5.03	6.27	4.88	6.08
Workers	2.90	3.62	3.29	4.10	3.82	4.76	3.92	4.88	4.34	5.41	4.21	5.25
Cadres	2.12	2.64	2.41	3.00	2.79	3.48	2.87	3.57	3.17	3.95	3.08	3.84
House-wife	3.35	4.17	3.80	4.73	4.41	5.49	4.52	5.63	5.01	6.23	4.86	6.05
50+ age cohort												
Peasants	4.38	5.23	4.52	5.40	4.95	5.91	4.92	5.88	4.98	5.96	4.54	5.42
Workers	3.92	4.68	4.04	4.82	4.42	5.29	4.40	5.26	4.46	5.32	4.06	4.85
Cadres	2.94	3.52	3.03	3.63	3.33	3.97	3.31	3.95	3.35	4.00	3.05	3.64
House-wife	4.28	5.12	4.42	5.28	4.84	5.78	4.81	5.75	4.87	5.82	4.44	5.30

Bibliography

BOOKS AND ARTICLES, IN ENGLISH

ACTION PACK, Distributed by the World Population Year Secretariat of the United Nations Fund for Population Activities, 1974.

AIRD, J. S., 'Population Policy and Demographic Prospects in the People's Republic of China', in Joint Economic Committee, Congress of the United States, *People's Republic of China: An Economic Assessment* (Washington DC, 1972), 220–331.

——— 'Fertility Decline and Birth Control in the People's Republic of China', *Population and Development Review*, 4 (2), 225–53 (1978).

——— 'Fertility Decline in China', in Nick Eberstadt (ed.), *Fertility Decline in the Less Developed Countries* (New York: Praeger, 1981), 119–227.

——— 'Population Studies and Population Policy in China', *Population and Development Review*, 8 (2), 267–97 (1982).

ALAM, I., and CASTERLINE J. B., 'Socio-Economic Differentials in Recent Fertility', *WFS Comparative Studies*, No. 33 (1984).

ANDORKA, R., *Determinants of Fertility in Advanced Society* (London: Methuen, 1978).

ARNOLD, F., and LIU ZHAOXIANG, 'Sex Preference, Fertility, and Family Planning in China', *Population and Development Review*, 12 (2), 221–46 (1986).

BANISTER, J., 'Recent Population Changes in China', in H. Hinton (ed.), *The People's Republic of China: A Handbook* (Boulder: Westview Press, 1979).

——— 'An Analysis of Recent Data on the Population of China', *Population and Development Review*, 10 (2), 241–71 (1984).

——— *China's Changing Population* (Stanford, Calif.: Stanford University Press, 1987).

——— and PRESTON, S. H., 'Mortality in China', *Population and Development Review*, 7 (1), 98–110 (1981).

BARCLAY, G., and COALE, A., *ET AL.*, 'A Reassessment of the Demography of Traditional Rural China', *Population Index*, 42 (4), 606–35 (1976).

BARY, T., *Sources of Chinese Tradition* (New York: Columbia University Press, 1960).

BAUM, J., 'Religion's "Blank Slate" is Crowded with Beliefs', *The Christian Science Monitor*, 15–21 Aug. 1988.

BEAVER, S. E., *Demographic Transition Theory Reinterpreted* (Lexington, Mass.: D. C. Heath and Company, 1975).

BEIJING REVIEW, 1967–88.

BERELSON, B., MAULDIN, W. P., and SYKES, Z., 'Conditions of Fertility Decline in Developing Countries 1965–1975', *Studies in Family Planning*, 9 (5), 89–147 (1978).

BERNSTEIN, T. P., *Up to the Mountains and Down to the Villages: The Transfer of Youth from Urban to Rural China* (New Haven: Yale University Press, 1977).

BIRDSALL, N., 'Analytical Approaches to the Relationship of Population Growth and Development', *Population and Development Review*, 3 (1), 63–102 (1977).

——— and JAMISON, D. T., 'Income and Other Factors Influencing Fertility in China', *Population and Development Review*, 9 (4), 651–75 (1983).

BOND, M. H. (ed.), *The Psychology of the Chinese People* (Oxford: Oxford University Press, 1986).

BONGAARTS, J., 'A Framework for Analysing the Proximate Determinant of Fertility', *Population and Development Review*, 4 (1), 105–32 (1978).

——— and GREENHALGH, S., 'An Alternative to the One-Child Policy in China', *Population and Development Review*, 11 (4), 585–618 (1985).

BRASS, W., *Methods for Estimating Fertility and Mortality from Limited and Defective Data* (Chapel Hill: Laboratories for Population Statistics, 1975).

CALDWELL, J. C., 'Toward a Restatement of Demographic Transition Theory', *Population and Development Review*, 2 (2), 231–66 (1976).

——— *Theory of Fertility Decline* (London: Academic Press, 1982).

——— and SRINIVASAN, K., 'New Data on Nuptiality and Fertility in China', *Population and Development Review*, 10 (1), 71–9 (1984).

CENTRAL COMMITTEE OF THE CHINESE COMMUNIST PARTY, *Decision of the Central Committee of the Chinese Communist Party Concerning the Great Proletarian Cultural Revolution* (Beijing: Foreign Languages Press, 1966).

——— 'Open Letter to All Party and Communist Youth League Members on the Question of Controlling China's Population Growth', BBC, *Summary of World Broadcasts*, 25 Sept. 1980.

——— *Resolution on Certain Questions in the History of our Party since the Founding of the People's Republic of China*, *Beijing Review*, No. 27 (1981).

CHANG, P. H., *Power and Policy in China* (University Park: Pennsylvania State University Press, 1975).

CHEN PI-CHAO, 'The Politics of Population in Communist China: A Case Study', Ph.D. diss. (Princeton University, 1966).

——— *Population and Health Policy in the People's Republic of China* (Washington, DC: Occasional Monograph Series No. 9, Interdisciplinary Communications Program, 1976).

——— *Rural Health and Birth Planning in China* (North Carolina, International Fertility Research Program, 1981).

——— 'Birth Control Methods and Organization in China', in E. Croll *et al.* (eds.), *China's One-Child Family Policy* (London: Macmillan, 1985), 135–48.

——— and KOLS, ADRIENNE, 'Population and Birth Planning in the People's Republic of China', *Population Report*, Series J, No. 25 (1982).

CHEN QUANGEN, 'Population Policies and Fertility Decline in China', M.Sc. diss. (University College, University of Wales, 1986).

CHEN YUN, *Chen Yun's Strategy for China's Development: A Non-Maoist*

Alternative, ed. N. R. Lardy and K. Lieberthal (New York: M. E. Sharpe, 1983).

CHINA POPULATION INFORMATION CENTRE, *Analysis on China's National One-Per-Thousand-Population Fertility Sample Survey* (Beijing, 1984).

CHU, L. L., *Planned Birth Campaign in China 1949–1976* (Honolulu: East–West Centre, Case Study No. 5, 1977).

CLELAND, J., and WILSON, C., 'Demand Theories of the Fertility Transition: An Iconoclastic View', *Population Studies*, 41 (1), 5–30 (1986).

COALE, A. J., 'The Demographic Transition', in *Proceedings of the International Population Conference 1973* (Liege: IUSSP, 1973), 53–72.

——— 'Population Trends, Population Policy, and Population Studies in China', *Population and Development Review*, 7 (1), 85–97 (1981).

——— 'A Further Note on Chinese Population Statistics', *Population and Development Review*, 7 (3), 512–18 (1981).

——— *Rapid Population Change in China 1952–1982* (Washington, DC: National Academy Press, 1984).

——— and CHEN SHENGLI, *Basic Data on Fertility in the Provinces of China, 1940–82* (Honolulu: East–West Population Institute, 1987).

——— and HOOVER, E. M., *Population Growth and Economic Development in Low-Income Countries* (Princeton, NJ: Princeton University Press, 1958).

——— and WATKINS, S. C. (eds.), *The Decline of Fertility in Europe* (Princeton, NJ: Princeton University Press, 1986).

COCHRANE, S. H., 'Effects of Education and Urbanization on Fertility', in R. A. Bulatao and R. D. Lee (eds.), *Determinants of Fertility in Developing Countries* (New York: Academic Press, 1983), ii. 587–626.

CROLL, E. J., 'The Chinese Household and its Economy: Urban and Rural Survey Data', *Contemporary China Centre Resource Paper*, (Oxford: Queen Elizabeth House, 1980).

——— 'A Conflict for Control of Marriage Patterns: Primary Groups versus Political Organizations', in S. L. Greenblatt *et al.* (eds.), *Organizational Behavior in Chinese Society* (New York: Praeger Publishers, 1981), 231–55.

——— *The Politics of Marriage in Contemporary China* (Cambridge: Cambridge University Press, 1981).

——— *The Family Rice Bowl* (London: Zed Press, 1983).

——— 'New Peasant Family Forms in Rural China', *The Journal of Peasant Studies*, 14 (4), 469–99 (1987).

DAVIN, D., 'The Single-Child Family in the Countryside', in E. Croll *et al.* (eds.), *China's One-Child Family Policy* (London: Macmillan, 1985), 37–82.

DAVIS-FRIEDMANN, D., 'Old Age Security and the One-Child Campaign', in E. Croll *et al.* (eds.), *China's One-Child Family Policy* (London: Macmillan, 1985), 149–161.

DAY, L. H., *Analysing Population Trends: Differential Fertility in a Pluralistic Society* (New York: St. Martin's Press, 1983).

DREYER, J., *China's Forty Millions* (Cambridge, Mass.: Harvard University Press, 1976).

DYSON, T., and MURPHY, M., 'The Onset of Fertility Transition', *Population and Development Review*, 11 (3), 399–440 (1985).

EASTERLIN, R. A., 'Modernization and Fertility', in R. A. Bulatao and R. D. Lee (eds.), *Determinants of Fertility in Developing Countries* (New York: Academic Press, 1983), ii. 562–86.

——— and CRIMMINS, E. M., *The Fertility Revolution: A Supply–Demand Analysis* (Chicago: The University of Chicago Press, 1985).

ECKSTEIN, A. (ed.), *Quantitative Measures of China's Economic Output* (Ann Arbor: University of Michigan Press, 1980).

EDITORIAL COMMITTEE, *1981 China's Official Annual Report* (Hongkong: Kingsway International Publications, 1982).

EDITORIAL COMMITTEE OF CHINA HANDBOOK SERIES, *Life and Lifestyle* (Beijing: Foreign Languages Press, 1985).

ELLIOT, F. R., *The Family: Change or Continuity?* (London: Macmillan Education, 1986).

FAIRBANK, J. K., and REISCHAUER, E. O., *China: Tradition and Transformation* (George Allen and Unwin Australia Pty. Ltd., 1979).

FEENEY, G., YU JINGYUAN, and CHI-HSIEN TUAN, 'Parity Progression Measures of Fertility in China', paper presented at the International Symposium on China's One-Per-Thousand National Fertility Sample Survey, Beijing, China, 14–18 Oct. 1985.

——— and YU JINGYUAN, 'The Effect of Son Preference on Fertility in China', paper presented at the 1986 annual meetings of the Population Association of America, San Francisco, Apr. 1986.

——— and YU JINGYUAN, 'Period Parity Progression Measures of Fertility in China', *Population Studies*, 41 (1), 77–102 (1987).

FRASER, S. E., *China: Population Education and People* (Canberra: School of Education, La Trobe University, 1987).

FREEDMAN, M., *Lineage Organization in Southeastern China* (London School of Economics Monographs on Social Anthropology, No. 18; London: Athlone, 1970).

FREEDMAN, R., 'Theories of Fertility Decline', in K. Mahadevan, P. J. Reddy, and D. A. Naidu (eds.), *Fertility and Mortality: Theory, Methodology and Empirical Issues* (New Delhi: Sage Publications, 1986), 30–6.

——— 'Fertility Determinants', in J. Cleland and C. Scott (eds.), *The World Fertility Survey: An Assessment* (London: Oxford University Press, 1987), 773–95.

——— *ET AL.*, 'Local Area Variations in Reproductive Behaviour in the People's Republic of China: 1973–1982', paper presented at the annual meeting of the Population Association of America, San Francisco, Apr. 1986.

GILLE, H., 'Policy Implications', in J. Cleland and J. Hobcraft (eds.), *Reproductive Change in Developing Countries* (Oxford: Oxford University Press, 1985), 273–95.

GOLDMAN, N., and HOBCRAFT, J., 'Birth Histories', *WFS Comparative Studies*, No. 17 (June 1982).

GOODSTADT, L. F., 'China's One-Child Family: Policy and Public Response', *Population and Development Review*, 8 (1), 37–58 (1982).

GREENBLATT, S. L., ET AL. (eds.), *Organizational Behaviour in Chinese Society* (New York: Praeger Publishers, 1981).

GREENHALGH, S., 'Fertility as Mobility: Sinitic Transitions', paper prepared for a Seminar on Societal Influences on Family Planning Programme Performance, Ocho Rios, Jamaica, 10–13 Apr. 1985.

—— 'Shifts in China's Population Policy: Views from the Central, Provincial, and Local Levels', *Population and Development Review*, 12 (3), 491–516 (1986).

—— and BONGAARTS, J., 'Fertility Policy in China: Future Options', The Population Council Working Papers, No. 127 (1986).

HANDWERKER, W. P., 'Culture and Reproduction: Exploring Micro/Macro Linkages', in W. P. Handwerker (ed.), *Culture and Reproduction: An Anthropological Critique of Demographic Transition Theory* (Boulder: Westview Press, 1986), 1–29.

HAN SUYIN, 'Population and Family Planning in the People's Republic of China', in *Family Planning in China* (Population Crisis Committee, Spring 1971).

HARTLEY, S. F., *Population: Quantity vs. Quality* (Englewood Cliffs, NJ: Prentice-Hall, 1972).

HEMMEL, V., and SINDBJERG, PIA, *Women in Rural China* (Studies on Asian Topics No. 7, Scandinavian Institute of Asian Studies, 1984).

HOBCRAFT, J., 'Family-Building Patterns', in J. Cleland and J. Hobcraft (eds.), *Reproductive Change in Developing Countries* (Oxford: Oxford University Press, 1985), 64–86.

—— 'The Proximate Determinants of Fertility', in J. Cleland and C. Scott (eds.), *The World Fertility Survey: An Assessment* (London: Oxford University Press, 1987), 796–837.

—— and LITTLE, R., 'Fertility Exposure Analysis: A New Method for Assessing the Contribution of Proximate Determinants to Fertility Differentials', *Population Studies*, 38 (1), 21–45 (1984).

—— *ET AL.*, 'Advances in the P/F Ratio Method for the Analysis of Birth Histories', *Population Studies*, 36 (2), 291–316 (1982).

HOHN, C., and MACKENSEN, R. (eds.), *Determinants of Fertility Trends: Theories Re-examined* (Liege: Ordina Editions, 1982).

HOLLERBACH, P. E., 'Fertility Decision-making Process: A Critical Essay', in R. A. Bulatao and R. D. Lee (eds.), *Determinants of Fertility in Developing Countries* (New York: Academic Press, 1983), ii. 340–80.

HOOK, B. (Gen. ed.), *The Cambridge Encyclopaedia of China* (Cambridge: Cambridge University Press, 1982).

HO PING-TI, *Studies on the Population of China, 1368–1953* (Cambridge, Mass.: Harvard University Press, 1959).

HOU WENRUO, 'Population Policy', in Liu Zheng *et al.*, *China's Population: Problems & Prospects* (Beijing: New World Press, 1981), 55–76.

JIANG ZHENGHUA, 'Reasons for Fertility Decline in China', paper presented at the Seminar on Fertility Transition in Asia: Diversity and Change, Bangkok, 28–31 Mar. 1988.

KANE, P., 'The Single-Child Family Policy in the Cities', in E. Croll *et al.* (eds.), *China's One-Child Family Policy* (London: Macmillan, 1985), 83–113.

—— *The Second Billion: Population and Family Planning in China* (London: Penguin Books, 1987).

KAUFMAN, J., *A Billion and Counting: Family Planning Campaigns and Policies in the People's Republic of China* (San Francisco: San Francisco Press, 1983).

KENDALL, M., 'The World Fertility Survey: Current Status and Findings', *Population Report*, Series M, No. 3 (1979).

KOLB, A., *East Asia: China, Japan, Korea, Vietnam: Geography of a Cultural Region* (London: Methuen, 1971).

KRAUS, W., *Economic Development and Social Change in the People's Republic of China* (New York: Springer-Verlag, 1982).

KUPINSKY, S., *The Fertility of Working Women* (New York: Praeger, 1977).

LANG, O., *Chinese Family and Society* (New York: Archon Books, 1968).

LAVELY, W. R., 'The Rural Chinese Fertility Transition: A Report from Shifan Xian, Sichuan', *Population Studies*, 38 (3), 365–84 (1986).

LEE HONG-YUNG, *The Politics of the Chinese Cultural Revolution* (Los Angeles and Berkeley: University of California Press, 1978).

LI BOHUA, 'Assessment of the Accuracy of a Sampling Survey', in China Population Information Centre, *Analysis on China's National One-Per-Thousand-Population Fertility Sampling Survey* (Beijing, 1984), 24–31.

LINDERT, P. H., 'Child Costs and Economic Development', in R. A. Easterlin (ed.), *Population and Economic Change in Developing Countries* (Chicago: The University of Chicago Press, 1980), 5–69.

LITTLE, R., 'Sampling Errors of Fertility Rates from the World Fertility Survey', WFS Tech. 1589 (1981).

LIU ZHENG, 'Population Planning and Demographic Theory', in Liu Zheng, Song Jian, and others, *China's Population: Problems & Prospects* (Beijing: New World Press, 1981), 1–24.

—— ET AL., *Population Theory in China*, translated and edited by H. Yuan Tien (London: Croom Helm, 1980).

—— SONG JIAN, and OTHERS, *China's Population: Problems & Prospects* (Beijing: New World Press, 1981).

LYLE, K., 'Planned Birth in Tianjin', *The China Quarterly*, No. 83 (Sept. 1980).

MABBETT, I. W., *Modern China: The Mirage of Modernity* (New York: St. Martin's Press, 1985).

MCCARTHY, J., 'Differentials in Age at First Marriage', *WFS Comparative Studies*, No. 19 (June 1982).

MCDONALD, P., 'Social Organization and Nuptiality in Developing Societies', in J. Cleland and J. Hobcraft (eds.), *Reproductive Change in Developing Counties* (Oxford: Oxford University Press, 1985), 87–114.

MACFARQUHAR, R., *The Origins of the Cultural Revolution*, Vol. 2: *The Great Leap Forward 1958–1960* (New York: Oxford University Press, 1983).

MCNICOLL, G., 'Institutional Determinants of Fertility Change', in C. Hohn and R. Mackensen (eds.), *Determinants of Fertility Trends: Theories Re-examined* (Liege: Ordina Editions, 1982), 147–68.

——— 'The Nature of Institutional and Community Effects on Demographic Behaviour: A Discussion', in J. Casterline (ed.), *The Collection and Analysis of Community Data*. (Voorbury, Netherlands: International Statistical Institute, 1985), 177–84.

MAO ZEDONG, 'The Bankruptcy of the Idealist Conception of History', in *Selected Works of Mao Tse-tung* (Beijing: Foreign Languages Press, 1969), iv. 451–9.

——— 'Be Activists in Promoting the Revolution', in *Selected Works of Mao Tse-tung* (Beijing: Foreign Languages Press, 1977), v. 486–8.

——— 'On the Correct Handling of Contradictions among the People', in *Selected Works of Mao Tse-tung* (Beijing: Foreign Languages Press, 1977), v. 384–421.

——— 'On the Ten Major Relationship', in *Selected Works of Mao Tse-tung* (Beijing: Foreign Languages Press, 1977), v. 267–88.

MARSHALL, M., *Organizations and Growth in Rural China* (London: Macmillan Press, 1985).

MASON, A., ET AL., 'Population Growth and Economic Development: Lessons from Selected Asian Countries', *Policy Development Studies*, No. 10, UNFPA (1986).

MATRAS, J., *Population and Societies* (Englewood Cliffs, NJ: Prentice-Hall, 1973).

MAULDIN, W. P., 'Population Trends and Prospects', *Science*, 209 (1980), 148–58.

——— 'The Determinants of Fertility Decline in Developing Countries: An Overview of the Available Empirical Evidence', *International Family Planning Perspectives*, 8 (1982), 119–27.

MOSER, L., *The Chinese Mosaic: The Peoples and Provinces of China* (Boulder: Westview Press, 1985).

NATIONAL CONGRESS OF THE PRC, *The Constitution of the People's Republic of China* (Beijing: Foreign Languages Press, 1983).

NEWELL, Co., *Methods and Models in Demography* (London: Belhaven Press, 1988).

NOTESTEIN, F. W., 'The Economics of Population and Food Supplies', *Proceedings of the Eighth International Conference of Agricultural Economists*, London, 1953.

NUGENT, J. B., 'The Old-Age Security Motive for having Children', *Population and Development Review*, 11 (1), 75–98 (1985).

ORLEANS, L. A., *Every Fifth Child: The Population of China* (London: Eyre Methuen, 1972).

——— *Chinese Approaches to Family Planning* (London: Macmillan, 1979).

PANNELL, C., and MA, LAURENCE, *China: The Geography of Development and Modernization* (London: Edward Arnold, 1983).

PARISH, W. L., and WHYTE, M. K., *Village and Family in Contemporary China* (London: University of Chicago Press, 1978).

PENG XIZHE, 'China's Regional Fertility Differences and Related Socio-economic Factors', M.Sc. diss. (London School of Economics, 1984).

——— 'Demographic Consequences of the Great Leap Forward in China's Provinces', *Population and Development Review*, 13 (4), 639–70 (1987).

——— 'Regional Differentials in China's Fertility Transition', paper presented at the Seminar on Fertility Transition in Asia: Diversity and Change, Bangkok, 28–31 Mar. 1988.

—— 'Fertility Transition in China and its Provinces since 1949', Ph.D. diss. (London School of Economics, 1988).

PEOPLE, 'China: Our Arduous Task', 11 (4), 1984.

POSTON, D. L., 'Patterns of Contraceptive Use in China', *Studies in Family Planning*, 17 (5), 217–27 (1986).

——— and BAOCHANG GU, 'Socioeconomic Development, Family Planning, and Fertility in China', *Demography*, 24 (4), 531–51 (1987).

POTTER, J. M., 'Land and Lineage in Traditional China', in M. Freedman (ed.), *Family and Kinship in Chinese Society* (Stanford, Calif.: Stanford University Press, 1970), 121–38.

POTTS, M., and SELMAN, P., *Society and Fertility* (Plymouth: Macdonald & Evans, 1979).

PYE, L. W., *China: An Introduction* (Boston: Little, Brown & Company, 1984).

QIAN XINZHONG, 'China's Population Policy: Theory and Methods', *Studies in Family Planning*, 14 (12), 302–17 (1983).

QIAO XINJIAN, 'Possible Obstacles to the Realisation of the One-Child Family', extended essay, David Owen Centre for Population Growth Studies, 1982.

RAVENHOLT, R. T., and CHAO, JOHN, 'Availability of Family Planning Services—The Key to Rapid Fertility Reduction', *Family Planning Perspectives*, 6 (4), 217–23 (1974).

REPETTO, R., 'Son Preference and Fertility Behaviour in Developing Countries', *Studies in Family Planning*, 3 (4), 70–6 (1972).

RINDFUSS, R., and MORGAN, S. P., 'Marriage, Sex, and the First Birth Interval: The Quiet Revolution in Asia', *Population and Development Review*, 9 (2), 259–78 (1983).

ROBINSON, J. C., 'Of Women and Washing Machines: Employment, Housework, and the Reproduction of Motherhood in Socialist China', *The China Quarterly*, No. 101 (Mar. 1985), 32–57.

SAICH, T., *China: Politics and Government* (London: Macmillan, 1981).

SALAFF, J., 'Youth, Family, and Political Control in Communist China', Ph.D. thesis (Department of Sociology, University of California, Berkeley, 1972).

SCHULTZ, T. P., *Economics of Population* (Reading, Mass.: Addison-Wesley, 1982).

SEN, A. K., *Poverty and Famines: An Essay on Entitlement and Deprivation* (New York: Oxford University Press, 1984).

SHARLIN, A., 'Urban–Rural Differences in Fertility in Europe during the Demographic Transition', in A. J. Coale and S. C. Watkins (eds.), *The Decline of Fertility in Europe* (Princeton, NJ: Princeton University Press, 1986), 234–60.

SHILS, E., *Tradition* (London: Faber & Faber Ltd., 1981).

SINGH, K., 'Statement Made at the World Population Conference', Bucharest (Aug. 1974), Mimeo.

SMITH, P. C., 'The Impact of Age at Marriage and Proportions Marrying on Fertility', in R. Bulatao and R. Lee (eds.), *Determinants of Fertility in Developing Countries* (New York: Academic Press, 1983), ii. 473–531.

——— SHAHIDULLAH, M., and ALCANTARA, A., 'Cohort Nuptiality in Asia and the Pacific: An Analysis of WFS Surveys', *WFS Comparative Studies*, No. 22 (Apr. 1983).

SNOW, E., *Red China Today* (London: Penguin Books, 1970).

——— *China's Long Revolution* (London: Penguin Books, 1972).

STATE STATISTICAL BUREAU OF PRC, *Statistical Yearbook of China, 1981* (English edition, Hongkong, 1981).

——— *China Urban Statistics, 1985* (London: Longman, 1985).

SU SHAOZHI, *Democracy and Socialism in China* (Nottingham: Spokesman, 1982).

SU WENMING (ed.), *Population and Other Problems* (Beijing: *Beijing Review* Special Feature Series, 1981), 35–57.

TAEUBER, I., 'The Families of Chinese Farmers', in M. Freedman (ed.), *Family and Kinship in Chinese Society* (Stanford, Calif.: Stanford University Press, 1970), 63–85.

THOMPSON, W. S., 'Plenty of People', *American Journal of Sociology*, 34 (1929), 959–75.

TIAN XUEYUAN, 'A Survey of Population Growth since 1949', in Liu Zheng *et al.*, *China's Population: Problems & Prospects* (Beijing: New World Press, 1981), 32–54.

TIEN, H. YUAN, *China's Population Struggle: Demographic Decisions of the People's Republic 1949–1969* (Columbus: Ohio State University Press, 1973).

——— 'Age at Marriage in the People's Republic of China', *The China Quarterly*, No. 93 (1983), 90–107.

——— 'Induced Fertility Transition: Impact of Population Planning and Socio-Economic Change in the People's Republic of China', *Population Studies*, 38 (3), 385–400 (1984).

——— 'Provincial Fertility Trends and Patterns', in E. Croll *et al.* (eds.), *China's One-Child Family Policy* (London: Macmillan, 1985).

TOWNSEND, J. R., *Politics of China* (Boston: Little, Brown & Company, 1980).

TREGEAR, T., *China, A Geographical Survey* (London: Hodder and Stoughton, 1980).

UNITED NATIONS DEPARTMENT OF ECONOMIC AND SOCIAL AFFAIRS, *Demographic Yearbook*, Annual, New York.

——— *Relationships between Fertility and Education: A Comparative Analysis of World Fertility Survey Data for Twenty-two Developing Countries*, ST/ESA/SER.R/48.

——— *World Population Prospects: Estimates and Projections as Assessed in 1984*, as *Population Studies*, No. 98 (1986).

WALKER, K. R., *Food Grain Procurement and Consumption in China* (London: Cambridge University Press, 1984).

WANG, J., *Contemporary Chinese Politics: An Introduction* (Englewood Cliffs, NJ: Prentice-Hall, 1980).

WANG KE, *ET AL.*, 'Demographic Transition and Current Population Situation of Chinese Tibetan', *Population Research* (English edition), 2 (3), July 1985.

WARE, H., *Women, Demography and Development* (Canberra: The Australian National University Press, 1981).

WARWICK, D., 'Culture and the Management of Family Planning Programme', *Studies in Family Planning*, 19 (1), 1–18 (1988).

WFS TECHNICAL BULLETINS.

WHYTE, M. K., and GU, S. Z., 'Popular Response to China's Fertility Transition', *Population and Development Review*, 13 (3), 471–93, (1987).

WOLF, A. P., 'The Preeminent Role of Government Intervention in China's Family Revolution', *Population and Development Review*, 12 (1), 101–16 (1986).

——— and HUANG CHIEH-SHAN, *Marriage and Adoption in China, 1845–1945* (Stanford, Calif.: Stanford University Press, 1980).

WORLD BANK, *World Development Report* (Oxford: Oxford University Press, 1984).

XIAO WENCHENG, LI MENGHUA, and WANG LIYENG, 'Changes in Total Fertility Rate since 1950s', China Population Information Centre, *Analysis on China's National One-Per-Thousand-Population Fertility Sampling Survey* (Beijing, 1984), 58–61.

XIAO ZHENYU, 'The Design of 1982's Fertility Sampling Survey in China', in China Population Information Centre, *Analysis on China's National One-Per-Thousand-Population Fertility Sampling Survey* (Beijing, 1984), 11–23.

XUE MUQIAO, 'China's Economy in Retrospect and Prospects, in G. C. Wang (ed. and tr.), *Economic Reform in the PRC* (Boulder: Westview Press, 1982), 11–20.

YANG, C. K., *The Chinese Family in the Communist Revolution* (Cambridge, Mass.: MIT Press, 1965).

YU, E. S. H., 'Overseas Remittances in South-Eastern China', *The China Quarterly*, No. 78 (1979), 339–50.

YU, Y. C., 'The Population Policy of China', *Population Studies*, 33 (1), 125–42 (1979).

ZENG YI, 'Marriage and Marriage Dissolution in China: A Marital Status Life Table Analysis', paper presented at the 20th general conference of IUSSP, Florence, Italy, June 1985.

——— 'Changes in Family Structure in China: A Simulation Study', *Population and Development Review*, 12 (4), 675–703 (1986).

ZOU PING, 'The Review and Discussion of Changes in China's Population Policy during the Early Years of the People's Republic', *Population Research (English edition)*, 4 (4), 1–8 (1987).

BOOKS AND ARTICLES, IN CHINESE

BAI JIANHUA, 'Woguo Chengxiang renkou de chuangkuang (Rural and Urban Population of China)', *Renkou Yanjiu (Population Research)*, Nos. 2 and 3 (1986).

CENSUS OFFICE OF LIANYUAN COUNTY, 'Analysis on Change in Family and its Impact', in *Renkou Tanshuo (Exploration on Population)*, Supplementary Issue (1984).

CHEN MUHUA, 'Shixian sige xiandaihua bixu youjihuade kongzhi renkou zengzhang (To Realize the Four Modernizations it is Necessary to Control Population Growth)', *Renmin Ribao (People's Daily)*, 11 Aug. 1979.

——— 'Fazhan renkou kexueuei kongzhi renkou mubiao fuwu (To Develop Population Science in the Service of Controlling Population Growth), *Renkou Yanjiu (Population Research)*, No. 3 (1981).

CHEN SHENGLI, 'Fertility of Women during the 42-Year Period from 1940 to 1981', 'An Analysis of a National One-Per-Thousand-Population Sample Survey in Birth Rate', *Renkou yu jingji (Population and Economy)*, Special Issue (1983).

CHENG DU, 'Woguo renkou zhengce de jige wenti jiqi jiejue tujing (China's Population Policy: Some Problems and the Prospects for their Solution)', *Wuhan University Journal, Social Sciences Edition*, No. 3 (May 1981).

——— 'Hubei nongcun shengyuli diaochao (Fertility Survey in the Rural Areas of Hubei Province)', in *Renkou Yanjiu (Population Research)*, No. 5 (1982).

CHENG FENGGAO, 'Anhui renkou xianzhuang de chubu fenxi (Preliminary Analysis of Current Situation of Anhui's Population)', in *Renkou (Population)*, No. 1 (1985).

CHINA POPULATION INFORMATION CENTRE, *Zhongguo renkou ziliao shouce (Handbook of Chinese Population Information*, 1985–1987 (Beijing).

CHINESE ACADEMY OF SOCIAL SCIENCE, *Zhongguo renkou nianjian (Almanac of China's Population)*, 1985.

DENG YAN, 'Dui wosheng renkou xingbiebi de fenxi (On the Sex Ratio of our Province)', *Renkou Tansuo (Exploration on Population)*, Supplementary Issue (1984).

DUN SONGTING, 'Dachengshi liudong renkou duiche chuton (Explore the Measures towards Floating Population in Big Cities)', *Zhongguo Chengshi Daobao*, 14 Jan. 1988.

EDITORIAL COMMITTEE, *Wenxian yu yanjiu (Document and Research)* (Beijing: People's Publish House, 1983).

EDITORIAL COMMITTEE, *Anhuisheng jingji nianjian (Economic Yearbook of Anhui Province), 1984.*

——— *Fujian jingji nianjian (Economic Yearbook of Fujian Province), 1985* (Fuzhou: Fujian People's Press, 1985).

——— *Zhonghua renmin gongheguo nianjian (1983 People's Republic of China Yearbook)* (Beijing: Xinhua, 1984).

——— *Zhongguo jiaoyu nianjian (Educational Yearbook of China), 1949–1981* (Beijing: Zhongguo Baike Qunsu Shubanshi, 1984).

——— *Zhongguo renkou chongshu (Chinese Population Monographs)*, Provincial Volumes: Beijing, Hebei, Shanxi, Tianjin, Jiangsu, Shanghai, Hunan, Jilin, Gansu, Guizhou.

——— *Zhongguo baike nianjian (Encyclopaedia of China) 1981* (Beijing: Encyclopaedia Publish House, 1981–3).

FALU YU SHENGHUO (Law and Life), Mar. 1986.

FAMILY PLANNING COMMISSION OF SHANDONG, *Shandongsheng renkou, jihuashengyu ji youguan jichu ziliao (Basic Information on Shandong's Population, Family Planning, and Other Related Matters)*, 1985.

FANG XIANGXIN, 'Shilun woguo nongcun jiating jiegou de fazhan qushi (On the Changes in the Family Composition in China's Rural Areas)', in *Xibei Renkou (Northwest Population)*, Mar. 1984.

FAN JINCHUN, 'Kongzhi renkou zengzhang gaohao shihua jianshe (Control Population Growth and Do Well in Building the Four Modernizations)', *Shihui kexue yanjiu (Social Science Research)*, No. 6 (1981).

FENG ZHONGHUI, 'Shaanxisheng yuling funu hunyin yu shengyu zhuangkuang (Marital Status and Fertility of Women of Childbearing Age in Shaanxi Province)', *Renkou Yanjiu (Population Research)*, No. 2 (1982).

FIVE CITIES FAMILY RESEARCH PROJECT GROUP, *Zhongguo chengshi jiating—wuschengshi jiating diaocha ziliao huibian (Family in China's Urban Areas: Collection of Data and Reports on a Family Survey in 5 Cities)* (Jinan: Shandong People's Press, 1985).

GAO ERSHENG, 'Shanghai shiqu shanshinian lai shengyulu de bianhua jiqi yingxiang yingsu (Change in Fertility Rate in Shanghai's Urban Areas and its Causes)', *Renkou Yanjiu (Population Research)*, No. 1 (1984).

GUI SHIXUN, 'Bashi niandai shanghai renkou tedian yu renkou pucha (The Distinguishing Features of Shanghai's Population in the 1980s and the Population Census)', *Jiefang Ribao*, 17 June 1982.

GUO NIANLAN and LI KEQIN, 'Time Distribution of Births', in *Population and Economy*, Special Issue (1983).

GU SUTANG (ed.), *Tianjin jingji gankuang (A General Survey of Tianjin's Economy)* (Tianjin: Tianjin People's Press, 1984).

HONG QI (RED FLAG), 1978–86.

HU HUANYONG, 'Zhongguo renkou de fenbu (The Distribution of Population in China)', in *Essays on China's Population Distribution* (Shanghai: Eastern Normal University Press, 1983).

——— and YAN ZHENGYUAN, 'Disequilibrium of Population Distribution between East and West China', in *Renkou (Population)*, No. 1 (1985).

——— and ZHANG SHANYU, *Zhongguo renkou dili (Population Geography of China)* (Shanghai: Eastern Normal University Press, 1986).

LIAOWANG (OUTLOOK WEEKLY), 1987–8.

LI CHENGRUI, 'Zhongguo renkou chushenglu he siwanglu de fazhan qushi (The Trends in the Birth-Rate and Death-Rate of China's Population)', *Renkou Yanjiu* (*Population Research*), No. 1 (1982).

LI HANBO, 'Guangdongsheng jihua shengyu gongzuo fazhan de jige jieduan (The Development Phases of the Family-Planning Programme in Guangdong Province)', *Guangdong Renkou (Guangdong Population)*, No. 2 (1984).

LI JIEPIN and QI YIJU, 'Shanghaishi jihuashengyu qingkuang fenxi (Analysis of the Family-Planning Programme in Shanghai)', *Renkou Kexue Congkan (Population Science)*, No. 1 (Sept. 1981).

LI MUZHEN, 'Zhongguo renkou wenti zhongdian zai nongcun (The Focal Point of China's Population Problem is in the Rural Areas)', *Renkou Yu Jingji* (*Population and Economics*), No. 6 (1982).

LIN FURUI and CHEN DAIGUANG, *Henan renkou dili (Population Geography of Henan)* (Zhengzhou, 1983).

LI RONGSHI, '1987 woguo renkou zhuangkuang fengxi (Analysis of China's Population Situation in 1987)', *Renkou Yanjiu* (*Population Research*), No. 1 (1988).

LIU JUNZHE, 'The Impact of Old Age Security on Family Planning', in *Xibei Renkou (Northwest Population)*, No. 1 (1984).

LIU SHUINIAN (ed.), *Liushi niandai guomin jingji tiaozheng de huigu (Recalling the Adjustment of the National Economy in the 1960s)* (Beijing, 1982).

LIU ZHENG, 'Chushenglu, shengyulu, zaishenchanlu (Birth-Rate, Fertility Rate, and Reproduction Rate)', *Renkou Yanjiu (Population Research)*, No. 2 (1981).

——— 'Zhongguo renkoukexue de fazhan yu chengjiu (The Development and Achievements in China's Population Science'), *Renkou Yanjiu (Population Research)*, No. 1 (1985).

LU YU, 'Shilun shengyu zhengce de kaixiaoko yu dudakou (Comment on the Population Policy of Blocking up the Big Breach whilst Opening a Small Hole)', *Shandong Renkou*, No. 3 (1984).

MA XIA, 'Zhongguo jiatinghu guimo he jiating jiegou fenxi (Analysis of Chinese Family Size and Composition)', *Renkou Yanjiu (Population Research)*, No. 2 (1986).

MA YINCHU, 'Xin renko lun (New Population Theory)', *Renmin Ribao (People's Daily)*, 5 July 1957.

NEW CHINA NEWS AGENCY, *Zhonghua renmin gongheguo dashiji (Chronology of Events in People's Republic of China)*, *1949–1980* (Beijing: Xinhua Press, 1981).

OFFICE OF POPULATION CENSUS OF GUANGDONG PROVINCE, *Guangdong renkou zhuangkuang fenxi yu yuce (Analysis and Projection of Population Situation in Guangdong Province)* (Guangzhou: Zhongshan University Press, 1985).

PLANNING COMMISSION OF GUANGXI AUTHONOMOUS REGION, *Guangxi quqing*

(A General Survey of Guangxi Autonomous Region (Nanning: Guangxi People's Press, 1985).

PLANNING COMMISSION OF HEILONGJIANG, *Fazhan zhong de Heilongjiang (Development in Heilongjiang), 1949–1983* (Haerbin: Heilongjiang People's Press, 1984).

POPULATION ASSOCIATION OF QINGHAI, *Qinghai shaoshu minzu renkou wenti tansuo (Exploration of Qinghai's Minority Population Problems)* Xining, 1984).

POPULATION DIVISION OF SHANGHAI ACADEMY OF SOCIAL SCIENCE, '1981 Shanghai renkou chushenglu huisheng yunyin de fenxi (Causes of Increase in Shanghai's Birth-Rate in 1981)', internal paper, No. 82109 (Apr. 1982).

PROPAGANDA DEPARTMENT OF THE PARTY COMMITTEE OF QINGHAI, *Qinghai 35 nian (Qinghai in the Past 35 Years), 1949–1984* (Xining: Qinghai People's Press, 1985).

QU YIBIN, 'Woguo renkou chushenglu mingixan huisheng de yuanying ji duiche tantao (Exploring the Cause of the Increase in Birth-Rate and the Measures to deal with it in China)', *Renkou Yanjiu (Population Research)*, No. 1 (1988).

RAN YUGANG and XIE QINBIN, 'Brief Analysis of Women in their First Marriage and the First Birth in Connection with Women', Special Issue of *Population And Economy* (Beijing, 1983).

REN LIZHONG, 'Hebeisheng jihuashengyu gongzuo sanshinian de huigu (Review of Family-Planning Programmes in Hebei Province in the Past 30 Years)', *Heibei Renkou (Hebei Population)*, No. 4 (1984).

RENMIN RIBAO (PEOPLE'S DAILY), 1957–62, 1977–87.

RESEARCH OFFICE OF THE PARTY COMMITTEE IN SICHUAN PROVINCE, *Sichuan shengqing (A General Survey of Sichuan Province)* (Chengdu, 1984).

SHEHUI KEXUE (SOCIAL SCIENCES), No. 1 (1984).

SI CHENGLI, 'Mao Zedong tongzhi dui jihuashengyu de gongxian (Comrade Mao Zedong's Contribution to Birth Control)', *Xibei Renkou (Northwest Population)*, No. 3 (1984).

STATE FAMILY PLANNING COMMISSION, *Quanguo jihuashenyu ziliao huibian (Collection of Family-Planning Statistics)*, 1983.

——— 'Quanguo qianfenzhiyi renkou shengyulu chouyang diaocha gongbao (Communique on the One-Per-Thousand Sample Fertility Survey of China's Population), *Renkou Yanjiu (Population Research)*, No. 3 (1983).

——— *Jihuashenyu tongxun (Newsletter of Family-Planning Work)*, 1985–6.

STATE STATISTICAL BUREAU, *Zhongguo tongji nianjian (Statistical Yearbook of China)* (Beijing, Annual, 1981–8).

——— *10 Percent Sampling Tabulation of the 1982 Population Census of the PRC* (Beijing, 1983).

——— *Gesheng, zizhiqu, zhixiashi, nongmin shouru, xiaofei diaozha ziliao huibian (Collection of Data on Peasants' Income and Consumption for Provinces, Autonomous Regions, and Major Cities)*, 1985.

STATISTICAL BUREAU OF ANHUI, *Anhui tongji nianjian (Statistical Yearbook of Anhui), 1984* (Anhui People's Press, 1984).

STATISTICAL BUREAU OF GUANGDONG, *Guangdong tongji nianjian (Statistical Yearbook of Guangdong, 1984.*

STATISTICAL BUREAU OF GUIZHOU, *Guizhou jingji shouce (Handbook of Guizhou's Economy), 1984* (Guizhou People's Press, 1984).

STATISTICAL BUREAU OF HEBEI, *Hebei jingji tongji nianjian (Statistical Yearbook of Hebei's Economy), 1985.*

STATISTICAL BUREAU OF HUNAN, *Hunansheng tongji nianjian (Statistical Yearbook of Hunan Province), 1983.*

STATISTICAL BUREAU OF JIANGSU, *Jiangsu tongji nianjian (Statistical Yearbook of Jiangsu), 1985.*

STATISTICAL BUREAU OF LIAONING, *Liaoning jingji tongji nianjian (Statistical Yearbook of Liaoning's Economy), 1984* (Shengyang: Liaoning People's Press, 1984).

STATISTICAL BUREAU OF NEI MONGGU, *Nei monggu tongji nianjian (Statistical Yearbook of Nei Monggu), 1984.*

STATISTICAL BUREAU OF SHANDONG, *Shandong tongji nianjian (Statistical Yearbook of Shandong), 1983* (Jining, 1983).

STATISTICAL BUREAU OF SHANGHAI, *Shanghai tongji nianjian (Statistical Yearbook of Shanghai), 1985.*

STATISTICAL BUREAU OF SHANXI, *Shanxi tongji nianjian (Statistical Yearbook of Shanxi), 1985.*

STATISTICAL BUREAU OF YUNNAN, *Yunnansheng guomin jingji tongji tiyao (Statistical Abstract of Yunnan's National Economy), 1949–1983.*

STATISTICAL BUREAU OF ZHEJIANG, *Zhejiang tongji nianjian (Statistical Yearbook of Zhejiang), 1984.*

——— *Zhejiang nongcun jingji nianjian (Yearbook of Zhejiang's Rural Economy), 1985.*

TIAN XUEYUAN, *Xinshiqi renkoulun (Population Theory in the New Era)* (Haerbin: Heilongjiang People's Press, 1982).

WANG DEYI, 'Xinhunyinfa he jihua shengyu (The New Marriage Law and Family Planning)', *Zhongguo Funu (Women of China)*, No. 11 (1980).

WANG WEI, 'Guanyu jihua shengyu gongzuo wenti (On Family-Planning Work)', *Handbook of Chinese Population Information, 1986*, 4–11.

——— 'Guanyu jihua shengyu gongzhou qingkuang de jianghua (A Speech on Family Planning), *Handbook of Chinese Population Information, 1987*, 13–19.

WU CANGPIN, 'Zhongguo shengyulu xunsu xiajiang de lilun jieshi (Theoretical Explanation of the Rapid Fertility Decline in China)', *Renkou Yanjiu (Population Research)*, No. 1 (1986), 11–16.

XIE CHENG, 'Youguan Youdai dusheng zinu jigi jiating zhengce wengti de tantao he jianyi (Remarks on Policies for Preferential Treatment Given to Only Children and their Parents)', *Renkou Yu Jingji (Population and Economy)*, No. 1 (1988).

XING LONG, 'Shanxi jindai renkou gao xingbili jiqi houguo (High Sex Ratio and its Consequences in Modern Shanxi Province)', *Renkou Yanjiu (Population Research)*, No. 5 (1986).

XUE MUQIAO, 'Guanyu gongzi wenti de tanhua (Talk on the Problem of Wage)', *Woguo dangqian de jingji wenti (Current Economic Problems in our Country)* (Beijing: People's Press, 1980), 122–38.

YANG DEQING, *Renkouxue Gailun (A General Introduction to the Study of Population)* (Hebei, 1982).

YANG JISHUN, 'Laoyou suoyang zai nongcun jihua shengyu gongzuo zhong de diwei he zuoyong (The Importance of Old-Age Security on Rural Family-Planning Works)', *Shandong Renkou (Shandong Population)*, No. 3 (1983).

YANG XIUYU, 'Yingxiang nongcun zhisheng yitai de yinsu fenxi (Factors Affecting Single-Child Policy in the Rural Areas)', *Renkou Tansuo (Exploration on Population)*, Supplementary Issue (1984).

YIE WENZHEN, 'Silun qiaoqu dui renkou kongzhi de libi (On the Advantage and Disadvantage of Population Control in Areas Where a Large Proportion of Families have Overseas Relatives)', *Fujian Renkou (Fujian Population)*, 1983.

ZHANG CHUNYUAN, 'Mao Zedong de renkou sixiang (Mao Zedong's Population Thought)', *Jingji Kexue (Economic Sciences)*, No. 6 (1986).

ZHANG LIZHONG, 'Jieyu, wanhun yu renkou zengzhanglu de xiajiang (Birth Control, Late Marriage, and the Decline in the Population Growth Rate)', *Renkou Yanjiu (Population Research)*, No. 1 (1980).

ZHANG NAIGONG and ZHOU NING, 'Wosheng sanshinianlai renkou fazhan de huigu he jingyan jiaoxun (Review and Lessons of Population Growth in the Past 30 years in our Province)', *Zhejiang renkou tongxun (Newsletter of Zhejiang Population)*, Feb. 1980.

ZHANG XINXIA, 'Jianguo yilai woguo shengyu zhengce de yanbian (The Evolution of our Country's Population Policy since the Founding of the People's Republic)', *Shandong Renkou (Shandong Population)*, No. 3 (1984).

ZHENG GUIZHEN, 'Shanlao zunlao shi kongzhi nongcun renkou de zhanlue cuoshi (To Support and Respect the Elderly is a Strategic Measure for Controlling Population Growth in the Rural Areas)', *Shehui (Society)*, No. 2 (1983).

ZHONGGUO FUNU, 1985–7.

ZHONGGUO QINNIAN, 1985–7.

ZHONGGUO QINNIAN BAO (Youth of China), July 1985–Dec. 1987.

ZHOU QING, 'Woguo xiandaihua guocheng zhong nongcunjiating guimo yu leixing jiegou (The Size, Type, and Structure of Rural Families in the Course of Modernization in China)', *Renkou Yanjiu (Population Research)*, No. 2 (1988).

ZHU CHUANYI, 'It is an Urgent Task to Establish a Social-Security System for the Rural Elders', *Laonian Wenti Yanjiu Ziliao (Research Information on Problem of Ageing)*, No. 54 (Nov. 1985).

Index

Index